Toward a Discipline of Nursing

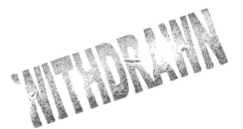
0443044384

Towards a Discipline of Nursing

Edited by

Genevieve Gray RN RM MSc (Nursing)(Manch.) Dip Adv Nsg St DNE(NSWCN) FCN(NSW) FRCNA

Rosalie Pratt RN RM MHPEd(NSW) BA(Macq.) DNE(Cumb.) FCN(NSW) FRCNA

Foreword by

Margaret Bennett RN RM IWC DipNEd BA BSc(Hons) PhD
Dean, School of Nursing, Phillip Institute of Technology, Bundoora

CHURCHILL LIVINGSTONE
MELBOURNE EDINBURGH LONDON MADRID NEW YORK AND TOKYO 1991

CHURCHILL LIVINGSTONE
Medical Division of Longman Group UK Limited

Distributed in Australia by Longman Cheshire Pty Limited,
Longman House, Kings Gardens, 95 Coventry Street, South
Melbourne 3205, and by associated companies, branches and
representatives throughout the world.

First published 1991
    Reprinted 1992

ISBN 0-443-04438-4

National Library of Australia Cataloging in Publication Data

    Towards a discipline of nursing.
        Includes index.
        ISBN 0 443 04438 4.

        1. Nursing–Australia. I. Gray, Genevieve. II. Pratt, Rosalie.
    610.730994

Produced by Longman Singapore Publishers (Pte) Ltd
Printed in Singapore

Foreword

This book represents a significant development in the history of nursing in Australia. By bringing together a number of Australian scholars to address the issues associated with the emerging discipline of nursing, many of the shackles holding back development in this country have been broken. The editors are to be congratulated on their foresight and courage in facilitating such timely change. Australian nursing is reaching new heights in its development as a substantive discipline.

The development of the discipline of nursing has some interesting parallels with the history of Australia's development as a nation. Although the land itself is thousands of centuries old, the development of modern Australia commenced with its European, largely British, colonization in the latter half of the 18th century. The land had much to offer. Indeed, as our national anthem indicates '...our land abounds in nature's gifts of beauty rich and rare...'. The original inhabitants of the land had survived on these natural resources for many centuries. With colonization, many of these natural resources were exploited. The combination of such riches, together with the development of knowledge and skill to utilize them, advanced Australia towards prosperous nationhood. Today Australia is recognized as a developed country, a nation in its own right, and proudly takes its place on the international scene, making significant contributions to world development. However, although Australia is moving towards nationhood, at this time the national identity is not always clearly evident; the philosophy is at times ambiguous; the characteristics of Australians are varied and inconsistent; and a body of knowledge that is recognized as Australian has only recently begun to emerge.

Despite the fact that the new colony was founded at a time when revolutions were in fashion, development towards nationhood occurred by evolution rather than revolution. There have been many factors that have facilitated Australia's evolutionary advancement towards nationhood. Not the least of these have been the characteristics of many Australians—their pioneering spirit with its desire to conquer adversity; their dogged determination to make the best of what was available; the brashness often associated with youth (the national anthem highlights the fact that '...we are young and free...'); the ability to absorb those of many different cultures into a single nation; and an ability to tolerate ambiguity.

There is, however, a negative side to the Australian character. Our history shows the systematic, and at times aggressive, rejection of all the wisdom and skill that the original inhabitants of this land had accumulated over the centuries. We are only now realizing how much they did have to offer. Our pioneers had to learn the hard way, often having to reinvent the wheel in order to survive the harshness of this land. Initially, we chose to emulate the 'mother country', trying to force-fit our way of life into a traditional British mould. However, immigrants from many other countries were attracted to our shores and, despite the richness that they had to offer, tensions developed. Bias and prejudice abounded, in relation to not only the more common negative 'isms' associated with such aspects as race, age, and science, but also the unique 'ockerism' prevalent in this country. This concept embodies a propensity to *knock* that which does not fit 'the arche-typal uncultivated Australian male' image as described by the Macquarie Dictionary (1981) ; and to cut the 'tall poppies' down to size. It is accom-panied by a large inferiority complex that too readily accepts that what is produced by others must be infinitely superior to that produced by Australians. Slowly, this is changing. Australians are now recognizing the richness of their diversity, especially their multiculturalism, and realizing that Australia does not have to import talent. It resides in its own citizens, be they indigenous or adopted. Further, the talent does not have to be exported to reach its full potential. Opportunities exist within Australia itself for maximum develop-ment. So too it is with nursing.

The 'nurturing' concept on which so much of nursing is based is as old as humankind. Modern nursing, as the Western world knows it, began with its Europeanization in the latter half of the 19th century, most noticeably through the efforts of Florence Nightingale and her disciples—six of whom were sent to the new southern colony in the 1860s. Nursing had enormous potential for development as a discipline in its own right. It too abounded with 'nature's gifts of beauty rich and rare', and it required not only knowledge and skill to harness these gifts, but the characteristics of true pioneers in order to move nursing towards discipline status.

Development within modern nursing has been by evolution, rather than by the revolution that Kuhn (1970) claimed had occurred in other disciplines. At its very foundation, modern nursing chose to ignore the wisdom and skill of those who had practised rudimentary forms of nursing through the ages. Our pioneers had to reinvent the wheel in order to establish the discipline of nursing. Only now are we coming to recognize the true value of the concepts associated with nurturing. Initially, our pioneers sought scientific recogni-tion, by emulating the discipline of medicine, attempting to force-fit the entire substance of nursing into the medical model. However, concepts, methods, and paradigms from other disciplines were attracted into nursing and, despite the richness that they had to offer, tensions developed. Rifts occurred between nursing practice and education, and between theory and practice, with competing paradigms and methodologies associated with research and theory development. 'Ockerism' was rife. The 'tall poppies' were cut to size. First British and later North American developments in nursing were considered highly desirable. After all, nothing good could come from Australian nurses.

Florence Nightingale recognized nursing's potential as a distinct discipline, suggesting that it was different from, but complementary to, medicine. However, it took many years before the discipline of nursing began to emerge as a separate entity in its own right with its own defined body of knowledge. Now a more clearly defined structure is beginning to emerge; the roles, functions, and characteristics of the practitioners are less ambiguous; conceptual schemata are becoming more cohesive, interrelated and internally consistent; and there is a concerted effort to pursue knowledge that is clearly identifiable as being nursing. A new maturity is developing in which it is recognized that the phenomena of nursing are complex and complicated, and will only be made known by using a variety of approaches. No one paradigm will reveal all that there is to know about nursing. The quest for scientific recognition is no longer being approached only from the traditional positivist tradition. Concepts such as caring, for too long undervalued and dismissed as women's work and therefore not worthy of scientific pursuit, are being recognized as integral to the substance of nursing, and are being explored with a variety of paradigms and methods. There is now an acceptance of diversity, a recognition of different points of view, and a tolerance of ambiguity. There is also a movement to find paradigms and methods that are not merely adapted from other disciplines but are developed from the practice of nursing itself. Thrown off are the beliefs that nursing is inferior to other disciplines, and that Australian nurses are not capable of making significant contributions to the discipline of nursing.

This book captures the essence of the debate about nursing as an emerging discipline, within an Australian context. It addresses the philosophies, methods and conceptual frameworks underlying nursing knowledge. It shows the journey that Meleis (1985) terms 'from can't to Kant' and beyond. It has a hard look at the theory-practice and the practice-theory-practice paradigms and in exploring concepts from critical theory and notions such as praxis and reflection, shows how theory can be generated from the experience of practitioners—from neophytes to experts. It also shows how such theory generation can be facilitated and how it can be used to change the practice of nursing. There is a strong theme of autonomy, both in education to produce self-directed students and in practice for self-care by clients. These Australian scholars also explore other paradigms, such as those associated with the feminist perspective and phenomenological philosophy and method. In this way, recognition is given to the importance of diversity in the pursuit of nursing knowledge.

The book also contains some warnings and challenges: it suggests guarding against the dismissal of paradigms dominant in the past; it warns against seeking new and unique knowledge in nursing for its own sake; it challenges the reader to look at what nursing ought to be, not what it is now; it stresses caution in the journey to discipline status, to avoid oppression and disintegration. Thus, all in all this collection of works from Australian scholars demonstrates a new maturity in Australian nursing. It will contribute to the wider, international debate about the very substance of nursing, and it will hasten the development of nursing towards a substantive discipline.

Melbourne 1991   Margaret Bennett

REFERENCES

Delbridge A (ed) 1981 The Macquarie Dictionary. Macquarie Library, St Leonards
Kuhn T S 1970 The structure of scientific revolutions, 2nd edn. University of Chicago
    Press, Chicago
Meleis A I 1985 Theoretical nursing: development and progress. Lippincott, Philadelphia

Contributors

Betty M. Andersen AM RN DSc(honoris causa) MA(Hons)Ed BA DipNEd FRSA FCN(NSW)
Professor of Nursing, Dean and Head of School of Nursing and Health Studies, University of Western Sydney, Macarthur

Amy Bartjes RN RM GNC PNC DipT(NEd) GradDipCD BEd MEd FRCNA
Senior Lecturer, School of Nursing Studies, The Flinders University of South Australia

Nina Bruni RN BA(Hons) MEdStds
Senior Lecturer, Department of Nursing Administration and Education, Phillip Institute of Technology, Bundoora

Elizabeth Cameron-Traub RN ICC Cert BA(Hons) PhD(Flinders) GradDipNursStud(Ed) (Armidale) FRCNA MCN(NSW) MAPsS
Professor of Nursing, Dean, Faculty of Nursing, University of Technology, Sydney

Helen Cox RN DipNEd BAppSci(Advanced Nursing)(La Trobe) FRCNA
Senior Lecturer, Faculty of Nursing, Deakin University, Geelong

Sue Crane RN BSc(Hons)(Liverpool) GerNursCert MRCNA
Lecturer/Clinician, Faculty of Nursing, Deakin University, Geelong

Elizabeth Davies RN BSc(GU) DipApSc(Nurse Education)(QIT) FRCNA
Head, Division of Nursing, Australian Catholic University, Queensland

Sheryl Delacour RPN DNE(Armidale) BA(UTS)
Lecturer, Department of Psychiatric Nursing and Mental Health Studies, Faculty of Nursing, University of Sydney

Carolyn Emden RN BEd GradDipEdCounselling MEd FRCNA
Senior Lecturer, School of Nursing Studies, Salisbury Campus, The University of South Australia

Merilyn Evans RN RM IWC BA DipEd(WA) MEdSt(Monash) FRCNA
Research Fellow, Centre for Research in Public Health and Nursing, La Trobe University (Abbotsford Campus), Melbourne

Sally Forsstrom RN BA(NSW) DNE(ACAE) FCN(NSW) FRCNA
Lecturer in Nursing Studies, Charles Sturt University, Riverina

Genevieve Gray RN RM MSc(Nursing)(Manch.) DipAdvNsgSt DNE(NSWCN) FCN(NSW)
FRCNA
Associate Professor and Dean, School of Nursing Studies, The Flinders
University of South Australia

Joanne Gray RN CM BHlthSci(Nursing)(RMIHE) MCNA MCN(NSW)
Lecturer in Nursing Studies, Charles Sturt University, Riverina

Pat Hickson RGON ICCert BA(SocSci)(Massey) MA(SocSci, Nursing)(Massey)
Lecturer/Clinician, Faculty of Nursing, Deakin University, Geelong

Colin Holmes RPN BA(Hons) TCert(Manc.) RNT MPhil
Lecturer/Clinician, Faculty of Nursing, Deakin University, Geelong

Jocalyn Lawler RN AssDipNursEd BSocSc MEd PhD FCN(NSW) FRCNA
Associate Professor of Nursing, Department of Nursing, University of New
England, Armidale

Judith Lumby RN ICCert DNE BA(UNE) MHPEd(NSW) FCN(NSW) FRCNA
Professor and Head, School of Nursing Health Studies, University of
Technology (Kuring-gai Campus), Sydney

Debbie Neyle RN BA(UNE) MScSoc(UNSW) ADNE(Armidale CAE)
Lecturer, Department of Life Sciences, Faculty of Nursing, University of
Sydney

Judith Parker RN BA(Hons) PhD
Professor, Department of Nursing, La Trobe University (Abbotsford Campus), Melbourne

Rosalie Pratt RN RM MHPEd(NSW) BA(Macq.) DNE(Cumb.) FCN(NSW) FRCNA
Associate Professor and Pro-Dean, Faculty of Nursing, University of Sydney

R. Lynette Russell RN RM DNE(NSW) BA(Hons) PhD FCN(NSW) FRCNA
Professor of Nursing and Dean, Faculty of Nursing, University of Sydney

Sally E. R. Sims BNurs MScNurs RGN NPNCert HVCert ONCCert
Formerly Lecturer, Department of Nursing, Australian Catholic University
(NSW Campus), North Sydney

Sandra Speedy RN BA(Hons)(Flinders) DipEd MURP(Adelaide) EdD(Rochester) FRCNA
Professor of Nursing and Dean of the Faculty of Health Sciences, University
of New England, Northern Rivers

Bev Taylor RN RM MEd(Deakin) FRCNA
Lecturer/Clinician, Faculty of Nursing, Deakin University, Geelong

Judith Townsend RN RM BAppSc DipEd MA(Education) FCN(NSW) FRCNA
Associate Professor, School of Nursing and Health Studies, University of Western Sydney, Macarthur

Sandra West RN MidCert IntCareCert BSc(Macq.) MCN(NSW)
Lecturer, Department of Life Sciences, Faculty of Nursing, University of Sydney

Lesley Wilkes RN CM RenalCert BSc(Hons) GradDipEd(Nurs) MHPEd MCN(NSW) FRCNA
Head, Department of Nursing, Australian Catholic University (NSW Campus), North Sydney

Contents

Prologue

Genevieve Gray   Rosalie Pratt

A JOURNEY

This book is in the nature of a journey—its ultimate destination, the discipline of nursing. The book was born of our time and place—the time of translation of Australian pre-registration nurse education into the tertiary sector. This is the context which gives broad meaning to the word discipline: a branch of learning demanding of those who would explore and extend a body of knowledge and ideas a rigorous intellectual and moral commitment.

Essentially, of course, it is a journey within a journey since nursing's evolution began in the mists of antiquity, thousands of years before the coining of the Latin word from which 'nursing' derives: 'nutrire—to nourish', with its acquired connotations of nurturing *and* education (Donahue 1985). Its many stages have reflected the various social contexts within which it has been practised, and represent not only responses to changing contexts, but also the reflection of nurse thinkers on what has gone before and the vision of nurse leaders on the many possible ways ahead. One such thinker and leader was Adelaide Nutting, who commented on knowledge and ideas in 1925:

> We need to realise and to affirm anew that nursing is one of the most difficult of arts. Compassion may provide the motive, but knowledge is our only working power. Perhaps, too, we need to remember that growth in our work must be preceded by ideas, and that any conditions which suppress thought, must retard growth. Surely we will not be satisfied in perpetuating methods and traditions. Surely we shall wish to be more and more occupied with creating them (Donahue 1985).

Thus it behoves us, on this journey-within-a-journey, to pause for reflection as we travel—reflection upon the discipline's heritage from the past; upon its possibilities for the future; and upon the meaning of its application to our particular context: Australian nursing as it approaches the 21st century. It behoves us, too, to recognize that it is the quality of the journey, not arrival at a destination, which is all important. 'It isn't the finding the truth that's so wonderful,' says Lydia in Belenky et al (1986). 'It is in the looking for it, the exploring, the searching. If you were ever to think that you've finally arrived at it, you've blown it.' Whilst we may never reach the place to which we

1

thought we were travelling, nevertheless in the 'ongoingness' we will celebrate another phase in nursing's evolution or 'convolution', as Meleis (1985) would have it.

A convolutional process of development allows for an explanation of competitions and collaborations, acceptances and rejections, cumulations and innovations, peaks and valleys, rejections and reconsiderations, development and evolution. Webster's Dictionary defines a convolution as a complex, twisting, winding form or design. Convolution is not a nonpattern or a negative pattern, rather it allows for pendulum swings and is explained as *a pattern in progress* (emphasis added).

Thus, in the concept of convolution we find a blending of imagery—a pattern *of* progress as we make our way (or ways) on a journey, together with a pattern *in* progress as a nursing tapestry is woven.

GENESIS

This book had its genesis in an idea generated from discussion in a variety of forums within the profession, over a number of years. Its time had arrived it seemed as nurse scholars began to write, or indicate a desire to do so, on themes associated with the development of the discipline of nursing—including its theoretical base, its research approaches, and its knowledge development—and thus to communicate with others their understandings of the discipline. The writings collected together in this publication can be seen themselves to be a prologue to Australian literature in the area of discipline development. Indeed it is considered that they may well contribute to debate and thought on a global scale.

The timing of this journey is significant in the historical context of nursing. The development of the profession in terms of its education, its practice, and its scholarship at a time of rapid transition in this country is indeed an achievement of some magnitude. Theory, scholarship, research, practice, and education are all addressed in the book as we proceed on our exploration. Each contributor brings a perspective and an understanding which gives meaning to the whole and offers 'unique ways of viewing the world' (Donaldson and Crowley 1978). Each perspective, as Belenky et al (1986) tell us, is 'in some sense irrefutably "right" by virtue of its existence'.

Through the combination of the works we have the same sense of weaving a tapestry that we first met when reflecting on Meleis's (1985) 'pattern in progress'. The framework for the book is our loom for creating a tapestry of the discipline of nursing. The threads and patterns of the tapestry are rich indeed, with a diversity of views on the elements of the discipline. The richness of our tapestry, and of our discipline, is dependent upon the diversity in its substance. There is no one 'right' colour or patterning of the threads, but you will find a degree of unanimity amongst the authors which allows a blending of the diversity of designs. Whether the tapestry will be completed during this journey; whether there will be particular segments of the tapestry yet to be woven or improved; or whether there is still space between the borders, will be for you to judge. The tapestry will portray a story which itself in time will be of historical importance to nursing in Australia.

In interpreting this tapestry you will call upon not only your reading from this journey but also your own experience. So often we neglect to draw upon this experience and yet as Alice Walker tells us 'the act of knowing from our own experience is so simple that many of us have spent years discovering it' (Aptheker 1989). Integrate with this experience the knowledge you intuitively feel is important. Throughout the journey you will be presented with different ways of thinking of and knowing about the discipline and the context within which it exists. Different world views will be brought to bear in the stories that are told. The authors have shared with you and each other their understandings in weaving this tapestry as an expression of ideas and thoughts, feelings, and beliefs.

NURSING

The image of tapestry evokes the complexity of nursing in terms of its component parts and the relationships among those parts, and of its relationships with the particular socio-historical contexts within which it is embedded. The definition of nursing as a discipline is in one sense a culmination of a long line of descriptors, many of which we are still debating—a vocation, a practice, an occupation, an industry, an art, a science, a craft, a profession.

A combination of one or more of those descriptors invites us to consider nursing as a 'practice discipline' or a 'professional discipline'. Either of those phrases suggests that the rich complexity which is nursing encompasses practice, theory, scholarship, research, and education. The essence of a discipline has to do with knowledge and ideas. For nursing these in turn have to do with application to and derivation from practice; with exploration and construction through scholarship, theory, and research; and with sharing, liberation, and creation through education, 'the mediating link' (Fuller 1978). Clearly, then, the component parts of nursing are inextricably interrelated, and any journey towards, and reflection upon, the discipline must address ideas and perspectives on any or all of nursing's interconnections. The ensuing debate, as it is portrayed in this book, represents what Belenky et al (1986) have called 'the opening of the mind and the heart to embrace the world [which] is characteristic...at the position of constructed knowledge'.

Nursing as art

What, then, are some of the ideas reflected in this debate about the development of the discipline? Perenially nursing has been described as 'both art and science'. In this book, Holmes bluntly challenges the extent to which we have even begun to explore the notion of nursing as an art—'where is the understanding of nursing as an art expressed in nursing theory?' On the other hand, Carper (1978) includes 'esthetics: the art of nursing' as the second of her four fundamental patterns of knowing in nursing. Lumby, too, in this book, draws persuasively on Donahue (1985) to suggest that ultimately it may be possible to demonstrate convincingly that nursing is indeed 'the finest art' and a voice from Australian nursing's past illuminates the metaphor.

In introducing the first Annual Oration of the New South Wales College of Nursing (1953), Agnes Mary Lions noted that the purpose of conducting such orations was 'to invite women...to present a word-picture of the lovely colour and pattern that is traced on the canvas of modern life by "human kindness skilfully administered"which is nursing. To emphasise the value of every minute particle of pigment, every tiny brushmark so that each member of our profession will be further convinced of the community's need of her' (Lions 1977). More recently another Australian (O'Brien 1990) has extended the concept of nursing as art to incorporate the notion of 'artistry' in nursing, which can 'be equated with the ability of nurses to view patients holistically and adapt their skill base to serve individual needs'.

Nursing as science

The concept of 'science' is fundamental to and integral with any notion of discipline on the one hand and practice on the other. Indeed a prevailing confusion of terminology sees it on occasion used synonymously with discipline. A consideration of nursing as science in a contemporary context leads inevitably to discussion of all of the previously designated component parts of nursing. The impassioned debate which surrounds the alternative paradigms and perspectives of science, enquiry, and theory development is fuelled by the very complexity of nursing—by the multitude interrelationships of those component parts; by its embedment in socio-historical context; and by its relational nature, that is, nursing's concern with interactions between people situated in particular environments. Thus concepts informing the debate include those of philosophy; history and context; positivist, interpretive, and critical praradigms; holism and reductionism; phenomenology; qualitative and quantitative research methodologies; image and gender.

Nurse scholars in other countries, engaged on their own travel towards the discipline, have contributed a variety of perspectives to the debate and provided illuminating ideas on the interrelationships among nursing's component parts. Thus Silva (1977), in addressing interrelationships between philosophy, science, theory, and research, has claimed that 'ultimately, all nursing theory and research is derived from or leads to philosophy...Philosophical introspection and intuition are legitimate methods of scientific inquiry...The time has come to value truths arrived at by intuition and introspection as much as those arrived at by scientific experimentation'. Silva was concerned that the proper end of nursing philosophy, science, theory, and research is the advancement of nursing knowledge, and that the only end for the advancement of nursing knowledge is its meaningfulness for nursing practice. Fuller's (1978) concern was similar, although she came from a different perspective. Discussing science, practice, and holism, she urged the development of knowledge within a 'substantive structure of biological, psychological, [and] sociological concepts related to the health of human beings', since 'the uniqueness of nursing may be found in its unusual and simultaneous concern with the relationship of these several dimensions to a condition of health'. Fuller perceived that science was the avenue to knowledge development, and that development within the structure which she proposed would have significant implications for theory, practice, and education.

> [The] focus...would be on the dimensions of the human being—the subject of nursing—and not on the profession of nursing itself. The question of what is nursing would then become irrelevant and be replaced by the question: What are the needs of human beings which might be met by nursing?...The results of our efforts should be manifested in the people we serve. If they do not benefit, if health care is not changed, we will have failed.

From a more phenomenological perspective, Tinkle & Beaton (1983) saw that a more convergent definition of science, in relation to synthesis of apparently opposing paradigms, had 'the potential to enhance the impact that nursing research has on health care delivery and social policy'. And Munhall (1982) cited Psathas (1973) in suggesting that 'phenomenological approaches shift allegiance to a valuing of enlargement rather than economy, complexity rather than simplicity, the lens rather than the hammer'.

The excitement of the Australian journey lies in the various ways that this book's authors address the same concerns, but from different perspectives. Thus, Emden sets the scene by pondering ways of knowing in nursing from historical and philosophical perspectives; Cameron-Traub proposes that nursing has a distinct philosophy, methodology and framework for interpreting its knowledge base; Russell wonders whether we are asking the right questions and provides an associated historical perspective; Townsend considers the development of learning/practice frameworks; and Sims and Davies address differing aspects of the relationship between theory and practice. Bruni considers nursing knowledge as a process of production; Speedy teases out the connections between feminist research and nursing theory, practice, and research; and Lawler searches for an Australian identity among the plethora of imported ideas which she perceives to have been, to date, dominating our intellectual progress. Both Wilkes and Bartjes offer views on phenomenology; Neyle and West point towards a scientific basis for nursing; Parker focuses on an understanding of being and nature;

Evans provides a moral analysis of reflective nursing practice; while Emden, Gray and Forrstrom, and Cox, Hickson and Taylor offer perspectives on the reflective practitioner and critical reflection. Crane, too, addresses the critical paradigm; Delacour considers the construction of nursing from the perspectives of ideology, discourse, and representation; and Holmes questions, in relation to theory, where we are going and what we have missed along the way.

Nursing as craft

Through all of this, inspiration for Australian nursing as a discipline lies in the awakening realization that nursing has the potential to encompass a diversity of seemingly conflicting beliefs, perspectives, and approaches, and to synthesize them in practice into a balanced harmony of knowledge and skills. It is axiomatic that the practice component of nursing is underpinned by knowledge and skills. With respect to the latter, O'Brien (1990) has proposed the concept of nursing 'craft' to define 'the body of skills based on established nursing knowledge about the general effect of applying such skills'. Moreover, O'Brien urges that there 'are elements of art, craft and science in all nursing activity'. As has been suggested, nursing activity is not confined to that component of nursing commonly called 'practice'. It embraces also components of theory, scholarship, research, and education. Thus the 'body of skills' incorporates not only those intellectual, interactive, and psychomotor skills which are prerequisites of the practice of clinical nursing, but also, for example, thinking and writing skills for scholarship and theory development; enquiry and reflection skills for research; and facilitation skills for education. According to this perspective, the craft of nursing is foundational to its discipline.

GROWTH OF THE DISCIPLINE

Growth of the discipline of nursing may be assessed by the development and explication of the body of knowledge which is unique to the profession of nursing. As Donaldson and Crowley (1978) point out, the 'professional nurse cannot put nursing into a societal context without knowledge derived from the discipline'. This body of knowledge is also essential for the education of practitioners for the profession of nursing.Nursing can be regarded as a professional discipline having a concern for human health and well-being, a blending of science and art, and a dialectic between theory and practice. A professional discipline's knowledge base is associated with the realm of practice. It is important to recognize the difference between a discipline and a profession. As Donaldson & Crowley (1978) state:

Although the discipline and the profession are inextricably linked and greatly influence each other's substance, they must be distinguished from each other.

Failure to recognise the existence of the discipline as a body of knowledge that is separated from the activities of practitioners has contributed to the fact that nursing has been viewed as a vocation rather than a profession. In turn, this has led to confusion as to whether the discipline of nursing exists.

The generation of this body of knowledge will involve both scholars and practitioners. Several authors in the book draw our attention to the vital nature of the contribution of practitioners to the discipline.

Research

Nursing research is for Margaret Bennett (1990) the vehicle by which the body of knowledge will be largely built up. She reminds us that a balanced, multiparadigm approach to nursing research is being advocated. 'The phenomena of nursing are', she says, 'too complex to be approached from one perspective only. It is time for nurses to have confidence to lead research into new paths and...help the human sciences...find the answers to questions which have evaded us for too long.'

Growth through research may be assessed in terms of methodological perspective; approach; 'fit' with nursing philosophy; quality of the research process; and influence on practice. Munhall (1982) asks 'are nursing philosophy and nursing research vis-a-vis the scientific method ideologically and philosophically opposed?' She reminds us that: 'Despite nurse researchers' humanistic intentions for their scientific endeavours, historically the intentions of scientists are considered incidental and not part of the scientific enterprise.' Several authors in this publication suggest that we need to recognize the humanistic intentions of nursing and ensure that our research enterprise is consistent with our orientation. Progress towards maturity of the discipline in this regard may well be judged by the strength of the argument which flows through much of this book. As Sarter (1988) suggests 'the dramatic increase in the use of qualitative research methods in nursing demonstrates that the old assumptions are under attack'. It would appear that in Australia the debate has shifted from that of qualitative versus quantitative research methods, to that of exploring and promoting the relative strengths of particular qualitative research approaches. In particular in this book phenomenology and critical theory are given substantial attention by the authors, which would appear to be an indication of the overwhelming orientation of the profession in this country at this time. It would seem that Australian nurse scholars have found, as Munhall (1982) states, that: 'Qualitative research methods, particularly in theory development, may be more consistent with nursing's stated philosophical beliefs in which subjectivity, shared experience, shared language, interrelatedness, human interpretation, and reality as experienced rather than contrived are considered.' Perhaps it is also an indication of the progress that has been made in the understanding and knowledge of the discipline, and in the recognition, as Cox, Hickson, and Taylor suggest, that the central business of nursing 'is practice and that the nature of nursing will be revealed by illuminating and articulating practice'.

Practice

The centrality of practice is also evident in the authors' contributions. The education, development, and growth of the practitioner and the identification of the knowledge embedded in their practice is of vital concern. Reflection upon practice and the unearthing of the intricacies of the 'dailiness' of our work can only result in the growth of the practitioner and knowledge of the discipline itself. The contribution that practitioners will provide through this reflection will vary depending upon their own stage of development. As they learn their craft and progress to competent and expert levels of practice, they will be able to bring artistry to bear and have access to the lived-experience which is necessary for the use of a phenomenological approach in understanding the lived-world of nursing.

Lawler suggests that the 'elements and essence of our discipline are already in existence and well established'. The work ahead is to illuminate and strengthen those features. In Lawler's view, and indeed in those of other authors e.g. Parker, Bartjes, Wilkes, the phenomenologists within the profession will provide the most productive illumination and there is already evidence of substantial work in this area in Australia.

ON OUR WAY...

Thus we embark on our journey of exploration, discovery, and growth towards a discipline of nursing in Australia. And 'journey', it seems, is indeed an apt metaphor. We will not travel undeviatingly along a highway or even along an arterial road. The way will be neither straight nor flat—in fact it may not be all on dry land. There will be byways and detours and multitude avenues; dead ends and bogs and the high seas; valleys and hills. And we will use a variety of modes of transport as befits such a scenario, to link the many staging posts. Somewhere along the way, although not necessarily at the end, will be a rise which commands a 360 degree view and a 'multiperspective (which) facilitates the development of rich, complex, practice theories that illustrate nursing's unique holistic view of people as they interact with their internal and external environments during health and illness' (Meleis 1985).

Early in our journey, Andersen 'maps the terrain'. At the final stage reached in this book, Lumby draws together the threads of the emerging discipline in Australia: praxis, reflection, rhetoric, and research. You are invited to join us as we travel on this nursing voyage, and are thereby empowered in our daily practice.

REFERENCES

Aptheker B 1989 Tapestries of life. Women's work, women's consciousness, and the meaning of daily experience. University of Massachusetts Press, Amherst

Belenky M F, Clinchy B M, Goldberger N R, Tarule J M 1986 Women's ways of knowing. The development of self, voice and mind. Basic Books, New York

Bennett M 1990 The tea-bag phenomenon. In: Conference proceedings: dreams, deliberations and discoveries. Nursing research in action. Royal Adelaide Hospital, Adelaide, p 1-10

Carper B A 1978 Fundamental patterns of knowing in nursing. In: Nicoll L H (ed) 1986 Perspectives on nursing theory. Little Brown, Boston, p 252-260

Donahue M P 1985 Nursing. The finest art. Mosby, St Louis

Donaldson S K, Crowley D M 1978 The discipline of nursing. Nursing Outlook 26(2):113-120

Fuller S 1978 Holistic man and the science and practice of nursing. In: Nicoll L H (ed) 1986 Perspectives on nursing theory. Little Brown, Boston, p 261-267

Lions A M 1977 Introductory address. First annual oration. In: Annual orations 1953-1976. The New South Wales College of Nursing, Sydney, p 12-13

Meleis A I 1985 Theoretical nursing: development and progress. Lippincott, Philadelphia

Munhall P L 1982 Nursing philosophy and nursing research: in apposition or opposition. Nursing Research 31(3):176-177, 181

O'Brien B 1990 Nursing: craft, science and art. In: Conference proceedings: dreams, deliberations and discoveries: Nursing research in action. Royal Adelaide Hospital, Adelaide, 306-312

Sarter B 1988 Metaphysical analysis. In: Sarter B (ed) Paths to knowledge: innovative research methods for nursing. National League for Nursing Pub. no 15-2233, New York

Silva M 1977 Philosophy, science, theory: interrelationships and implications for nursing research. In: Nicoll L H (ed) 1986 Perspectives on nursing theory. Little Brown, Boston, p 563-568

Tinkle M B, Beaton J L 1983 Toward a new view of science: implications for nursing research. Advances in Nursing Science 5(2):27-36

1. Ways of knowing in nursing

Carolyn Emden

Serious students in the nursing discipline quickly find themselves drawn into a study of the history of ideas. To understand some of the origins and processes of human thought is an important hallmark of scholarship and a recognition of the centrality of philosophy to all fields, including nursing. Current interest by nurses in the potential of reflective practice is an indicator of nursing's quest for self understanding, as is an unprecedented interest in research and the generation of nursing knowledge. This discussion deepens nursing's search for meaning through an exploration of some key philosophic ideas on which nursing inquiry draws, sometimes unknowingly. As such, it is of fundamental interest to researchers in the field of nursing. As in all pieces of writing, the works on which the chapter draws are selected (as are the personal insights derived from them) and consequently the discussion presented here represents just one facet of how the topic could be addressed. The philosophic ideas within this discussion arise largely from 'modern philosophy', that is philosophy of the 17th century onwards. This thinking is built heavily on 'ancient philosophy' particularly that of early Greek philosophers. While equally compelling to the discussion at hand, space does not allow consideration of these more ancient ideas here. Reading and writing such as this reminds one how vast is the realm of human meaning and indeed how little one truly understands.

The discussion in this chapter therefore becomes an exchange of ideas between writer and reader, a discourse by which both can learn. The discussion takes as its focus Jürgen Habermas's theory of cognitive interests and the three sciences it proposes: the empirical-analytic; the historical-hermeneutic, and the critical. From a brief introduction to these sciences, the discussion moves into an historical overview of their origins: the work of the logical positivists and the Vienna Circle; the work of Husserl and his followers in the phenomenological tradition; and the origins and ideas of the Frankfurt School. Further contemporary schools of thought also are touched upon. Readers hopefully will be challenged to consider how the traditions of nursing research are influenced by the thinking of past and current philosophers and how the discipline of nursing may wish in turn to influence the evolving history of human ideas.

THEORETICAL FRAMEWORK

Jürgen Habermas's theory of cognitive interests (1987) seeks to systematically analyse the 'connections between knowledge and human interests' and was first expounded by Habermas at an inaugural address at Frankfurt University in June 1965 and first published in German text in 1968. McCarthy (1978), who has undertaken an extensive study of Habermas's work, suggests that *Knowledge and Human Interests* is Habermas's most difficult text for Anglo-American readers to comprehend. Not only is it Habermas's first attempt to systematically present his position but it is the way in which his thinking is so deeply rooted in German philosophy that makes understanding difficult. Certainly the work has generated considerable debate and controversy among philosophers and social theorists, as evidenced by editors Thompson & Held (1982) in their text *Habermas: Critical Debates*. In a postscript to a second printing of *Knowledge and Human Interests*, Habermas (1987) replies to some of his critics, and comments that the work generated such 'unexpectedly intensive and far-ranging discussion' and raised so many questions that he would need to write a new and different book if he were to deal fully with them. While acknowledging the importance of criticisms of *Knowledge and Human Interests* Habermas nevertheless chooses to uphold the 'systematic conception of the book'. It is to this original conception that the discussion now turns.

Origins of theory of cognitive interests

The origins of Habermas's theory lie in an historical tracing of epistemological ideas, particularly from the European philosophers Husserl, Kant, Hegel through to Marx and Freud. Habermas's own ideas are profoundly influenced by the writings of these philosophers but he experiences deep dissatisfaction with them all, referring to them as 'abandoned stages of reflection' (1987). The arguments against each of these influencing forces (largely to do with their inherent positivism) are of minor concern here, but more important are the essential features of Habermas's theory.

Essential features of the theory

Essentially, Habermas (1987) proposes that there are different categories of inquiry which give rise to different sciences according to different interests: 'There are three categories of inquiry for which a specific connection between logical–methodological rules and knowledge–constitutive interests can be demonstrated...the approach of the empirical-analytic sciences incorporates a *technical* cognitive interest; that of the historical-hermeneutic sciences incorporates a *practical* one; and the approach of the critically oriented sciences incorporates the *emancipatory* cognitive interest...'

Habermas states these interests 'have their basis in the natural history of the human species'; that the knowledge they give rise to 'serves as an instrument and transcends mere self-preservation' and that 'knowledge-constitutive interests take form in the medium of work, language, and power' (1987).

Habermas's concept of 'interest'

The concept of *interest* is the most central (and potentially difficult) in Habermas's theory: 'While "interest" is a literal translation of the German '*Interesse*', its use invites misunderstanding because, in contemporary English, "interests" are usually attributed to private individuals or politically motivated groups.' Habermas's 'interests' refers rather to *cognitive interests*: they are cognitive (or knowledge-constitutive) interests because they 'shape and determine what counts as the objects and types of knowledge' (Bernstein 1976).

Habermas thus locates three 'anthropologically deep-seated interests of the human species' whose basis follows from an understanding of humans as both tool making and language using beings.

Humans must produce what is required in confrontation with nature through the manipulation and control of objects. Humans must also communicate with one another through the use of intersubjectively understood symbols within communities. The species thus has an interest in the creation of knowledge which enables it to control objects and to communicate. From this it follows, in Habermas's account, that there must be a third fundamental human interest, namely, the interest in the reflective appropriation of human life without which the interest bound character of knowledge could not itself be understood. This interest is based in the human capacity to act rationally, to be self-reflective and self-determining. The species thus also has an interest in the creation of knowledge which furthers autonomy and responsibility (*Mundigkeit*). It is an emancipatory interest (Roderick 1986).

Habermas thus argues that the natural sciences are 'fundamentally and structurally oriented towards the production of technically useful knowledge' (Roderick 1986). It is important to appreciate that Habermas is not criticizing or denigrating this type of knowledge. His primary objection is 'the ideological claim that this is the *only* type of legitimate knowledge, or the standard by which all knowledge is to be measured' (Bernstein 1976).

The cultural sciences, unlike the natural sciences which grasp reality with regard to technical control, grasp interpretations of reality with regard to subjectivity and mutual understanding. Habermas thus argues that the cultural sciences are fundamentally and structurally oriented towards the production of mutual understanding and agreement.

The third emancipatory interest argued for by Habermas secures freedom from self-imposed constraints and distorted communication:

It is apparent that history embodies unreason in the form of domination, repression, and ideological constraints on thought and action...If the rational capacity of humans is to function truly, a particular type of knowledge becomes necessary to overcome and abolish these constraining conditions. This form of knowledge is self-reflection...Thus, self-reflection can, by revealing the structure of distortions, aid human beings in overcoming them (Roderick 1986).

Habermas's ideas will emerge in various ways throughout this discussion. At this point it should be appreciated how the discussion derives from his theory, that is, an historical tracing of ideas of the three major sciences: empirical-analytic (or positivist), historical-hermeneutic (or interpretive), and social action (or critical). Such an attempt appears relatively novel in the literature, thus heightening the need for critical readership and ongoing scholarship in this area.

THE NATURE OF PHILOSOPHY

Before proceeding further, it may be useful to capture a sense of what is meant by 'philosophy', and also in a very general way, the progression and focus of philosophy over time. On reading the history of philosophy, it quickly becomes apparent that the work of philosophers has changed markedly with time. It appears early philosophers were concerned with all that concerned humanity: the nature and structure of the earth and skies; the origins and purposes of human beings; the best ways to conduct human affairs; the meaning and importance of religion; and so on. 'Philosophy' naturally incorporated science and theology right up to the 17th century, while in later centuries philosophy became somewhat distinct from them. Bertrand Russell suggested in 1946 that the business of philosophy is the study of questions that fall between the dogma of religion and the reason of science: 'Is the world divided into mind and matter?...Has the universe any unity or purpose?...Are there really laws of nature?...Is there such a thing as wisdom?...'In 1976, Lacey stated that it is an embarrassment for professional philosophers that their field cannot be defined: 'What is philosophy?' is itself a philosophical question. A contemporary philosopher, Richard Bernstein talks about the 'scandal of philosophy' being the assumption that there is a 'proper object' of philosophy and suggests we abandon the idea that philosophy 'knows something about knowing, language, or thought that nobody else knows' and admit that philosophy is 'just another voice in the conversation of mankind' (1983).

At another level, on reading philosophy and its history, one becomes entangled in the 'humanness' of the philosophers themselves: their achievements and disappointments, foibles, family and health problems, passions and aspirations. It emerges that philosophy is a very human endeavour, reflective of its historical and social contexts. It clearly is apparent that philosophy, as it is recorded, has been the business of men. One can therefore ponder whether philosophy to date largely represents the thoughts and attitudes of just half the species. These gender issues are being increasingly taken up by feminist philosophers and addressed in important texts such as *Discovering Reality: Feminist Perspectives on Epistemology, Metaphysics, Methodology, and Philosophy of Science* (Harding & Hintikka 1983).

Despite its ambiguities and shortcomings, philosophy continues to occupy scholars, students and laypersons, and in its own way, to provide a meaningful thread to the history of human ideas. As such, it serves to anchor, in meaning, the thinking of *all* spheres of human activity and endeavour. Philosophy arguably becomes a legitimate foundational body of knowledge upon which all fields may draw—and indeed to which all fields ultimately contribute by virtue of their self understanding. In this sense of philosophy, the discussion resumes with a tracing of ideas about Habermas's first science.

POSITIVIST SCIENCE

Positivism has become a difficult term to define. It cannot be identified by its current adherents because there do not appear to be any. As Norman Stockman suggests, 'a positivist is not a nice thing to be, and nobody will own up to being one' (1983). He further suggests that attempts to identify the 'central tenets' of positivism have run into difficulties because of its many different usages and interpretations over time. Anthony Giddens (1977) believes positivism has become more a term of abuse than a philosophical term indicating that a thoughtful exploration of its origins is warranted.

Historical origins

Historically, positivism originated with the work of Comte (1798-1857) who proposed a 'positive philosophy' to replace the 'negative' thinking of the past, particularly theological and metaphysical speculation. Although Comte's views were influenced by others before him, such as Saint-Simon, the term positivism was his invention (as also was the word 'sociology'). Comte (in O'Connor 1964) advanced the notion that all knowledge comprises a hierarchy of six sciences (mathematics, astronomy, physics, chemistry, biology, and sociology) which are irreducible to one another, and yet all founded on systematic observation. For Comte, the new certainty, or 'scientific outlook', replaced all prior philosophic thinking. His views were to have considerable impact, not so much in France, but in other European countries, Britain, and North and South America. Even though positivism as a movement had died away by 1881, a small remaining group of disciples celebrated the Festival of Humanity in London that year. Essential themes of Comte's thinking were to persevere however, and eventually emerge in the highly influential work of the Vienna Circle (Giddens 1977).

The Vienna Circle

Ernt Mach is attributed with being the link between positivism and the Vienna Circle. Successors to his professorship of philosophy at the University of Vienna included Moritz Schlick, appointed in 1922, who became the leader of a group of philosophers who shared a common method to their diverse fields of mathematics, sociology, history, and law. The group became known as the Vienna Circle and its philosophy 'logical positivism'. The main task of logical positivism was to eliminate metaphysical elements from the sciences and to show that all the sciences, including the human sciences, are reducible to the method of induction. They developed the 'verification principle' which holds that something is meaningful only if it can be ultimately observed through the senses. Wittgenstein was an important early influence on the Circle, while Popper was a later significant fringe member. The Circle published widely and generated sympathetic groups in Europe, Britain, and the United States. After Schlick's death in 1936 the Circle did not meet regularly and had disbanded entirely by 1938, due to the political situation in Vienna. Members dispersed to Holland, England, and the United States, where they continued individual work.

Ashby (in O'Connor 1964) suggests that the logical positivists brought an interest in cooperation and a spirit of optimism to philosophy. While aspects of their doctrine have been rejected and many of their philosophical problems are still unresolved, (for example, 'what is meant by saying that a statement is empirically confirmable, or that one statement may be evidence for another?'), their rigorous approach contributed much to the understanding of philosophical questions.

Critics of positivism

Karl Popper

Logical positivism was soon, however, to attract major critics, one of the first and most devastating being the Austrian philosopher, Karl Popper (1902–). Although Popper's major work, *The Logic of Scientific Discovery* (1934), was considered by the Vienna Circle to be basically in accord with its own thinking, Popper insisted his position was contrary to any form of empiricism or positivistic philosophy (Giddens 1977). Giddens summarizes the most distinctive contrasts of Popper's work to positivism: '... his complete rejection of induction...his substitution of falsification for verification...his defence of tradition...and his replacement of the logical-positivist ambition of putting an end to metaphysics by revealing it as nonsense, with the aim of securing criteria of demarcation between science and pseudo-science'.

Popper's rejection of induction is fundamental to his position. To him, scientists do not 'observe', but 'conjecture'. These conjectures may come from anywhere, including intuition and imagination, but are always used for the purpose of falsification. 'The crucial feature of the scientific method then is not that it seeks to confirm scientific generalisations by collecting particular instances which confirm those generalisations, but rather that it actively seeks to falsify and refute the conjectures or hypotheses put up to explain natural phenomena' (Charlesworth 1982). On this basis, Popper rejected Marxist and Freudian theories because their proponents resisted attempts to falsify the theories (Charlesworth (1982).

Popper introduced a creative and imaginative element to the scientific process that was to appeal to many scientists. However, his theory of science suffers internal contradictions (for example, many theories survive even in the presence of falsifying evidence) and has not maintained its importance, despite efforts by Lakatos, one of Popper's followers, to rewrite the theory in more acceptable terms. Finally, it is noteworthy that while Popper distinguishes between science and pseudo-science, he does not reject the latter as meaningless (Charlesworth 1982).

Thomas Kuhn

A further major critic of positivism is Thomas Kuhn (1922-) who produced his major work *The Structure of Scientific Revolutions* in 1962. In the course of preparing a series of lectures at Harvard University on 17th century mechanics, Kuhn was led to his startling thesis that the history of science is not evolutionary, but revolutionary. Examining Aristotle's theory of motion, it appeared simple and false—until Aristotle's meaning of motion was understood. Similarly, Newton's meaning of motion was quite different to Kuhn's meaning. Thus Kuhn conceives science, not as progressing steadily over time, but from time to time undergoing revolutions, whereby old ideas are overturned by new ideas. Each period of relative stability is dominated by a 'paradigm' or model which guides scientific activity of the time, until a 'paradigm shift' occurs. Times of 'normal science' involve largely ordinary work, or 'mopping up operations' between big breakthroughs. Kuhn emphasizes that science is a 'social activity', both between scientists themselves and within the wider context of society, leading to considerable further work in the area of sociology of science (Charlesworth 1982).

Bernstein (1983) suggests that Kuhn's work raises prominent questions, such as: 'What is it that constitutes a scientific community? How are norms embodied in the social practices of such communities, and how do such communities reach objective-intersubjective-agreement?' As pointed out by Charlesworth (1982), the 'humdrum business' of Kuhn's science is a far cry from Popper's 'dramatic conjecturing', reminding readers that the nature of science is indeed unclear.

The Frankfurt School

In addition to the major critiques of positivism by Popper and Kuhn, the Frankfurt School has also been strongly critical of positivist thinking. The

Frankfurt School (Institute of Social Research) was founded in Frankfurt in 1923 under the guidance of Max Horkheimer, and comprised individuals from many fields including philosophy, sociology, economics, and psychology (Thompson & Held 1982). Interestingly, both the Frankfurt School and the Vienna Circle were meeting around the same time, resulting in numerous 'onslaughts' particularly by the Frankfurt members. Giddens (1977) suggests the situation has become more fluid in recent times with younger Frankfurt philosophers attempting to make connections between different schools of thought.

Antipositivism of the Frankfurt School operates at epistemological and sociological levels. Epistemologically, positivism's identification of certainty with sense experience was accepted by the Frankfurt School as adequate for the natural sciences, but not for the social sciences, because reflection is disavowed. Sociologically, not only is positivism the 'unreflectively dogmatic doctrine of the unity of science', but it is also found in separatist theories of historical and hermeneutic sciences. Frankfurt scholars argue that different modes of experience provide access for different realities—'sensory experience' for natural reality, and 'communicative experience' for social reality (Stockman 1983).

Positivism can thus be appreciated as a movement that enjoyed considerable respect and prestige for a short while before experiencing, over time, quite devastating attacks from several philosophical fronts. It continues to flourish through debate and discussion and much research, despite an apparent lack of proponents. It is important to note that Habermas does not dismiss positivism as having no value or place in the generation of knowledge—clearly it has an important place in his theory of cognitive interests. What he objects to most vehemently is 'scientism' or the belief of science (positivism) in itself to provide all the answers required by human beings. This position leads to the historical tracing of ideas about Habermas's second science: interpretive science.

INTERPRETIVE SCIENCE

Positivist science had achieved such success by the end of the 19th century that philosophy also was considered to be properly concerned with empirical statements and logic. Ethical, religious, and metaphysical concerns were put aside while logical positivism flourished (Stewart & Mickunas 1974). The phenomenological movement was a reaction against these extremes and of profound interest to Edmund Husserl (1859-1938) who contributed probably more than any other philosopher to its development. Husserl trained initially in mathematics, logic, and psychology before concentrating on phenomenological philosophy and particularly the significance of the 'lived-world'. The movement he founded deserves attention in some detail here.

Phenomenology

Husserl uses three metaphors to describe the attitude necessary for phenomenological inquiry: 'the phenomenological reduction' or narrowing of attention to what is essential; 'the phenomenological epoche' or suspension of judgement; and 'bracketing' or 'placing the natural attitude towards the world in brackets' (Stewart & Mickunas 1974). The later work of Husserl and that of Kierkegaard and Nietzsche led to a further movement of existential phenomenology and three emphases: the importance of the body; freedom and choice; and intersubjectivity, or the recognition of others' humanity. Both Jean-Paul Sartre and Martin Heidegger followed Husserl. Heidegger developed a new set of categories for understanding reality, especially the notion of Being, while Sartre rigorously analysed the nature of consciousness, largely through literary works.

Phenomenology may be regarded as a different way of looking at traditional philosophical problems such as the concept of the self, freewill, one's body, perception, values, language, and metaphysics. The phenomenological perspective on these problems is aptly described by Stewart & Mickunas (1974) to whose ideas I am indebted in this section.

Major concepts

The concept of the self is a major theme in philosophy, especially since Descartes. Consciousness, for phenomenology, is regarded as an activity that is directed beyond itself (intentionality). It is not experienced as a 'thing' among other things; the self cannot be separated from its conscious activity. This position is contrary to behaviourist positions which hold that consciousness is a response to outside stimuli and forces.

Freewill, from the phenomenological point of view, is not a separate faculty or a particular characteristic; it is rather a complex of conscious activities. Deliberation involves considering a range of possibilities (not just a choice between fixed options) whereby 'I am' becomes as important as 'I will'.

The meaning of body is limited in the English language because there is only one word, body, to describe its different realities. Body tends to be understood only in the scientific sense of a physical object, whereas in German and French, different words distinguish between the body which one lives, and the body which one encounters. This fundamental distinction in phenomenology has led to the use of the English terms 'lived experience' and 'lived body' to capture the phenomenological meaning of body. The lived-body therefore becomes the centre for all experience; the source of all motivation for action; the means by which consciousness experiences the world; a backdrop to the current project; and the avenue to awareness of others as embodied consciousness. In other words, 'the body cannot even be considered apart from the perspective offered by the body' (Stewart & Mickunas 1974).

Perception, for the phenomenologist, does not separate the act of perception and the object being perceived, but sees them as continuous. Traditionally, the empirical concern is to do with how individuals experience or perceive the real world. 'For the phenomenologist, the perceived world is the real world' (Stewart & Mickunas 1974).

Values are generally regarded as being subjective and based on life's needs and what gives pleasure and pain. Phenomenology challenges this view by claiming the subjectivity argument is based on a spatio-temporal conception of objectivity. Phenomenology holds, on the other hand, that 'every conscious state is conscious of something' and that 'different levels of conscious experience have different areas of objectivity' (Stewart & Mickunas 1974). Phenomenological understanding of values goes far beyond the notion of values as simply expressions of like and dislike, to central beliefs in freedom and choice, and respect for others.

Language, from the phenomenological view, includes 'all the ways consciousness expresses its relation to the world' (Stewart & Mickunas 1974). Written language can only be understood in its context and according to its meanings, never in isolation. Focusing on formal language systems provides only a limited understanding of the infinite number of meanings of language, according to phenomenology.

Metaphysics, or the 'ultimate nature of reality', is made explicit in phenomenology by the contention that 'reality is as it is experienced'. The ultimate question of metaphysics can be considered as the question of Being. Since Plato, Being has been regarded as an 'entity among entities', whereas Heidegger and the phenomenological tradition regard Being as belonging to all entities and expressed according to the lived-experience of the moment (Stewart & Mickunas 1974).

Application and ongoing tasks

Stewart & Mickunas (1974) outline some of the ways phenomenology has been applied in the fields of psychology (for example, by Victor Frankl and Rollo May); religion (for example, by Paul Tillich, Martin Buber, and Gabriel Marcel); the social sciences (for example, by Alfred Schutz); and the natural sciences. (The authors point out that in English 'science' tends to be regarded as referring to the natural or physical sciences, whereas in German *Wissenschaft* refers to both the natural and social sciences.) Phenomenology is particularly useful for determining the value of the natural sciences—their own methods being incapable of this.

In discussing the ongoing tasks of phenomenology, Stewart & Mickunas (1974) suggest that there is 'no *one* single phenomenological method' and that the extent to which phenomenology's method can be formalized depends on the area being investigated. One of the ongoing tasks of phenomenology is therefore the elaboration of the phenomenological method. The process of phenomenological analysis and the areas open to phenomenological analysis are also of ongoing interest. Phenomenology sees as one of its major tasks the analysis of the assumptions underlying the various human sciences and their methods, that is, of providing them with a way of understanding themselves better. Stewart & Mickunas believe phenomenology has succeeded in 'broadening the scope of philosophy to emphasize all human concerns'. Hermeneutics provides one way of finding multiple expressions of meaning or interpretation and can be considered an extension of the phenomenological method.

Hermeneutics

Solomon (1988) outlines the origins of hermeneutics (as a means of biblical interpretation) by Freidrich Schleiermacher, who worked with Hegel at the University of Berlin in the early 1900s. Dilthey picked up the work later in the century and insisted that all texts and human activities should be subject to rigorous interpretation on the basis of their intrinsic meanings. Heidegger extended the tradition but considered Dilthey too Cartesian (that is, too adherent to Descartes's mind/body dualism) in restricting interpretations to texts and human activities. He believed the human and natural sciences, indeed the whole world, were filled with such meanings and should similarly be interpreted. One of Heidegger's students Hans-Georg Gadamer proceeded to a life-long study of hermeneutics and became a key figure in the field. His major work *Truth and Method* was published in German in 1960 and in English in 1975.

Solomon (1988) goes on to point out some of the similarities between the ideas of Gadamer and Habermas—despite the long running and public differences between the two. Both are concerned with historical and social contexts, life's practical aspects; and rejecting scientism and Cartesian dualisms. However, Habermas does not agree with the 'universal consensus' that Gadamer believes possible through hermeneutics, nor does he believe that it is adequate just to elicit meanings in life—there must also be criticism of these meanings. Such a notion brings the discussion around to consideration of Habermas's third science: critical science, which acknowledges the enormous contribution and importance of the interpretive approach, but claims to go beyond its limits.

CRITICAL SCIENCE

Critical theory is generally regarded as emerging in Germany when the Frankfurt School was founded, with Horkeimer, Ardorno, and Marcuse as its prominent early members, and Habermas its most influential contemporary member. Brian Fay (1987) points out however, that there are many other critical theories than those emanating from the Frankfurt School, and for this reason he chooses to use the term 'critical social science' rather than 'critical theory'. Fay (to whose work *Critical Social Science* I am indebted in this section), suggests that critical social science carries a 'vision of existence' and is a medium by which many people 'express their most profound longings'. In this sense, it fulfils a role for some that is similar to the role of religion for others: it is the 'modern humanist conception of human possibility'.

Fay proposes that a critical social theory is one which will 'simultaneously *explain* the social world, *criticize* it, and *empower* its audience to overthrow it'. Such theories therefore enable individuals to understand how their society functions, ways in which it is unsatisfactory, and the means to bring about desired change. They are at the same time scientific, critical, and practical. Fay refers to 'explanations' in terms of basic principles subject to public evidence; by 'critical' he means sustained negative evaluation on the basis of explicit criteria; and by 'practical' he means transformation by way of self-knowledge. Fay acknowledges that the notion of a theory being scientific, critical, and practical all at once, flies in the face of much long standing philosophy—philosophy which he believes should be called into question.

Processes of critical social science

The essential processes of critical social science are enlightenment, empowerment, and emancipation. A critical theory therefore needs to be able to offer: '... a critique of the self-understandings of the members of its audience...a demonstration of the crisis nature of the workings of the society under discussion; and an identification of those aspects of this society which need to be changed if the crisis is to be resolved in a positive way for its audience' (Fay 1987).

Fay proposes that a fully developed critical theory must in fact consist of a complex of four related theories, each of which comprises further sub theories. The four theories comprise:

1. A theory of false consciousness which demonstrates how the self-understandings of a group of people are false and/or incoherent.
2. A theory of crisis which spells out how a particular society is dissatisfied and in crisis.
3. A theory of education which offers an account of the conditions necessary for enlightenment.
4. A theory of transformative action which details a plan of action for social transformation.

It is only when the entire structure above is intact, according to Fay (1987); 'that a theory can explain, criticize, and mobilize in the way a critical social science must'. Such a scheme also serves as a standard against which to compare other theories. For example, Fay cites the most frequent criticisms of Habermas's work as relating to it being academic and utopian and thus not meeting all requirements of his four-fold scheme.

Fundamental values

Critical social science, according to Fay , rests on the fundamental values of 'rational self-clarity' and 'collective autonomy', with 'happiness' being a further important value. Rational self-clarity is the 'essential ingredient' of enlightenment and amounts to people knowing the 'true nature of their existence' and being able to 'discern their genuine needs and capacities'. Collective autonomy is the essential ingredient of emancipation and amounts to people having the will and the power to direct their own lives. The other necessary part of critical social science, happiness, is taken by Fay to mean 'a mental state in which people are pleased with their lives as a whole'. Fay suggests that these values of critical social science are inspired largely by the thinkers of the Enlightenment, especially Rousseau.

Fay's account of the foundations of critical social science makes compelling reading and tends (along with reading of other writers in the area) to engender feelings of hope and anticipation about the potential of society and groups within it (for example, nursing). This is of course one of Fay's central and most intriguing points—that critical social science provides a secular means to salvation: 'Such a science is the continuation in another guise of the traditional ideas of salvation through illumination' (Fay 1987). To those interested in the history of ideas this proposition makes good sense: human beings have always sought a way out of the human condition, but for the greater part of history through metaphysical belief rather than through the power of human reason.

Critique of critical social science

As with all great cycles of thought, it appears critique is inevitable. While many writers are still predicting highly optimistic outcomes for critical theory and critical social science (for example, it is likely Carr & Kemmis (1983) have inspired thousands of teachers and others by their influential work *Becoming Critical: Knowing Through Action Research*) Fay addresses its weaknesses at length.

Fay (1987) finds weaknesses in critical social science in terms of its practicality and its integrity as an ideal. Both these weaknesses derive from a problem with the ontology of critical social science, rather than its epistemology, that is, with matters relating to Being rather than knowledge. Fay states most objections are epistemological: that a theory cannot be both scientific and political. However he considers he has successfully countered this argument and is more concerned with the ontology of 'activity' which underlies critical social science—that is, a conception of human beings 'who broadly create themselves on the basis of their own self-interpretations'. Fay believes this conception is far too limiting and that humans are also 'embodied, traditional, historical, and embedded creatures' and that this complexity creates powerful barriers to enlightenment and empowerment. Thus the limitations of human reason threaten the practicality of critical social science, that is, its ability to be a 'practical force for changing the social world it confronts'. Critical social science thus becomes utopian.

The integrity of critical social science as an ideal is similarly threatened by the limits of human reason to 'reveal to humans definitively who they are' or 'produce judgements which all members of a group must accept' (Fay 1987). Fay believes critical social science overstates the power of reason and consequently its ideals—rational self-clarity, collective autonomy, and happiness—are unpersuasive. Furthermore, and more worryingly, Fay reminds readers of revolutions inspired by critical theories which have only succeeded in replacing one kind of oppression with another: the terrible irony of promising to set people free and ending up enslaving them. The 'one-sidedness' of critical social science is partly to blame for such degenerations into oppression according to Fay, the over emphasis on the power of reason. He believes there is much good to be retained in critical social science, but proposes that future work must take into account deep changes in conception that include an ontology of embodiment, tradition, historicity and embeddedness. Otherwise: '... such a science is an instance of the ancient dream of a world where people live in harmony, united by a single faith and will which controls the conditions of their existence without deception about themselves or others'. We need to recognize that: '...this dream contains the seeds which, in certain circumstances, can lead to its own destruction: the paradise it promises fails to do justice to the inherent ambiguity of all human actions and relations, and to the limits of human reason and power' (Fay 1987).

In view of critiques on critical social science such as Fay's, one may well ask: What else? What next?

OTHER CONTEMPORARY SCHOOLS

In a contemporary exploration of the self since 1750, Solomon (1988) touches upon other schools of continental thought not mentioned to date but which may attract increasing attention. They emanate largely from France and include post modernism, structuralism, post structuralism, and deconstructuralism.

Claude Levi-Strauss (1908–), an anthropologist, represents the French reaction against modernism—from Descartes to Sartre and the German thinkers between. This reaction was dubbed post modernism. Strauss utterly rejects the Cartesian notion of the subjective self and replaces it with a theory called structuralism which is based ultimately in language and the human brain. Solomon (1988) suggests Strauss may have done no more than reintroduce old ideas in a more scientific form but adds that he shows an 'appreciation of cultural differences that is immensely refreshing after three centuries of chauvinist talk about "man"'.

The further reaction against Strauss is accordingly called post-structuralism and is currently maintained by Michel Foucault and Jacques Derrida. Foucault is a radical historian who is concerned with the place of power in knowledge. He rejects the term structuralist, referring to his own historical method as 'archaeology'. Unlike the structuralist interest in a general theory of human nature, Foucault believes the human sciences will eventually disintegrate, and prefers to study the 'seemingly aimless, shifting behavior that betrays the ultimate meaninglessness of human activity' (Solomon 1988).

Derrida does not share Foucault's sense of danger, and indeed seems more concerned with a sense of philosophical play, particularly on words. Solomon suggests Derrida is a serious scholar who knows the philosophical tradition he criticizes—its just that he finds it pretentious and 'pumped up with a confidence it cannot possibly sustain'. His style is not to offer counter hypotheses to traditional ideas but rather to attack and retreat, a way of doing philosophy he calls deconstruction. Solomon suggests Derrida's ways are 'truly perverse' and that only time will tell if he drops out of the story of modern European philosophy and if Foucault drops out as well. He concludes his history with the humbling reminder that 'the intellect is prone to self-aggrandizement, and that intellectual arrogance will always take a fall'.

An American viewpoint

In closing this 'What else? What next?' discussion, it is useful briefly to consider the work of Richard Bernstein, a contemporary American philosopher. Bernstein is steeped in the interpretive and critical traditions, having for many years travelled regularly to Europe to confer and teach with his philosophical counterparts there, especially Gadamer, Habermas, and Rorty. His project is interesting because it represents another perspective on where current philosophic thought is located. In the philosophical tradition, Bernstein has studied the works of philosophers before him in great depth before consolidating his own thoughts. In his earlier work, *The Restructuring of Social and Political Theory* (1976) he argued that a new 'sensibility' was emerging which contained elements of the empirical, interpretive, and critical schools of thought. In his more recent text *Beyond Objectivism and Relativism* (1983) Bernstein has continued to find common themes between disparate schools of philosophic thought, particularly objectivism and relativism.

Bernstein uses the terms objectivism and relativism in a broad sense. By objectivism he means 'the basic conviction that there is or must be some permanent, ahistorical matrix or framework to which we can ultimately appeal in determining the nature of rationality, knowledge, truth, reality, goodness, or rightness' (1983). By relativism he means that 'there can be no higher appeal than to a given conceptual scheme, language game, set of social practices, or historical epoch...there is no substantive overarching framework...no universal standards that somehow stand outside of and above these competing alternatives' (1983).

Bernstein explains how the themes of objectivism and relativism have pervaded philosophical thinking from the time of Plato; he believes the debates are more fierce at present than ever before because of the 'growing apprehension that there may be nothing—not God, reason, philosophy, science, or poetry—that answers to and satisfies our longing for ultimate constraints, for a stable and reliable rock upon which we can secure our thought and action' (1983).

The way ahead

Bernstein is not concerned with taking sides on the either/or debate (the Cartesian legacy) but rather with his conviction that the great debates are being played out and that a new understanding is emerging. Ultimately, he believes we are faced with the practical (not theoretical) task of 'furthering the type of solidarity, participation, and mutual recognition that is founded in dialogical communities' (1983). He is calling for a way of thinking (practical rationality) that will help us understand our human situation. Undistorted debate and dialogue, and community life, clearly are very important to Bernstein's vision for the future—and to this discussion. A brief examination of nursing's quest for understanding and meaning will bring the discussion to a close.

NURSING'S QUEST FOR MEANING

Members of all disciplines are faced with philosophical challenges: defining their field; clarifying the origins and nature of knowledge in their field; and determining how best to go about the practice of their field. (As we have seen, philosophers themselves share these challenges.) Behind these concerns lie the big philosophical questions: What is knowledge? Where does it come from? What matters most? Discrete fields, such as nursing, are not alone in their search for meaning: one study which explored epistemological questions with academics in the fields of music, theology, education, town planning, dentistry, and nursing found some startling commonalities. For example, all highlighted difficulties in defining the parameters of their fields (as exemplified by the following extract):

...education is a very fuzzy field...it is so big it's difficult to think of the whole...it has no clear boundary, although some may attempt to carve out a unique field of study;...town planning is actually a lot of different fields...that's its problem, it tries to claim more territory than it can deliver on...it doesn't have well defined boundaries or a core;...religion has so many different branches and facets...there's no single theme or unifying factor, it's a very wide field;...dentistry uses knowledge from many other fields although there is some unique knowledge in relation to materials research;...the field of music overlaps with the field of opera and theatre...nursing is not explicit...we can't pin nursing down...it's hard to agree on any area that is absolutely nursing unique...(Emden 1988).

As we move into a discussion pertaining specifically to nursing, it is worth remembering that disciplinary boundaries may be more blurred than is generally assumed.

Nursing's scholarly evolution

Afaf Meleis (1985) has written at length about the scholarly origins and evolution of nursing. She suggests that nurses have always tended to be influenced by the 'philosophical underpinnings' of their time, and because nurses have tended to study within the paradigms of other disciplines, their theories have reflected a range of perspectives and premises. For example, in a study of twenty six nursing theorists, it was found that their underlying philosophical assumptions could be clustered into those that were concerned with humanistic nursing as an art and a science (Nightingale, Henderson, Abdellah, Hall, Orem, Adam, Leininger, and Watson); those that focused on interpersonal relationships in nursing (Peplau, Travelbee, Orlando, Wiedenbach, King, Riehl-Sisca, Barnard, and Erickson, Tomlin and Swain); those that dealt with systems (Johnson, Roy, and Neuman); and those concerning energy fields (Rogers, Fitzpatrick, Newman and Parse) (Marriner 1986).

Meleis (1985) refers to nursing's development as a discipline as being a 'convolutionary process' (as distinct from Kuhn's 'revolutionary' theory of science), a process that allows for 'an explanation of competitions and collaborations, acceptances and rejections, cumulations and innovations, peaks and valleys, rejections and reconsiderations, development and evolution'.

Meleis acknowledges that nursing has been, and to a large extent still is, heavily influenced by the scientific or positivist approach to inquiry and that this limited view has hindered nursing's development (1985). Criticism of nursing's reliance on inappropriate and outmoded notions of epistemology has been documented by many authors including Thompson (1985), Watson (1985), Pearson (1989), Allen (1985), Brown (1989), Webster and Jacox (1985), and Emden (1988). Most of the authors take readers beyond the shortcomings and limitations of positivism, to the possibilities and potential of the interpretive and critical approaches to inquiry. Indeed numerous nursing research papers can now be found reflecting phenomenological methodologies and, although fewer, increasing reports of critical inquiries in nursing. Some authors propose combining approaches to inquiry, while others propose that it is more important for nursing to discover meaning through philosophy than through theory or research. One research report extract exemplifies this:

> Nursing is close to losing its humanity unless we recognize the danger of treating it as a science; an excessive belief in empirical research is a threat and highlights the urgent need for a philosophical examination of nursing [using philosophical methods]; other fields are also showing a renewed interest in fundamental issues of meaning: nursing academics must join this search with extraordinary courage—or perish (Emden & Young 1987).

In the study concerned, this was the highest ranking participant statement concerning the issue: 'Nursing should develop its own unique research tradition'—an issue which proved highly controversial (Emden & Young 1987). Support for the statement from senior nursing academics of the time around Australia highlights the importance of the current discussion, which certainly is concerned with fundamental issues of meaning and a philosophical examination of nursing. Just as the debates have continued for centuries in Western philosophy, so will they continue between and among nursing scholars. From nursing's relatively short existence to date, history may distil few significant milestones of thought other than a contribution to the conversation of humankind. In Bernstein's (1983) view, it is primarily through discourse such as this that we shall advance.

The value of discourse

Discourse broadens our intellectual horizons. For example, it is becoming increasingly apparent that nursing is concerned not just with Western philosophy and thinking, but with world views and practices. Leininger (1978) has written at length about her aspirations for nurses to practise transcultural nursing, many of which are still to be realized. Perhaps it is not until we come to terms with the philosophical underpinnings of transcultural nursing that such practice will be possible. The work of Fritjof Capra (1985) is useful here. In *The Tao of Physics* he explores the parallels between the world views of Western physics and Eastern mysticism. Capra points out that the central aim of both Eastern and Western civilisation was very similar: 'seeing the essential nature of all things', and that Western philosophy is only just beginning to recover from the Cartesian division of the mechanistic world view, and to return to the idea of unity. Other fields are also exploring new horizons: Rupert Sheldrake (1988) seriously challenges traditional scientific thinking in the field of biology—a bastion of scientism; Marilyn Ferguson (1987) reports on a major project involving many fields and persons engaged in 'social transformations'. These and many other projects provide a source of inspiration and encouragement to nurses who wish to break new intellectual and philosophic ground, and to tackle professional projects in fresh and innovative ways. Such is the climate of possibility in nursing today. Establishment by nurses of the Centre for Human Caring at the University of Colorado in Denver, Colorado is one realization of nursing's potential. The mission of the Centre is to advance the art and science of human caring knowledge, ethics, and clinical practice in nursing and health sciences. As such it is likely nursing will be the leading field in the generation of caring knowledge—knowledge that will be valuable to many fields (Watson 1990).

CONCLUSION

Hopefully this discussion has challenged readers to consider further some key historical and contemporary themes of Western thought. By gaining a sense of the history of human ideas one can more readily recognize some fundamental ways of knowing that underlie human inquiry or, in Habermasian terms, recognize cognitive interests and their consequences. Such an appreciation by nursing scholars should arguably lead to inquiry in which research problems and questions are addressed by the most appropriate methodologies. Indeed, the potential of different approaches to inquiry to produce different kinds of knowledge may not be fully understood without such an appreciation. Therefore I submit, and would welcome reply, that the discipline of nursing will be strengthened and enhanced by scholars who bring to their work an appreciation of the history of human ideas, as well as a sensitive awareness of different cognitive interests and their consequences. Beyond this discussion, the challenge remains for the themes of Western thought to be brought into context with historical and contemporary Eastern thought—thus broadening and further deepening nursing's quest for meaning. Continuing discourse between nursing scholars themselves and between nursing scholars and scholars in other disciplines ensures this quest is ongoing.

REFERENCES

Allen D G 1985 Nursing research and social control: alternative models of science that emphasize understanding and emancipation. Image: The Journal of Nursing Scholarship XVII (2): 58-64
Bernstein R J 1976 The restructuring of social and political theory. Harcourt Brace Jovanovich, New York
Bernstein R J 1983 Beyond objectivism and relativism. Basil Blackwell, Oxford
Brown J 1989 Emancipation through praxis: the reflective relationship between theory and practice. In: Koch T (ed) Theory and practice—an evolving relationship. Monograph: School of Nursing Studies, Sturt, South Australian College of Advanced Education, Bedford Park
Capra F 1985 The tao of physics: an exploration of the parallels between modern physics and Eastern mysticism, 2nd edn. Shambhala, Boston

Carr W, Kemmis S 1983 Becoming critical: knowing through action research. Deakin
    University Press, Geelong
Charlesworth M 1982 Science, non-science and pseudo-science—and Feyerabend on
    defining science. Deakin University Press, Geelong
Emden C, Young W 1987 Theory development in nursing: Australian nurses advance global
    debate. The Australian Journal of Advanced Nursing 4 (3):22- 40
Emden C 1988 Nursing knowledge: an intriguing journey. The Australian Journal of
    Advanced Nursing 5 (2): 33-45
Fay B 1987 Critical social science. Polity Press, Cambridge
Ferguson M 1987 The aquarian conspiracy: personal and social transformation in our time.
    Tarcher, Los Angeles
Gadamer H G 1975 Truth and method. Sheed & Ward, London
Giddens A 1977 Studies in social and political theory. Hutchinson, London
Habermas J 1987 Knowledge and human interests (Translated J Shapiro). Polity Press,
    Oxford
Harding S, Hintikka M (eds) 1983 Discovering reality: feminist perspectives on epistemol-
    ogy, metaphysics, methodology, and philosophy of science. Reidel, Dordrecht
Kuhn T S 1962 The structure of scientific revolutions. University of Chicago Press, Chicago
Lacey A R 1976 A dictionary of philosophy. Routledge & Kegan Paul, London
Leininger M 1978 Transcultural nursing: concepts, theories and practices. Wiley, New York
McCarthy T 1978 The critical theory of Jürgen Habermas. MIT Press, Cambridge
Marriner A 1986 Nursing theorists and their work. Mosby, St Louis
Meleis A I 1985 Theoretical nursing: development and progress. Lippincott, Philadelphia
O'Connor D J 1964 A critical history of Western philosophy. Macmillan, Houndmills
Pearson A 1989 Translating rhetoric into practice: theory in action. In: Koch T (ed) Theory
    and practice—an evolving relationship. Monograph: School of Nursing Studies, Sturt,
    South Australian College of Advanced Education, Bedford Park
Popper K 1968 The logic of scientific discovery. Hutchinson, London
Roderick R 1986 Habermas and the foundations of critical theory. Macmillan, Houndmills
Russell B 1946 History of Western philosophy: and its connections with political and social
    circumstances from the earliest times to the present day. George Allen & Unwin,
    London
Sheldrake R 1988 The presence of the past: morphic resonance and the habits of nature.
    Collins, London
Solomon R C 1988 Continental philosophy since 1750: the rise and fall of the self. Oxford
    University Press, Oxford
Stewart D, Mickunas A 1974 Exploring phenomenology: a guide to the field and its
    literature. American Library Association, Chicago
Stockman N 1983 Antipositivist theories of the sciences: critical rationalism, critical theory
    and scientific realism. Reidel, Dordrecht
Thompson J B, Held D (eds) 1982 Habermas: critical debates. Macmillan, London
Thompson J L 1985 Practical discourse in nursing: going beyond empiricism and histori-
    cism. Advances in Nursing Science 7 (4): 59-71
Watson J 1985 Reflections on different methodologies for the future of nursing. In:
    Leininger M (ed) Qualitative research methods in nursing. Grune & Stratton, Orlando
Watson J 1990 Human science and human care. Two-day seminar conducted by School of
    Nursing Studies, Sturt, South Australian College of Advanced Education, Bedford Park
Webster G, Jacox A 1985 The liberation of nursing theory. In: McCloskey J, Grace H K
    (eds) Current issues in nursing, 2nd edn. Blackwell Scientific Publications, Boston

2. An evolving discipline

Elizabeth Cameron-Traub

Nursing has been an evolving discipline for well over a century. The foundation stone for a discipline of nursing was laid in the Nightingale era when this nursing leader argued that nursing knowledge and practice were different from that of medicine. Differentiation between nursing and medicine is upheld by nurses today on the grounds that, for nursing, interpersonal interactions are the primary focus, whereas technological intervention is the main focus of medicine (Chinn & Jacobs 1987).

Philosophical and practice-orientated dispositions in nursing today are grounded in centuries of folk caring and healing, helping and sharing between people in the context of human and social existence. The emergence of nursing as a discipline, however, is attributed to changing societal needs and the unique interplay of art and science in nursing (Doheny et al 1982). Disciplines are 'created by the development of knowledge, including theory' (Chinn & Jacobs 1987). Following recognition that nursing practice must derive from sound and relevant educational preparation, the requisite knowledge base for nurses has been broadened and deepened, and has become increasingly inclusive of material originating from various disciplines. Only in recent years has the formalization of a knowledge base in, rather than for, nursing been given due attention. The rapid expansion of nursing theory over the past three decades, given the emergence of nursing science in the 1950s (Choi 1989), has added weight to nursing's claim for recognition as a practice discipline in its own right. Although achievement of this goal still seems some decades away, nursing should be well along the evolutionary path as a new identifiable discipline by the turn of the next century.

As members of the nursing profession, nurses are collectively charged with the task and responsibility for developing appropriate knowledge for nursing practice. Since development of a knowledge base is closely associated with education for the profession and academic research and scholarship, the complete transfer of nursing education to the higher education sector in Australia should enhance the opportunity for Australian nurses to contribute to the development of the discipline of nursing.

According to Donaldson & Crowley (1978) a discipline has a 'unique perspective, a distinct way of viewing all phenomena, which ultimately

31

defines the limits and nature of its inquiry'. Therefore, the evolutionary process for nursing must be characterized by a uniqueness of vision and purpose, a balance between hindsight and foresight, conviction and flexibility, and initiative and constraint. As with the evolution of other aspects in nursing academe (Cameron-Traub 1986) this process will necessitate discarding inappropriate or obsolete knowledge and discovering and creating new knowledge. At the same time nurses will carry forward valued concepts and principles in nursing which are essential ingredients for the integrity, authenticity, and respectability of the discipline. Continuing expansion and refinement of nursing knowledge by interactive processes of conceptualization, formalization, empirical evaluation, critical appraisal, and dissemination amongst members of the discipline will optimize the evolution of nursing knowledge as a valued and useful endeavour.

In this chapter some of the issues underpinning processes in the formalization of nursing knowledge, and further development of a discipline of nursing, are considered. Some key elements for achievement of social and academic merit for nursing theory are identified, together with frameworks for evaluation of theoretical activities.

SOCIAL RELEVANCE OF NURSING

In the last few decades nursing has been gathering a diverse literature which attests to its concern for philosophical debate, methodological discussions, divergent theoretical trends, and search for strategies to promote academic endeavours. There has been a continuing pursuit by nurse academics for clarification of the nature of nursing. However, nursing knowledge and theory development has not been clearly linked with professional practice, despite the fact that the context of health care is the garden in which nursing must bloom as a reputable and significant professional discipline.

Styles (1982) states that 'in the pursuit of academic respectability, or a deeper commitment to securing a firm scientific foundation for practice, or both, we in nursing have devalued the service ideal to raise an intellectual one'. Johnson (1978) claims that there is an interdependence between the focus of a profession's concern with scientific pursuits and the social function of the profession. She states that 'if nursing's social responsibility had been clearly and precisely formulated as an ideal goal in patient care many years ago, perhaps we, too, would have been building upon previously established theory'. Instead our nursing heritage of practical experience and personally transmitted knowledge has now to be transformed into formal knowledge for a disciplinary base.

As a practice discipline responsible for rendering a service to the community, we must not lose sight of the fact that development of the discipline of nursing cannot be divorced from our social commitments as a profession. Menke (1990) exhorts nurse scholars to continue the pursuit of knowledge in order to develop 'a highly organised, cumulative, specialised field'.

Achievement of this goal would help to free nursing from some of the societal and multidisciplinary constraints which have impinged on, and determined, the context, scope, and justification for nursing practice. Past and present constraints on practice need not constrain and mould the development of knowledge for the future, providing that nursing's academic growth and its growth as a social and community service are closely linked and complementary.

Johnson (1978) suggests three social criteria by which theoretical formulations of nursing may be evaluated. The first criterion is social congruence which addresses the extent to which nursing decisions and actions will be consistent with social expectations. The second criterion of social significance is concerned with evaluation of the impact of nursing on the life or well-being of persons receiving nursing care. Does nursing make a difference to patient outcomes or is it really inconsequential? The third criterion, social utility, addresses the relevance and usefulness of a nursing theory to practice, education, and research.

Recognition and acceptance of nursing as a discipline may be determined primarily in academic circles. However, given its practice foundation and service responsibilities, the real test of nursing knowledge will be evaluated in the professional context. By taking extant knowledge into the field for testing, evaluation, and ultimately application as a guide to practice, congruence between academic and social perspectives should be optimized. Nursing will spearhead its evolution as a discipline by maximizing development of a knowledge base which has relevance to varied nursing practice contexts, and has the flexibility, depth, and breadth to meet new and changing social needs.

FOUNDATIONS OF THE DISCIPLINE OF NURSING

Development of a discipline of nursing is inextricably linked with formal development of a body of knowledge pertaining to nursing's concerns. Underpinning development of nursing knowledge are three components which should differentiate the discipline of nursing from other disciplines, including those of other health professions. These essential and interactive ingredients for disciplinary pursuits are (1) an identifiable philosophy, (2) at least one conceptual framework (or perspective) for delineation of what are nursing concerns and what are not, and (3) acceptable methodological approaches for the pursuit of knowledge. Each of these elements should be consistent with beliefs and values about nursing which are held by members of the profession.

Nursing as a concept

Concepts associated with nursing as a professional discipline probably have particular meanings for nurses, which may or may not be shared with others.

As the discipline becomes established and consolidated, dissemination of pertinent information to non-nursing constituents of society should facilitate broader comprehension of nursing as an academic and community process. Nevertheless, understanding of a concept of nursing may depend on what one assumes about concepts.

Rodgers (1989) suggests that a concept may be construed as an entity, a disposition, or an evolutionary phenomenon. If nursing were considered to be an entity, something which has some measure of constancy, there would have been virtually no change in nursing practice, beliefs, and values since nursing was first identified as a specific activity. Alternatively, nursing may be considered a dispositional concept, whereby nursing is seen as predisposing its members to act in certain ways. Consistent with ethical theory, Packard & Ferrara (1988) suggest that nursing is a 'moral idea, which obligates and inspires right action to serve the good' and, therefore, nurses are predisposed 'to know and to do right things for other people'. As a dispositional concept the uniqueness of nursing would be clarified by definition of attributes or principles which constitute or give rise to a 'nursing disposition' in behaviour. Finally, nursing may be conceptualized as an evolving phenomenon. From this perspective, the main thrust to development of nursing knowledge would come from the perceptions, expectations, and aspirations of members of the profession, nurse academics, and nurse practitioners alike. Definitions of nursing may well be linked with complementary role development for other health professions, but nursing would be differentiated by its unique approach to practice and its significant contributions to human concerns. Nurses in the future should carve out for themselves an innovative nursing role (Sovie 1978) and a crucial role in health care (Schlotfeldt 1978). Awaiting a definitive nursing theory or revolutionary changes in societal expectations of nursing may decrease the likelihood that nursing will achieve its potential for actualization as a practice discipline. An evolutionary view of the concept of nursing should stimulate optimal development for the profession and the discipline, facilitating linkages between them.

Philosophical basis of nursing

Threads in the evolution of nursing as a practice discipline are undoubtedly linked with philosophical perspectives on nursing practice and theory. Formal development of a body of nursing knowledge and theoretical expositions therein could hardly proceed without some degree of coherence in values and beliefs concerning the nature of nursing, what it is, and what it could (or should) be.

Recent writers identify a number of elements to do with the focus or purpose of nursing. Nursing is about persons and human dignity (Fry 1989), about caring (Watson 1987), about interpersonal processes (Peplau 1987), about acceptance of others and commitment to them (Fry 1989). Nursing is about being capable and purposive (Styles 1982), about helping (Murphy 1978), about humanistic helping (La Monica 1983), about treatment of potential or actual health problems (Gordon 1987), about holism, holistic health, and holistic practice (Kramer 1990). From this sample of views alone there are several identifiable themes: a human or person oriented theme; a theme suggesting nursing action (i.e. nurses do something); a theme about assisting people; and a theme about implications of nursing for health, or even life and life experiences.

Johnson (1968) describes three types of knowledge pertinent to nursing: knowledge of order; knowledge of disorder; and knowledge of control. Each of these areas of knowledge are consistent with Nightingale's school of thought which was strongly focused on environmental elements as potentially disruptive influences which would impede the course of natural reparative processes. Building on the assumption that humans are instruments of nature, nursing knowledge would include information about the ordered existence of people, the potential effects of disorder (e.g. wars, disease) and implications for human existence, and possible control processes which would circumvent trends toward disorder (Roy 1983).

Summarizing extant views on nursing Donaldson & Crowley (1978) propose that the following phenomena are of concern to nursing: (1) the principles and laws pertaining to processes of life; (2) the pattern of human-environmental interaction in critical life events; and (3) the processes which could effect positive changes in relation to health status. These focuses for nursing are consistent with the idea that nursing is an interactive human process whereby a person entrusted to nursing care will be protected, nurtured, sustained, and moved toward a more optimal health status, perceived well-being, and actual well-being.

Although nursing terminology has changed over the past century, the core of nursing thought today has strong similarities to ideas from earlier times. The perspective on nursing's domain of action has been broadened, and greater clarity of purpose has been achieved. As Peplau (1987) says, the nurse is the keeper of the purpose of the relationship between the nurse and the person receiving nursing care. Last century the purpose may have been mainly protection from forces tending to produce disorder. Today the purpose in nursing philosophy focuses more overtly on enhancement of life experiences and well-being. This changed perspective is consistent with societal humanistic movements, recognition and respect for the dignity of life, and increasing regard for people from different cultural backgrounds (c.f. Leininger 1978).

Some of the concepts of interest to nurses today are clearly related to intangible phenomena. Sarter (1990) identifies a number of themes which have recurred in nursing literature: process, consciousness, openness, harmony, noncausality, space-time and pattern. If these themes reflect evolving nursing philosophy then nursing as a discipline in the future has the potential to present a unique perspective on meanings of health, life and well-being, and nursing's relationship to these phenomena. Nursing theory may also go further than current health-related concerns; it may provide a rich source of information to understand processes and experiences of human existence, and how nursing actions may enhance them.

Nursing world views: evolutionary frameworks

Nursing rhetoric has not been constrained by divergent theories of the philosophy of science, competing world views or evolving conceptualizations about the nature of nursing. Discourse has been characterized by openness, flexibility, and a willingness to facilitate exposure to alternate and even conflicting points of view.

When disciplines have a metaparadigm it represents and serves as 'a gestalt, a global perspective, a total world view or a cognitive orientation which is held by the majority of the members of a discipline or scientific community' (Hardy 1983). Given the variety of theories which have been generated in nursing literature, it is as if theorists are searching for the best (and perhaps only) perspective, rather than building on previous efforts or working collectively toward a unified theoretical framework. Flaskerud & Halloran (1980) suggest that nurses have concentrated on the differences between theories rather than on possible similarities or areas of agreement.

Hardy (1983) argues convincingly that nursing is in a preparadigmatic stage of development, wherein the discipline tolerates diversity in theory development and methodological approaches. Individualistic enterprises in the formalization of nursing knowledge may result in some discontinuity along an evolutionary path until there is reasonable consensus, evidenced by collective patterns of disciplinary thought and action. It would be reasonable to assume that, as nurses, we must share some kind of gestalt about nursing. Perhaps explication of this global perspective will become more evident as nursing theories evolve. Such a perspective may already be guiding theory development consistent with extant nursing philosophy.

Four elements have been identified as components of a possible metaparadigm for nursing—the concepts of person, health, environment, and nursing which are consistent with Nightingale's perspective on nursing. Newman (1983) states that 'the domain of nursing has always included the nurse, the patient, the situation in which they find themselves, and, the purpose of being together, or the health of the patient'.

There are a number of difficulties with the proposal that these four elements constitute a metaparadigm for nursing practice, research, and education. The first three elements (i.e. person, health, and environment) could apply to a number of other disciplines, including medicine. Although necessary as a differentiating element, the concept of nursing may not be sufficient to signify nursing's world view unless it is clearly independent of other areas of health care practice. Secondly, a metaparadigm, like a metalanguage, should define the area(s) of concern for nursing rather than depend on the concept of nursing itself as a differentiating feature. Some concepts may indeed be shared with other disciplines, however, either there must be unique elements, or a unique configuration of elements which will pertain only to nursing and serve to describe its practical and theoretical orientation. Finally, there is little evidence to suggest that nursing theories have been derived from a singular world view suggested by a metaparadigm of person, health, environment, and nursing. These four components have been given differential interpretation, emphasis, and saliency in different theories (Marriner-Tomey 1989). In a review of nursing articles Deets (1990) found no support for the paradigm as a guide to nursing research or scholarship. It is unlikely, then, that this framework has guided theory or research activities so far.

Progress in the development of nursing theory has been achieved through deliberative and self-conscious processes (Johnson 1978). Although divergent approaches have been taken, there has been some measure of consensus between groups of nurse writers regarding their cognitive orientations for formalising nursing knowledge. Theories in nursing have been grouped by different criteria, often according to their underlying conceptual model (e.g. systems model). One method of classifying theories has produced four groups: philosophy, interpersonal relationships, energy field, and systems theories (Choi 1989, Marriner-Tomey 1989). A different approach was taken by Meleis (1985) who classified nursing theories into three groups according to their focus on needs, interpersonal processes, or outcomes. In general, the focus for theory development has involved alternative conceptualizations of nursing as meeting patients' needs, interactive processes of the nurse-patient dyad, outcomes for the patient, or influences on human-environment patterning. These themes have continued through the last four decades as new theorists propose their models.

As the collective product of many nurse theorists, a framework comprising the elements outlined above could represent a synthesis of extant nursing views, and hence a collective, nursing world view. If indeed a perspective for nursing can be drawn from these phenomena, then concerns for nursing would be associated with the following areas:

1. Antecedents to practice: Human needs and nursing competencies which are consistent with nursing practice as a social phenomenon.
2. Processes in practice: Meaningful interchange between the nurse and the person, including goal-directed action, in the context of the nursing relationship.
3. Consequences of practice: Outcomes of the nurse-person interchange which have significant implications for the person's current and future life patterns.

Each of these three areas can be identified only with the discipline of nursing, since this concept is integral to and underlies each of them. The focus of the framework is associated with the purpose and process of nursing. What is it about the person and the nurse that brings them together in a nursing relationship, how is nursing carried out, and what effect does nursing have? Finally, there is no separation of the nurse and patient into discrete elements; the elements are related to phenomena rather than possible entities.

As a conceptual framework for nursing research, education, and practice, the above elements may be used for nurses to generate questions and seek answers in any (or all) areas of concern to nursing. Moreover, the framework would be consistent with theories which give different weight to these elements. Future theories may be developed which could, under this formulation as a metaparadigm, facilitate formal linkages between aspects of all three areas, thereby providing comprehensive accounts about nursing practice.

Methodological perspectives

It is perhaps in the methodological area that nursing is clearly characterized as an eclectic discipline. Vigorous debate has continued over the past two decades about competing philosophies of science and their methodological implications for development of nursing as a research-based discipline.

Considering alternate possible scientific paradigms with different methodological implications (i.e. quantitative versus qualitative approaches), Menke (1990) concludes that it is too early to judge the strength of nursing's allegiance to either approach. As an alternative Stember & Hester (1990) propose a transcendent paradigm. They argue that the approaches may be considered complementary and that either method is not logically dependent on a prevailing paradigm.

Sarter (1990) argues that inductive and deductive approaches to theory development are each essential for completion of the scientific process. They are 'complementary and equally important phases of nursing science. Whether one begins with experience or with theory, the circle must be completed'. An inductively developed theory must be tested for its generalizability to a population of interest whereas theory developed initially by a deductive method must be tested for its relevance to the real world. Undoubtedly, nurse researchers will follow in the footsteps of their teachers, however, as long as methodological tolerance prevails, the discipline of nursing may be built on a combination of approaches to scientific endeavour. Hence, research questions and acceptable answers will continue to be diverse, following from the differential perspectives of nurse researchers who hail from different schools of philosophical and scientific thought.

DEVELOPMENT OF NURSING KNOWLEDGE

Traditionally, formal development of knowledge may flow from either of two perspectives. These are idealism (rationalism) or materialism (empiricism), whereby knowledge is either derived from mental events or from the five senses, respectively (Bishop 1989a, Sarter 1990). In the following discussion, the approach stemming from idealism is termed the conceptual approach, whereas the one linked with materialism is identified as the empirical approach. Consistent with opposing philosophical theories, it is assumed that either approach may be used independently of the other, that there is no necessary link between them, and that, in the purest non-interactive or non-integrated forms, each approach is suitable for generating new knowledge.

Conceptual approach

The conceptual approach is a primary one for philosophical discourse. It focuses on the acquisition and verification of knowledge by various specifiable mental activities. This approach includes identification of relevant phenomena, definition of concepts, relationships between concepts, and postulation of assumptions, premises, constructs, and hypotheses. Suggested methods for theory construction to guide the would-be nurse theorist include various forms of logic such as deduction, induction, or retroduction (Bishop 1989b), and attendance to principles for theory organization and evaluation (Chinn & Jacobs 1987, Keck 1989, Marriner-Tomey 1989).

Empirical approach

The empirical approach has its foundation in a school of philosophical thought which argues that the only true knowledge is that which is derived from experience. Although opposed to the view that knowledge can be developed by mental activity alone, the main philosophical disagreement appears to be based on the sequence in which the activities of conceptualization and observation should take place. In general an empirical approach requires that conceptualization of phenomena be developed following observation. Only through the senses can knowledge (about the world) be acquired. Once sensory data has been collected then concept identification and organization may be conducted. Various mental activities such as analysis, synthesis, and evaluation may be performed on these data, however, conceptual processes must not go beyond what has been gained from experience. Inference may be made, but only in so far as it is consistent with sensory data.

Origins of nursing theory

It is difficult to determine the extent to which nurse theorists have taken a conceptual or empirical approach to theory development. Most of the theorists have had lengthy experience in nursing, many in combinations of practice, education, and academic activities in relation to nursing. Various theorists have based their work on an analysis and synthesis of nursing practice, however, traces of thinking from other disciplines are evident in their expositions. In particular, some concepts, principles, or processes originate from theories in other disciplines. For example, such concepts found in nursing theories include conservation (Levine), stressors (Neuman), anxiety (Peplau), adaptation (Roy), and principles of helicy and resonancy (Rogers) (George 1985). These theories of nursing are no less creative because of the adaptations made to nursing. On the contrary, theorists have used an accepted 'theory-model' building approach, whereby theoretical formulations for nursing are based on a model which appears to fit the phenomena of interest (Chinn & Jacobs 1987). What is then required is testing of the new theory in the context of the alternate discipline (i.e. nursing) to ascertain its relevance and accuracy as an account of most (or all) nursing phenomena. This testing process would require conceptual appraisal, and also empirical validation of the theory for and in nursing as suggested by Klein (1978).

Some nurse theorists have taken account of observational data from clinical practice, thereby combining conceptual and empirical approaches. Orlando's theory is an instance in which refinement of the theory was based on clinical observation over a period of time (Marriner-Tomey et al 1989). Other theories in nursing would have been mainly derived from conceptualization of phenomena relating to nursing practice. For example, theories proposing that nursing is concerned with meeting specific needs of people (e.g. the theories of Henderson & Abdellah et al, in George 1985) are highly consistent with long held views about nursing, that its purpose is to help and assist people who have nursing needs associated with a health disorder.

Regardless of the potential origins of a theory of nursing, it is clear that the theorist carried out an analysis of nursing for the purpose of delineating important elements of practice in order to provide an understanding of the concept and processes of nursing. In doing so, a primary activity would have been that of conceptualization, a mental process for the development of knowledge from ideas about nursing and nursing phenomena. Some of these ideas may well have come from an analysis of the theorist's concept of nursing, derived either directly from his/her own experience or indirectly from the oral or written discourse of nursing colleagues.

Conceptualizations of phenomena in nursing must be linked with experience in some way. Refinement of one's interpretation of a concept, demonstrated by an ability to correctly identify exemplars of that concept, occurs within the context of the individual's experience. However, once defined by the person the concept must also be verified as similarly meaningful to others so that the product of conceptualization is understood by those communicating with the individual. For theories developed and published in nursing literature, this process is undertaken by other writers in the field. Nevertheless, these conceptualizations of nursing should also be meaningful to practitioners who may never take to writing formal appraisals of nursing theories.

A number of nursing theories have been tested for their application to nursing practice in varied contexts of care (Riehl & Roy 1980). Theories which have been clinically validated should be useful for explaining and guiding nursing practice, and will be essential for consolidation of nursing as a practice discipline. However, the interactive process of theory to observation and back to theory has not been systematically used as a basis for theory development or evaluation (Meleis 1985).

Interactive approaches and implications

Theoretical formulations may be evaluated according to the extent to which a conceptual or an empirical approach has been successfully utilized in theory development. Conceptual merit and empirical merit may be construed as two dimensions and measured according to criteria such as those advocated for analysis and evaluation of theory (e.g. Chinn & Jacobs 1987). Criteria for evaluation of conceptual merit would be simplicity, structural and semantic clarity, and structural and semantic consistency. Empirical merit would be judged by the generality of the theory to account for a range of empirical nursing phenomena, its empirical applicability as a guide to nursing practice, and its significance as a contribution to nursing research and practice.

Table 2.1 shows an orthogonal arrangement for the two dimensions of conceptual and empirical merit, each with two levels (i.e. high/low). Thus, a theory evaluated on each dimension may fall into one of the four cells, designated as an optimistic, idealistic, realistic, or cynical theory.

Table 2.1 Categories for theory evaluation according to levels of conceptual and empirical merit

EMPIRICAL MERIT	CONCEPTUAL MERIT	
HIGH	HIGH 'OPTIMISTIC' Consistent Clear Valid Applicable Useful	LOW 'REALISTIC' Inconsistent Unclear Valid Applicable Limited use
LOW	'IDEALISTIC' Consistent Clear Invalid N/applicable Limited use	'CYNICAL' Inconsistent Unclear Invalid N/applicable Not useful

The most encouraging category for a theory to be assigned to upon evaluation would be the optimistic category. Such a theory would have scored highly on both the conceptual and empirical dimensions, and thus would be appropriate and useful for development of nursing theory and its application to practice.

An idealistic theory would be one with a high level of clarity and logical or internal consistency but which has little relationship to nursing phenomena in the real world. A realistic theory would be the reverse, having relevance to nursing as it is perceived or experienced, but having minimal significance for the advancement of nursing knowledge due to a low level of conceptual merit.

The least useful theory would be one evaluated as low on both dimensions. Such a theory may be described as cynical and it would be an inappropriate guide for either nursing research or practice. The theory would need considerable conceptual and empirical development in order to raise it to the level of an idealistic or realistic theory evaluation.

Many nursing theories are suggestive of what *ought to be* in nursing, rather than what *is* (Meleis 1985). If they are conceptually sound then these theories may well be more idealistic than realistic, according to the above model for evaluation. A healthy dose of idealism may not be a disadvantage if, and only if, nursing as a profession has aspirations to approximate the goals for nursing proposed by an idealistic theory. In this case the idealistic theory could be moved to the optimistic category if it proposed effective strategies for eliminating phenomena of real-world nursing which detracted from the empirical merit of the theory. Theories in the realistic category, judged as having low conceptual merit arising from problems such as a lack of internal consistency, would need to be strengthened by clearer conceptualization (e.g. clarification of concepts and relationships). A realistic theory may be a fragmented representation of reality; it may contain elements which seem to match those of real-world nursing, however, a full account of nursing phenomena would be lacking due to gaps in the theoretical exposition.

FOCUSES IN NURSING THEORY

Traditional scientific approaches may be useful only as general guides to theory development. Within a discipline specific approaches to theory and research generally evolve and serve to focus members of the discipline on areas of interest. So far there has been a variety of theoretical approaches specific to nursing, as discussed earlier. The two approaches selected for analysis in this paper are (1) a focus on the nurse's role function (i.e. functional approach); and (2) a focus on person outcomes (i.e. pragmatic approach). These approaches are consistent with the position that nursing theory should be linked with nursing's social responsibility as a professional discipline.

Functional focus

Doheny et al (1982) state that a role involves actions of an individual in a particular setting and is linked with specific expectations, values, and feelings. They suggest that elements of the nurse's role are coordinator, counsellor, caregiver, educator, collaborator, patient advocate, change agent, and consultant. Each of these elements may be associated with identifiable functions, for example, 'giving medication' may be an aspect of the role of 'caregiver'.

Few major nursing theories have specifically focused on the role of the nurse. Role functions may be inferred, however, from the theorist's perspective on nursing. For example, theories based on the concept of patient's needs imply that the main nursing function is to alleviate or meet nursing-related needs. Meleis (1985) infers from needs theories the roles of 'problem solver', 'performer' of nursing problem related activities, 'knowledge-giver', or 'temporary self-care agent'. Systems or outcomes theories suggest that the function of the nurse is to produce suitable outcomes for the patient, consistent with the given theory. Roles suggested in various extant theories may include 'external manipulator', 'controller', 'conservator', 'healer without touch', or 'pace-setter' (Meleis 1985). Interpersonal or interaction theories are mainly concerned with the process of nursing in the context of the nurse-patient relationship. Possible roles suggested by interaction theories are 'goal-attainer', 'nurturer', 'helper', or 'meaning-finder' (Meleis 1985). One interpersonal process model of nursing which does specify elements of the nurse's role is that proposed by Peplau. The nurse is postulated to move between six different roles (i.e. teacher, surrogate, resource person, counsellor, leader, and technical expert) (Belcher & Fish 1985).

Although nursing theories have generally not prescribed roles for the nurse, some writers are seeking clearer delineation in this area, especially given the notion of expanding the role for nurses in recent times (e.g. Tomich 1978). Is it enough to infer role elements from a nursing theory, or should there be some theoretical explication which can demonstrate congruence of theory with the service function of nursing in the community? A functional focus for theory development would provide clarification of relevant and useful role elements for describing, guiding, and explaining actual and potential nursing practice.

Pragmatic focus

Expected nursing outcomes for persons receiving nursing care have not usually been identified in nursing theories, except in general theoretical terms. Patient outcomes following needs theories are inferred when the person's nursing needs are met, that is, the outcome of nursing practice is essentially removal of a need. In the case of theories based on a systems model, outcomes are expressed in terms of concepts of the model, for example, strengthening the 'lines of defence' for a person in relation to health matters (Neuman's theory), restoration of balanced function to specific behavioural subsystems (Johnson's theory), or adaptation to the situation (Roy's theory) (George 1985).

Theoretical expression of outcomes is to be expected since they should be consistent with the perspective and terminology of the theory. However, this approach does leave room for large variations in interpretations of nursing outcomes. Without clear linkage with behavioural exemplars it would be difficult to ensure adequate testing of some theories. The task of operationalizing variables for measurement of theory related outcomes would be assisted when the theory explicates relevant aspects of patient behaviour. In this respect some of the outcomes (or systems) models would have a distinct advantage for empirical validation and application to practice.

Overall, nursing theories vary in the extent to which they provide a balance between functional and pragmatic approaches to theory formulation. Falco (1985) argues that an apparent focus on the nurse in some early theories was reactionary, and designed to elucidate nursing functions as opposed to those of medicine. Subsequent movement away from this focus on the nurse may also have been related to a belief that the proper concern of nursing is the patient rather than the nurse. Nevertheless, one half of the nursing dyad is the nurse who, within the limits of his/her knowledge and constraints deriving from the health care system and societal expectations, must function in order to effect appropriate nursing outcomes for persons cared for. An assumption that patient or person outcomes can be expressed independently of the nurses role function may be unwarranted and even false. Clearly, this argument suggests that the author assumes a systems model for nursing practice, whereby the nurse enters the person's world (i.e. input) and at the time of the nurse's exit, (if not before), there should be some identifiable outcomes (i.e. output) for the persons concerned (Cameron-Traub 1988). This assumption may not be tenable to a process theorist. However, it is consistent with the metaparadigmatic view proposed earlier in this paper.

Interactive approaches and implications

The two perspectives of 'nurse's role' and 'patient or person outcomes' may be considered in an interactive manner, as was done for the conceptual and empirical approaches. What happens when a dimension for a functional approach (i.e. focus on nurse's role) is linked with that for a pragmatic or useful approach (i.e. focus on person outcomes)? By considering a diagrammatic representation of these two dimensions in an orthogonal arrangement, (i.e. assuming that they may be conceptualized and measured independ-

TABLE 2.2 Categories for nursing practice associated with theories evaluated on functional (nurse's role) and pragmatic (person outcomes) dimensions

PRAGMATIC FOCUS	FUNCTIONAL FOCUS	
	HIGH	**LOW**
HIGH	'EMPOWERED'	'SERENDIPITOUS'
	Shared focus	Patient focus
	Defined roles	Unclear roles
	Defined outcomes	Defined outcomes
	Effective	Effective
	Efficient	Inefficient
LOW	'INEFFECTIVE'	'IRRELEVANT'
	Nurse focus	Non-focused
	Defined roles	Unclear roles
	Unclear outcomes	Unclear outcomes
	Ineffective	Ineffective
	Efficient	Inefficient

ently) as shown in Table 2.2, four categories of nursing theory may be hypothesized. These categories have been identified as empowered, ineffective, serendipitous, and irrelevant nursing.

If a theory were to be evaluated as having clearly addressed the role of the nurse (i.e. high functional) and also having given attention to specifiying outcomes for the patient, then this category of theory should lead to conjunctive or empowered nursing practice. This would be the only category for a theory of nursing which would strengthen or enhance nursing practice due to comparably high levels on each dimension. Alternatively, theories having a relative imbalance between the focus on role and outcomes could result in either ineffective or serendipitous practice. Ineffective nursing would be associated with a theory which was evaluated as low on the pragmatic dimension but high on the functional dimension. Nursing practice based on such a theory may enable fulfilment of expected or prescribed nursing-related roles, but it would be ineffective (or at best indeterminate) as far as defining or facilitating specifiable outcomes for the patient. Theories which explicate desired patient outcomes (i.e. high pragmatic), but pay little attention to functional aspects of the nursing role (i.e. low functional), would be associated with serendipitous nursing. Nursing practice through nursing-role functions may be linked with outcomes for the person receiving care, but the theory would not be able to describe, explain, or predict these linkages. Finally the category for theories addressing neither the nurse's role nor person outcomes would constitute disjunctive or irrelevant nursing. Since theories in this category would not be consistent with either primary focus of the nurse-person dyad, it is likely that these theories would be of little use for nursing practice or research.

COMPREHENSIVE APPROACH TO THEORY DEVELOPMENT

Theory development in nursing should be optimised when a combination of approaches, as discussed above, are used. There are strengths in combining conceptual and empirical approaches, and also by addressing both functional and pragmatic perspectives in nursing theory. The following analysis of how nursing theories may be associated with nursing practice suggests that a comprehensive approach to theory development would be most likely to encourage formulation of a theory relevant to all aspects, nursing practice, education, and research.

If a theory were evaluated favourably on two of the four dimensions (i.e. conceptual or empirical merit and functional or pragmatic focus), this theory could be assigned to one of the four categories shown in Table 2.3. The categories, namely, ideational, operational, intentional, or consequential, are interpreted in terms of theoretical implications for nursing practice.

Ideational practice would be linked with a theory based on conceptual-functional approaches. Such a theory would provide a blueprint for practice according to role definition, suggesting how nurses should carry out nursing consistent with theoretically prescribed behaviour.

An operational perspective for practice, arising from an empirical-functional theory, would allow for contextual influences or moderators to be taken into account by the nurse. The theory would provide clear guidelines relating to the nurse's role function. However, due to the empirical nature of the theory, there would be theoretical consideration of how practice may be modified given variations in contextual factors. In this case, practice would be contingent upon theoretical interpretation of real-world phenomena.

The third category for nursing practice is characterized as intentional practice, since a theory assigned to this cell would provide guidelines for purposive action in its application to practice. The conceptual-pragmatic

Table 2.3 Categories for nursing practice associated with combined approaches in theory development

NURSING FOCUS	PHILOSOPHICAL BASIS	
FUNCTIONAL	CONCEPTUAL 'IDEATIONAL' Idealised Process oriented Roles defined Pre-planning Prescription	EMPIRICAL 'OPERATIONAL' Observed Process oriented Roles defined Context dependant Contingency
PRAGMATIC	'INTENTIONAL' Idealised Product oriented Outcomes defined Goal-direction Purposiveness	'CONSEQUENTIAL' Observed Product oriented Outcomes defined Goal-attainment Causality

theoretical approach associated with this category would involve proposal of expected or desired outcomes so that goal-directed nursing actions could be determined. This theory would not provide a blueprint for action, but would focus on potential outcomes, leaving it to the nurse's discretion to determine how these outcomes could be effected.

A theory assigned to the consequential category for nursing practice would be based on an empirical-pragmatic approach. Focusing on outcomes as observed in real-world nursing, such a theory would provide an account of practice in terms of goal attainment. Based on sound empirical information this theory should facilitate assessment of the nursing situation and introduction of theoretically based specific nursing actions in order to produce specified outcomes for the person receiving nursing care. Thus, this theory would be based on a notion of causal relationships between nursing actions and nursing outcomes.

CONCLUSIONS

A discipline of nursing has to be constructed toward actualization of nursing's academic and professional aspirations and potential. As a professional discipline nursing must constitute a branch of specialized and socially significant knowledge integral to and demonstrated in nursing practice. The evolutionary path and pattern for nursing in the future will be shaped by interactions of nursing theory and changing patterns and processes in the context of practice. Harmony and balance between academic and practice orientations, idealistic and realistic perspectives, and functional and pragmatic viewpoints will be essential for fulfilment of nursing's potential.

Coordinated strategies for development of nursing knowledge will be required. Building on the strengths of nursing's distant philosophical and recent theoretical heritage continuity in the development of the discipline will be facilitated as new options and pathways are explored and achievements consolidated. Nursing can be construed as an evolutionary phenomenon and as having an historically determined conceptual framework which could serve as a metaparadigm for research, education, and practice. An evolutionary view of nursing together with theoretical precision and methodological tolerance should facilitate optimal development of the disciplinary base for nursing practice into the coming century.

Clarification of nursing's concerns and purpose will be enhanced by a combination of approaches to theory development and evaluation. Conceptual, empirical, functional, and pragmatic approaches may be selectively and exhaustively combined so as to encourage formalization of a comprehensive, sound and socially relevant knowledge base which, in turn, will strengthen nursing practice.

The concept of nursing itself will evolve as a distinctive and relevant knowledge base is established and as practice by members of the profession is enhanced. The challenge facing nurses and nursing in the future is establishment of formal linkages between parameters of the nursing role and its outcomes, between academic and service achievements, and between theoretically engendered research and informed nursing practice.

REFERENCES

Belcher J R, Fish L J B 1985 Hildegarde E. Peplau. In: George J B (ed) Nursing theories, 2nd edn. Prentice-Hall, Englewood Cliffs
Bishop S M 1989a History and philosophy of science. In: Marriner-Tomey A (ed) Nursing theorists and their work, 2nd edn. C V Mosby, St Louis
Bishop S M 1989b Logical reasoning. In: Marriner-Tomey A (ed) Nursing theorists and their work, 2nd edn. C V Mosby, St Louis
Cameron-Traub E 1986 From tutor sister to nursing academic. Proceedings of the 8th National Conference of the College of Nursing, Australia, Darwin
Cameron-Traub E 1988 I have a dream for nursing. Proceedings of the 3rd Annual Conference, Australian Nurse Teachers Society (NSW), Sydney
Chinn P L, Jacobs M K 1987 Theory and nursing, 2nd edn. C V Mosby, St Louis
Choi E C 1989 Evolution of nursing theory development. In: Marriner-Tomey A (ed) Nursing theorists and their work, 2nd edn. C V Mosby, St. Louis
Deets C A 1990 Nursing's paradigm and a search for its methodology. In: Chaska N L (ed) The nursing profession: turning points. C V Mosby, St. Louis
Doheny M O'B, Cook C B, Stopper Sr M C 1982 The discipline of nursing. Robert J Brady, Bowie
Donaldson S K, Crowley D M 1978 The discipline of nursing. Nursing Outlook 26:113-120
Falco S M 1985 Faye G. Abdellah. In: George J B (ed), Nursing theories, 2nd edn. Prentice-Hall, Englewood Cliffs
Flaskerud J H, Halloran E J 1980 Areas of agreement in nursing theory development. Advances in Nursing Science 3:1-7
Fry S T 1989 Toward a theory of nursing ethics. Advances in Nursing Science 11(4):9-22
George J B (ed) 1985 Nursing theories, 2nd edn. Prentice-Hall, Englewood Cliffs
Gordon M 1987 Nursing diagnosis process and application, 2nd edn. McGraw-Hill, New York
Hardy M 1983 Metaparadigms and theory development. In: Chaska N L (ed) The nursing profession : a time to speak. McGraw Hill, New York
Johnson D E 1968 Theory in nursing: borrowed and unique. Nursing Research 17:206-209
Johnson D E 1978 Development of theory : a requisite for nursing as a primary health profession. Nursing Research 23:372-377
Keck J F 1989 Terminology of theory development. In: Marriner-Tomey A (ed) Nursing theorists and their work, 2nd edn. C V Mosby, St.Louis
Klein J F 1978 Theory development in nursing. In: Chaska N L (ed) The nursing profession: views through the mist. McGraw Hill, New York
Kramer M K 1990 Holistic nursing: implications for knowledge development and utilisation. In: Chaska N L (ed) The nursing profession: turning points. C V Mosby, St Louis
La Monica E L 1983 The nurse as helper: today and tomorrow. In: Chaska N L (ed) The nursing profession: a time to speak. McGraw Hill, New York
Leininger M 1978 Transcultural nursing: concepts, theories, and practices. John Wiley, New York
Marriner-Tomey A 1989 Introduction to analysis of nursing theories. In: Marriner-Tomey (ed) Nursing theorists and their work, 2nd edn. C V Mosby, St Louis
Marriner-Tomey A, Mills D I, Sauter M K 1989 Ida Jean Orlando (Pelletier). In: Marriner-Tomey A (ed) Nursing theorists and their work, 2nd edn. C V Mosby, St Louis
Meleis A I 1985 Theoretical nursing. J B Lippincott, Philadelphia
Menke E M 1990 Rhetoric and reality in the development of nursing knowledge. In: Chaska N L (ed) The nursing profession: turning points. C V Mosby, St. Louis
Murphy J F 1978 Toward a philosophy of nursing. In: Chaska N L (ed) The nursing profession: views through the mist. McGraw Hill, New York

Newman M A 1983 The continuing revolution: a history of nursing science. In: Chaska N L (ed) The nursing profession: a time to speak. McGraw Hill, New York

Packard J S, Ferrara M 1988 In search of the moral foundation of nursing. Advances in Nursing Science 10(4):60-71

Peplau H E 1987 Interpersonal constructs for nursing practice. Nurse Education Today 7:201-208

Riehl J P, Roy C 1980 Conceptual models for nursing practice, 2nd edn. Appleton-Century-Crofts, Norwalk

Rodgers B L 1989 Concepts, analysis and the development of nursing knowledge: the evolutionary cycle. Journal of Advanced Nursing 14:330-335

Roy C R 1983 Theory development in nursing: proposal for direction. In: Chaska N L (ed) The nursing profession: a time to speak. McGraw Hill, New York

Sarter B J 1990 Philosophical foundations of nursing theory. In: Chaska N L (ed) The nursing profession: turning points. C V Mosby, St Louis

Schlotfeldt R M 1978 The nursing profession: vision of the future. In: Chaska N L (ed) The nursing profession: views through the mist. McGraw Hill, New York

Sovie M D 1978 Nursing: a future to shape. In: Chaska N L (ed) The nursing profession: views through the mist. McGraw Hill, New York

Stember M, Hester N K 1990 Research strategies for developing nursing as the science of human care. In: Chaska N L (ed) The nursing profession: turning points. C V Mosby, St Louis

Styles M 1982 On nursing—toward a new endowment. C V Mosby, St.Louis

Tomich J H 1978 The expanded role of the nurse: current status and future prospects. In: Chaska N L (ed) The nursing profession: views through the mist. McGraw Hill, New York

Watson J 1987 Nursing on the caring edge: metaphorical vignettes. Advances in Nursing Science 10(1):10-18

3. The nature and relevance of theory for practice

Sally E. R. Sims

Nursing is both a science and an art. The art of nursing encompasses intuitive, expressive, subjective, creative, humanistic, and holistic dimensions (Jennings 1986). While at first sight science and theory may appear to be incongruent with the human focus of nursing because 'dispassionate and insensitive images may prevail when science is mentioned' (Jennings 1986), the emergence of nursing as a scientific discipline in its own right is essential for the advancement of nursing as a profession. Professional advancement depends upon accurate definition of patient problems for which nurses are uniquely responsible, and the development of a scientific knowledge base guided by conceptual models and theories which reflect the reality of nursing.

As nursing establishes itself alongside other disciplines, it is important that nurses keep their minds open to bold, creative and imaginative ways of developing and using nursing theory. Different theories of nursing will lead to profound differences in the delivery of patient care. It is therefore important that nursing theory is considered of value to all nurses and not merely the domain of a few.

THE DISTINCTION BETWEEN NURSING THEORY AND NURSING MODELS

The terms nursing theory and nursing model are frequently used loosely and interchangeably. As McFarlane (1976) has pointed out, there is considerable semantic confusion in the nursing literature in this area. A theory is a proposed explanation or hypothesis that describes the relationship between or among concepts. A concept is 'an abstract notion or idea often conveyed by a simple word, although the features of the concept may be extremely complex' (Chapman 1985). Concepts may be described as 'the bricks from which theories are constructed' (Hardy 1974). In addition to a set of well defined concepts, a theory must have a set of propositions that specify the relationships between the concepts and hypotheses which are derived from the theory to test the relationships between the concepts and propositions.

Pain is an example of a concept which is abstract and conveys much more than the word alone. Pain is a complex phenomenon with physiological,

51

psychological, spiritual, and social components. A number of theories have been postulated to explain pain and its perception. These include the Gate Control Theory (Melzack & Wall 1965), the Pattern Theory and the Specificity Theory. It is commonly believed that knowledge, especially scientific knowledge, is permanent. However, theories are dependent upon the state of knowledge at a given time. All knowledge has a hypothetical status and may be disproved at a later stage. The Gate Control Theory of pain, for example, has superseded the Specificity Theory because it is now known that pain signals do not travel from a specific nociceptor to a pain centre in the brain.

A model is not the same as a theory. A model is an outline or representation of reality. For example, a diagram of the brain and nervous system may be used to represent the working of the Gate Control Theory of pain. Models can be broadly classified into analog, iconic, and symbolic models (Hardy 1974). An analog model (or analogy) draws resemblances between theory and the subject matter. For example, the analogy of a mechanical pump may be used to explain the workings of the heart. Iconic models are used if a direct representation of the subject matter is wanted, for example, a model of the heart built to scale. Symbolic models represent phenomena figuratively. For example, car drivers are familiar with the symbols associated with the highway code.

Models can be further categorized according to the dominant thought processes used to develop the model (e.g. logistic method) and according to their theoretical base (e.g. developmental, systems, behavioural, interactional) (Stevens 1984).

Lancaster & Lancaster (1981) suggest that all theories are models because they purport to represent some aspect of reality. However, the converse is not true. All models are not theories because many models do not have all the requisites of theoretical construction. Kristjanson et al (1987) point out that the majority of theoretical advancements in nursing fall into the conceptual model category because they do not provide the level of specificity required to derive and test hypotheses found in theories. A conceptual model for nursing practice has been defined as 'a systematically constructed, scientifically based, and logically related set of concepts which identify the essential components of nursing practice together with the theoretical bases for these concepts and the values required in their use by the practitioner' (Riehl & Roy 1980). Approximately forty conceptual models representing the reality of nursing have been created (McKenna 1989). These models provide a view of what nursing is or could be, while theory provides the workings within the model. The theoretical foundations of some of the major conceptual models are summarized in Table 3.1.

In addition to making the distinction between nursing theory and models, it is important to distinguish between the nursing process and models of nursing. Although the nursing process is described by some as a model (Ziegler at al 1986), Aggleton & Chalmers (1986) argue that it is not a model

Table 3.1 The theoretical foundation of some of the major nursing models

Theoretical foundation	Nursing model
1. Developmental theory	
Focuses on the stage, direction and potential for human growth and motivation.	Peplau H (1952) Henderson V (1986)
2. Systems theory	
Both people and their environment are open systems in relationship with each other. A change in one system influences the other.	Roy Sr C (1976) Parse R (1981) Neuman B (1982)
3. Interactional theory	
Emphasizes relationships between people and the roles they play in society.	Orlando I J (1961) King I M (1971) Travelbee J (1966)
4. Behavioural theory	
Individuals normally learn to function in society by their own efforts and carry out their own activities of living and self care requirements.	Rogers M E (1970) Orem D E (1971) Roper et al (1980) Johnson D E (1980)

For a more detailed description of the theoretical foundations above, see Thibodeau (1983) and Chapman (1985)

rather a set of systematic steps that can be used in planning and delivering care. Commonly the nursing process consists of five steps: assessing, diagnosing, planning, implementing, and evaluating (Ziegler et al 1986). Models of nursing attempt to explain and describe nursing and comprise more than a set of systematic steps.

Chapman (1985) suggests that many nurses believe that the isolation of concepts, the proving and testing of theory, and the use of models is an unnecessary complication in nursing. However, theory development is at the crux of nursing's evolution as a scientific discipline (Jennings 1987). Theories and models are essential if nursing is to develop a sound knowledge base which advances understanding of nursing and guides practice, education, and research. Theory provides a framework for action and helps to eliminate care which is based on trial and error. It enables the nurse to explain patient need and behaviour, to plan to meet these needs, and to predict the likely outcome. Models outline the elements, process, and goals of nursing.

Theory development involves searching for answers which clarify the nature of nursing and in turn clarify the focus of nursing, i.e. the independent role of the nurse. Independent nursing functions are those activities nurses initiate and perform under their own professional licence (Ziegler et al 1986). If nursing has no unique function then the activities of nursing may be divided up and taken over by skilled technicians (Weatherston 1979) or may be carried out on the orders of others. It is therefore important that nursing develops its own body of knowledge. It is often believed that 'there can be no theory of nursing in the sense of theory belonging to nursing because all of the theory applied to nursing is borrowed from other disciplines' (Weatherston 1979). Indeed, the majority of theories used to describe and guide nursing practice do arise from other disciplines such as psychology, biology, and sociology. In addition, theories incorporated into nursing models are also for the most part borrowed from other disciplines. However, it can be argued that once such theories have been adapted to the context of nursing, they become nursing theory because they comprise shared knowledge used in a distinctive manner. It is when borrowed theoretical concepts are used before their relevance to nursing has been determined and without modification, that problems arise.

There are many different sources of knowledge in nursing. 'The crucial notion is that different ways of thinking about people, health, the environment and nursing influence how care is carried out' (Aggleton & Chalmers 1989). Nursing must decide how it defines people, health, the environment, and nursing and how its practice differs from other disciplines. While there is currently little agreement in this area, there is a growing consensus that nurses are concerned with people, health, the environment, and nursing (Fawcett 1984). These four concepts have been identified as nursing's general paradigm. A paradigm singles out the phenomena which a discipline deals with in a unique manner and 'is a way of looking at the phenomena that fall within a discipline' (Thibodeau 1983). In an evolving discipline such as nursing, it is important to encourage the development of alternative ways of looking at this paradigm and indeed alternative paradigms before adopting

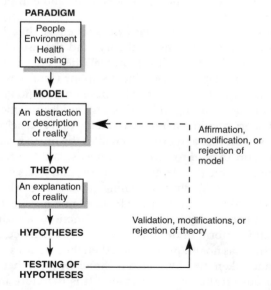

Figure 3.1 The relationship between the nursing paradigm, models and theories of nursing

a dominant theoretical stance. As McFarlane (1976) indicates, nursing must be aware of 'grasping any structural security that is not reflected in the reality of nursing'. Figure 3.1 illustrates the relationship between paradigms, models, and theories in nursing.

LEVELS OF THEORY

Theories may be classified in many different ways. One useful classification divides theories into different levels and their corresponding purposes (Thibodeau 1983). Levels of theory are identified somewhat differently by different authors (Jacox 1984, Riehl & Roy 1980). The most frequently cited classification, however, is Dickoff & James' (1968) hierarchy. They propose four levels of theory:

1. Factor isolating (lowest)
2. Factor relating
3. Situation relating
4. Situation producing (highest).

Factor isolating theory is the simplest structural level of theory. It is descriptive theory which is used to categorize, classify, or name elements. The theory does not explain what is being described, it merely asserts what is (Stevens 1984). Nursing diagnosis is an example of first level theory development. The purpose of nursing diagnosis is to allow groups of signs and symptoms of interest to nurses to be classified or named (Ziegler et al 1986). McFarlane (1977) has suggested that much of nursing theory has not progressed beyond the level of identifying concepts (Orem 1971, King 1971). Factor relating theories comprise the second level of theory. Their purpose is to state and explain correlations between concepts and variables. Theory at this level is explanatory. It attempts to identify how or why the elements of a theory relate to each other.

The third level of theory according to Dickoff & James (1968) is situation relating. Theory at this level is predictive. Predictive theory moves beyond explanation to predict specific outcomes, for example, a pressure area assessment tool. However, it does not tell one specifically what to do. The fourth level of theory, situation producing or prescriptive theory, informs what is to be done. This type of theory prescribes how an individual must act in order to bring about a desired result (Thibodeau 1983). The respective purpose of each level of theory is summarized in Table 3.2 on page 56.

Dickoff & James's (1968) hierarchy provides a guide for theory development, each level serving as the basis for the next level of theory building. Since theories are concerned with a wide range of very specific issues, theories at each of the different levels are needed to deal with all the concepts of interest to a discipline. Dickoff & James (1968) point out that in a practice discipline such as nursing, prescriptive theories are essential to identify clearly the goals to be achieved and the activities required to achieve the

Table 3.2 The purpose of each level of theory

Level	Purpose
1. Factor isolating	1. Naming or labelling, classifying or cataloguing
2. Factor relating	2. Depicting or describing, relating
3. Situation relating	3. Prediction
4. Situation producing	4. Prescription of activity

goals. The specific aim of prescriptive nursing theory is to base all interventions on a tested body of knowledge. It is ethically questionable to carry out activities which are not theoretically sound. It is therefore essential that practice innovations are subjected to scientific rigour before being implemented. Nursing is only now beginning to realize the need for research studies that build on one another from the descriptive theory stage to that of clinical evaluation (Fawcett 1984).

APPROACHES TO THEORY DEVELOPMENT

Theories are not discovered, they are created. Theory building is a creative, intellectual exercise that can be carried out by anyone with sufficient imagination (Polit & Hungler 1983).

However, an understanding of the analytical thought processes involved in theory development is essential if theory is to be logically constructed. Logic involves orderly reasoning. In its broadest sense, logic is the study of the structure and principle of reasoning (Flew 1979). Theories must follow the principles of logical reasoning and the relationships between concepts must be consistent. Logical analysis is concerned with whether the reasoning behind arguments is sound. Broadly speaking, there are two main approaches to logical analysis in theory development, induction, and deduction.

The inductive method of theory development uses observations of specific instances to formulate theory. The fundamental principle of induction is that the more frequently a situation or occurrence is observed, the more likely there will be a similar situation or occurrence in the future (O'Hear 1980). Having formulated the theory it is then verified by research. The following is an example of inductive logic:

- Morphine is an opioid which relieves chronic cancer pain
- Diamorphine is an opioid which relieves chronic cancer pain
- Oxycodone is an opioid which relieves chronic cancer pain
- All opioids relieve chronic cancer pain.

This inductive argument actually proves to be false since not all opioids relieve chronic cancer pain. For example, pethidine does not. However, by making the pattern of recurring phenomena explicit, knowledge can be generated. Induction is therefore grounded in experience and inductive theory development is the activity of generating theory from practice. Figure 3.2 summarizes the inductive method of theory development.

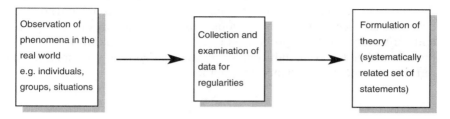

Figure 3.2 Inductive method of theory development

Deductive theory development is the inverse of the inductive method. The deductive process begins with a theory which is then tested. The theory is validated if instances cannot be found to contradict it (Thibodeau 1983). The process of deduction therefore involves progression from the general to the particular. The following is an example of deductive logic:

- A is larger than B
- B is larger than C
- It can be deduced that A is larger than C.

Such deduced statements are then tested by research. An applied science such as nursing uses the deductive method to apply borrowed theoretical concepts from other disciplines to the practice of nursing (McFarlane 1977). Field (1987) points out that the nursing process is a special case of problem solving using the deductive method. The nursing process is a systematic way of collecting data which is analyzed in order to develop tentative hypotheses about patient needs so that a plan of care can be formulated. Early in the assessment process, the nurse formulates a diagnosis concerning the patient's problems based on the incomplete data available at that stage.

Evidence is then sought in order to substantiate or disprove the initial diagnosis. Each hypothesis is tested and evaluated, firstly to confirm its presence and secondly to determine its extent and cause. This is the hypothetico-deductive method of clinical reasoning (Jones 1988). Figure 3.3 summarizes the deductive method of theory development.

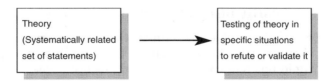

Figure 3.3 Deductive method of theory development

More recently a third method of theory development has been identified. Fawcett (1984) refers to this as retroduction, a combination of induction followed by deduction. This strategy starts with a series of observations thought to be related. Regularities among the observations are looked for in order to make sense of the observations. Finally, the validity of the concepts and verification of the hypothesized relationships, in situations other than those in which they were induced, is carried out. Figure 3.4 summarizes the retroductive method of theory development.

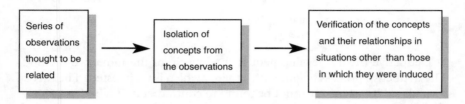

Figure 3.4 Retroductive method of theory development

By using the nursing process in conjunction with a nursing model, Aggleton & Chalmers (1986) suggest that nurses can use retroduction to evaluate nursing models critically and generate nursing theory. They argue that by systematically assessing patients using a nursing model, nurses can detect irregularities among the observations made and develop the beginnings of inductively generated theory. Having implemented the theory according to a clearly defined plan, it is then possible to evaluate the outcomes which allows a preliminary testing of theory to take place. The nursing process provides nurses with a framework which facilitates and encourages logical analysis in the giving of care. This approach should not, however, remove the continued need to speculate and postulate about truths and the application of truths. In addition to developing the skills of logical analysis, nurses need to develop the skills of scepticism. Garforth (1971) describes scepticism as 'relentless questioning forcing an individual to clarify his position or relinquish it'. Scepticism forces individuals to consider the content of their arguments more carefully, a process fundamental to both theory development and the research process.

THE RELATIONSHIP BETWEEN THEORY AND PRACTICE

Stevens (1984) indicates that the term practice is often equated with the practical and theory with the impractical, thus negating its importance. Operating within this framework theory and practice never meet because theory, by definition, does not relate to practice. Carr & Kemmis (1986) contend that the assumption that theory is non-practical and practice is non-theoretical is entirely misguided since one can no more practice without reflecting upon (and hence theorizing about) what one is doing, than theorists can produce theories without engaging in activities distinctive of their practice.

In order to examine the role of theory in practice, it is important to clarify what is meant by practice. In the context of this discussion practice refers to clinical practice, research, and education. Theory, clinical practice, research, and eduction are inextricably linked, and the major relationships that exist between them will be considered under the following headings:

1. The contribution of clinical practice and research to theory development
2. The validation of theory through critical evaluation and research
3. The application of theory in clinical practice and education.

THE CONTRIBUTION OF CLINICAL PRACTICE AND RESEARCH TO THEORY DEVELOPMENT

McFarlane (1977) reminds us that nursing is a practice discipline and therefore any theory of nursing must be intimately related to practice. She states that theory grows out of practice. One observes, names and clarifies nursing experience, and develops nursing concepts. Concepts play an important role in the development of knowledge promoting the organisation of experience and facilitating communication about phenomena (Rodgers 1989). Concept analysis is one method of concept clarification. Rodgers (1989) describes concept analysis as 'primarily a means of identification, not imposing any strict criteria, expectations, or view of reality on the concept, but simply seeing what is common in the existing use of the concept'. She describes the following phases (not steps as concept analysis does not proceed in a linear fashion):

1. Identify and name the concepts of interest
2. Identify surrogate terms and relevant uses of the concept
3. Identify and select an appropriate sample for data collection
4. Identify the attributes of the concept
5. Identify the references, antecedents and consequences of the concept if possible. (Identifying the references clarifies the situations under which the concept is appropriate; antecedents are the events or phenomena that are generally found to precede an instance of a concept; consequences follow an occurrence of the concept.)
6. Identify concepts that are related to the concept of interest
7. Identify a model case of the concept.

Concept analysis is one way in which nursing can develop its knowledge base and clarify its conceptual foundation. The observation, naming, and classification of nursing concepts and experiences can also be carried out using the grounded theory approach (Glaser & Strauss 1967). This is an inductive research process which generates theory from facts obtained within the natural setting of the phenomenon being observed.

The major assumption of grounded theory and other phenomenological research processes is that knowledge and social facts are best obtained when the researcher gets inside the natural setting and attempts to understand the phenomenon in the same way as the subjects. Theory generated from this methodology results in theory which is reality based. Dickoff et al (1968) warn against the development of 'armchair theories' in nursing. These are theories which are not grounded in reality and which researchers knowingly or unknowingly have set out to verify without raising doubts about whether these theories reflect the reality of nursing or not (Duffy 1985). The aim of theory is to enhance our understanding of, and to guide nursing practice. Armchair theories therefore have little value for a practice discipline such as nursing. The practitioner who is immersed in the reality of nursing and who brings existing practice to conceptual awareness (through reflecting on practice, for example) develops theory which has direct relevance to practice.

Personal knowledge is perhaps one of the least recognized but most important sources of knowledge in nursing practice. It is generally accepted that all nurses have a personal conception in their minds regarding the nature of nursing. These values and beliefs have been referred to as the practitioner's 'personal nursing model' (Clarke 1986). Hardy (1986) suggests that the wholesale adoption of nursing models has deflected the focus from developing more simple theories which may be of more significance to practitioners. Meleis & Price (1988) urge nurses to study the theoretical ideas that have emerged from local theorists rather than believing without question that 'what is imported has more value'.

There is a wealth of knowledge that could be gained from observing and reflecting upon practice and analyzing the reasons underlying apparently intuitive decisions. The intuitive practitioner arrives at answers or performs actions with little awareness of the thought processes involved. Nursing needs to develop ways of bringing intuitive action to the level of perceptual awareness. Benner (1984) argues that perceptual awareness is crucial to good judgements and that judgement for experienced nurses begins with vague hunches and global assessments that initially bypass critical analysis. The experienced nurse sees the situation as a whole and only later do the parts become evident. If the experienced nurse's knowledge is to be tapped, it needs to be made explicit.

Other ways in which nursing knowledge is developed from practice include tradition, trial and error, and authority. Tradition refers to practices that lack scientific evidence but are accepted as truths. The ritual monitoring of vital signs at prescribed periods of time is an example of a nursing activity based on tradition (Ziegler et al 1986). Trial and error is another way in which nursing knowledge has evolved in the past. This method of knowing is derived from trying different courses of action until one appears to work. Another source of knowledge is authority. An authority is an expert in a given area. Unless nursing develops its own area of expert knowledge it will be controlled and directed by others. As nursing moves towards a more scientific base, it must move away from knowledge centred on tradition, trial and error, and authority, and must fully utilize the relationship between practice and theory.

THE VALIDATION OF THEORY THROUGH CRITICAL EVALUATION AND RESEARCH

If a theory is to be useful for practice, it must be valid. That is, it must provide evidence of accurately representing the reality of nursing. Attempts to falsify the conclusions drawn from a theory must be made, and the theory modified, rejected, or accepted in light of the conclusions. There are two main ways in which this can be done, through research and through evaluation of the theory using an accepted framework.

Research can be defined as 'the rigorous application of the methods of science in order to obtain reliable and valid knowledge about reality' (Chinn & Jacobs 1983). The scientific approach involves systematically collecting and comparing data in order to describe, explain, and predict. It is the most powerful method of theory validation. It must be stressed that a theory can never be proved or confirmed. No theory is ever final and verified. There always remains the possibility that a theory will be modified or discarded (Polit & Hungler 1983).

Evaluation of theory to determine the extent to which its structure meets accepted criteria, begins with a description of its components. Once a theory has been thoroughly described, it can be evaluated or judged against stated criteria.

Fawcett (1984) points out that existing frameworks for describing and evaluating nursing theory (for example, Duffey & Muhlenkamp 1974, Stevens 1984, Meleis 1983) reflect the confusion that exists between nursing theory and conceptual models of nursing. Chinn & Jacobs (1983) have produced a framework for the description and evaluation of theory that assists the individual to answer the question, 'Is this a theory?'

The following areas are addressed in their framework for the description of theory.

Framework for the description of theory

1. Concepts: number; relationships; arrangements; scope; degree of abstraction.
2. Definitions: how the concepts are defined.
3. Goals: why the theory is formulated; goals for nursing, patient, society; scope of the theory.

4. Relationships: major relationships within the theory.
5. Structure: how ideas are organized.
6. Assumptions: those underlying the theory and whether they are explicit or implicit.

In summary, the five criteria Chinn & Jacobs (1983) use to evaluate theory are as follows.

Framework for the evaluation of theory

1. Clarity: the lucidity of the theory.
2. Simplicity: the number of structural components and relationships within the theory.
3. Generality: the scope of events covered by the theory.
4. Empirical precision: the extent to which concepts within the theory are grounded in observed or observable reality.
5. Desirable consequences: the extent to which theory results in or produces valued nursing knowledge.

Fawcett (1984) has developed a framework for the analysis (description) and evaluation of nursing models. This framework facilitates a detailed examination of the model and enables the individual to draw conclusions regarding the model's validity. In this way, it is possible to determine which model is most appropriate for a given nursing environment. Fawcett's (1984) framework addresses the following issues.

Framework for the analysis (description) of theory

1. The way in which the model has evolved.
2. The type of analytical thought processes utilized.
3. The concepts and propositions; in particular, those relating to the person, environment, health, and nursing.
4. The areas of nursing concern identified by the model.

Framework for the evaluation of theory

1. The extent to which the assumptions are explicit.
2. The comprehensiveness of the concepts and propositions.
3. The logical congruence of the propositions and assumptions.
4. The social congruence of the model, in particular the relationship of nursing to a wider society.
5. The value of the model's contribution to nursing knowledge and the extent to which it provides guides for practice, education, administration, and research.

The process of testing a theory through research begins with the formulation of research hypotheses (predictions about the relationship between variables if the theory were correct). The hypotheses are then tested by comparing the findings of the research with the relationships predicted by the hypotheses.

The research design is usually experimental because experiments have the greatest potential for controlling variables which might provide alternative explanations for the findings obtained. The process of testing a theory is deductive in nature because it begins with a general statement derived from the theory and progresses to the testing of hypotheses specific to a given situation.

Research therefore contributes to theory development in two ways, by generating theory and by testing theory. The research design and analytical thought processes must be consistent with the theory generating or testing orientation of the research. Duffy (1985) points out that in nursing, experimental (quantitative) research designs are frequently attempted whereas grounded theory and other qualitative research designs are less often considered. She suggests that this is because qualitative research methods have been relegated to the role of secondary significance and quantification of data has emerged as the true scientific methodology and the preferred way of knowing. More recently the need for an eclectic approach to data collection (the use of a variety of research methods) has been emphasized (Webb 1989). Webb writes that methodological eclecticism involves using different methods in parallel, rather than in series as previously advocated.

While theory and research guide and inform each other, it has been suggested that research and theory need not be related. The argument usually presented is that research may arise from an 'open question' which has no theoretical basis and that research findings stand free of 'facts'. However, as Schwab (1964) argues, even the questions asked by the researcher originate in a theoretical framework (whether or not the researcher recognizes it) and knowledge obtained through inquiry is not knowledge merely of the facts, it is of the facts interpreted. Interpretation depends upon the theoretical framework used. For this reason, it is important that research studies contain an explanation of where the study fits into the building and testing of theory.

Polit & Hungler (1983) suggest that the following questions should be asked when evaluating the theoretical underpinnings of a research report:

1. Does the report attempt to link the problem with a theoretical or conceptual framework?
2. Is the theoretical framework tied to the problem in a natural way or does the link seem contrived?
3. Would an alternative conceptual framework be more appropriate?
4. Are the deductions from the theory or conceptual framework logical?

Historically, much of the research in nursing has comprised descriptive research and accumulated knowledge has been poorly linked to theory. As

Polit & Hungler (1983) state, 'the time is ripe for the discipline [of nursing] to enter a new phase in which theory development and testing are major goals'.

THE APPLICATION OF THEORY IN CLINICAL PRACTICE AND EDUCATION

The development of theory is not an end in itself. Theory must ultimately be of some utility (Polit & Hungler 1983). There are five main ways in which theory guides clinical practice:

1. Creating different ways of looking at particular phenomena; providing a guide for assessment
2. Interrelating concepts in such a way as to summarize existing knowledge; providing a rationale for interventions
3. Explaining how concepts are related and predicting the nature of relationships under specified circumstances; providing criteria for evaluation
4. Stimulating creative thinking, new approaches and behaviour
5. Facilitating socialization into nursing by identifying the phenomena of the discipline, promoting coherence of purpose, and promoting communication.

The methodology which enables nurses to apply theory in practice is the nursing process. Ziegler et al (1986) describe the interface between nursing knowledge and the nursing process in the following way: 'Nursing theory guides assessment by describing which characteristics are to be assessed and how these characteristics cluster together to form patterns of behaviour'. Theories guide diagnosis by describing the norms against which the client's patterns of human response are within the normal range, potentially outside the normal range, or actually outside the expected values. Theory then provides the explanation for the client's response and serves as the base for the aetiology component of the nursing diagnosis statement. As Aggleton & Chalmers (1986) state, the nursing process by itself is, 'essentially an empty approach to care'. It does not tell nurses what to assess, how to plan and intervene, or how or when to evaluate. They illustrate how nursing models can act as guidelines for the use of the nursing process through organization of the database. This varies according to which model is used, for example, the focus of assessment using Roy's (1976) model is adaptation and using Orem's (1971) model, self-care.

Nurses who are able to apply theory to practice in this way operate from a logical base and are more likely to consider interrelationships between data. Novice nurses begin by operating from sets of rules such as these, while expert nurses no longer need to rely on them to connect understanding as it has become internalized. While the nursing process and nursing models are valuable tools for organizing care, it is important that the collection of objective data is not over emphasized at the expense of subjective data. Objectivity can lead to generalizations, subjective data is needed to provide insight into the patient's perceived experience. Nursing education plays a vital role in developing the skills necessary to create, criticize, and use nursing theory. Nursing theory and nurse education interact in two ways. Nursing theory is the subject matter in nursing curricula and together with educational theory, nursing theory organizes and designs the curriculum (Stevens 1984). In the past the nursing curriculum has been based on the medical model. Using the medical model, disease is the focus of the curriculum and the interdependent rather than the independent role of the nurse is stressed. The nursing domain is perceived as a subset of medical intervention. A curriculum designed to develop the independent role of the nurse must focus on nursing theory.

Meleis & Price (1988) suggest that there are four main ways in which nursing theory can be incorporated into a nursing curriculum:

1. In the curriculum as a whole by utilizing a theoretical framework for the curriculum. The model or framework guides the selection of subjects studied
2. As a self contained course
3. Integrated theory and clinical practice. Courses which focus on theories that describe clinical practice
4. Integrated approach to teaching theory.

In addition, Meleis & Price (1988) propose five components of theoretical nursing to be included in the curriculum:

1. Historical analysis and critique of the theoretical development of the discipline
2. Identification and use of the parameters and boundaries of the nursing domain
3. Use of nursing theory where appropriate
4. Awareness of process and strategies that could be used in the development of theoretical nursing
5. Development and testing of theories.

It is commonly agreed that nurse education is best carried out when the theoretical base and practical relevance of what is being taught is made explicit. When the model on which the curriculum is organized is not made explicit, the student is likely to learn in a disassociated manner or develop personal concepts of nursing as the framework for acquiring nursing knowledge. The use of nursing models assists the nurse to distinguish between the medical and nursing database. Nurses need to collect data pertinent to the medical diagnosis in order to carry out their interdependent functions. However, if nurses are to perform an independent role, they must not restrict their database to this area only. The parameters of the nursing database therefore need to be made explicit during nurse preparation. While the use of models or theoretical frameworks in education facilitates explanation of the independent role of the nurse in a more comprehensive and structured way, it is important to be aware that a particular model represents the subjective views of those who constructed it. Models if rigidly adopted restrict questioning and change, and models promote the use of specialized concepts and jargon which may create a distance between carer and consumer and between professions (Hardy 1986). These arguments should not stand in the way of the development of nursing models. As Thibodeau (1983) points out, nursing needs several well developed models. Several models provide healthy competition and the impetus for theory development. In addition, a diversity of nursing models enables nurses to explore phenomena in different ways and from different viewpoints. A pluralistic, eclectic approach is needed to embrace the complexity of human behaviour.

Although nurses are more informed about nursing theory and how it relates to practice, there are still areas of divergence between theory and practice, including language and vocabulary which constrain the clear communication of concepts, and divergence between the 'reality' of nursing and the 'ideal' that is taught by nurse educators (Miller 1985). In addition, a philosophical divergence exists between those who believe in induction and those who consider deduction the most appropriate methodology for theory development and research. It could be argued that we unwittingly perpetuate the notion that practice and theory are separate by continuing to use phrases such as the 'translation of theory in practice', 'closing the gap between theory and practice', 'integrating theory in practice', and so on.

The emergence of nursing as a discipline in its own right rests upon the development of stronger links between the many facets of nursing and nursing theory. If nurses are to be able to define the areas for which they are uniquely qualified to offer solutions, they must have a research based, discipline specific knowledge base, which is structured around an appropriate conceptual framework. Stronger links between practice and theory could be achieved through:

1. Greater personal involvement in the development of nursing theory
2. Implementation of strategies to bridge the education and service sector
3. Collaborative research between nurse clinicians and academic researchers in nursing.

REDUCING THE PRACTICE-THEORY GAP

Taking each of the above areas, a number of strategies which may reduce the practice-theory gap and facilitate integration of theory in practice, will be discussed.

Personal involvement in the development of nursing theory

Models of nursing and nursing theory are frequently studied and then forgotten, or studied but not well utilized in practice. Students are often told to memorize a model of nursing without necessarily understanding that practice will vary according to the model or theory put into operation, and that models and theories are not ends in themselves; they are developed to answer questions, describe events, predict consequences, and prescribe action. Jennings (1987) points out that clinical nurses must have a sense of theory devleopment as a process not as a product. As Bronowski (1978) states, 'science and therefore theory is an ongoing process not an isolated product, it is not a set of findings but the inquisitive search'. One important way in which nurses can be actively involved in theory development is through exploring the processes involved in clinical decision making. Through exploring methods of clinical reasoning, such as those discussed by Jones (1988), both expert and novice nurses could contribute to the development of practice theories of nursing by verbalizing how they use theoretical knowledge to derive logical and valid patient problems and plan patient care.

Another example of personal involvement in theory development is matching one's own philosophy of nursing with an acknowledged model of nursing (Pearson & Vaughan 1986). This involves considering the underpinnings of a given model and how the description of nursing, health, person, and environment compares with one's own ideas. Powell (1989) believes that many nurses have 'theories in use' which are different to their 'professed theories'. They are often unaware of the theories they use and therefore unable to describe them. The development of reflective techniques would promote a greater understanding of personal beliefs and practices and would enable nurses to learn from experience rather than by experience. Other strategies which facilitate active involvement in theory development include publishing, journalling, academic debate, research, and workshops which involve participants in activities such as:

1. Reflecting upon a nursing activity and isolating its components, then devising a model that represents the activity. This should include the essential features (concepts) of the activity and the relationships between them.
2. Selecting a discipline (e.g. biology, psychology, sociology) and discussing the contribution it makes to nursing's knowledge.
3. Designing nursing care plan documentation based on a chosen nursing model.
4. Identifying and explaining the models that underlie course curricula.

Strategies to bridge the education and service sectors

The movement of nurse education into the tertiary sector has highlighted the importance of maintaining strong links between the education and service sectors. Where links between the two are poor, the greater the probability that the gap between theory and practice will widen.

Nurse educators must be able to act as role models for the real world of nursing. Unfortunately the majority of nurse educators have little clinical responsibility and inevitably lose some of their clinical expertise over time. Joint education/service appointments are one way of bridging the service sector and tertiary education. Crane (1989) has described the role of joint appointee at Deakin University, Victoria, as that of expert clinician, clinical theorist, practical teacher, and clinical researcher who engages in clinical practice, management, teaching, and research. However, the process of setting up joint appointments is often difficult and includes issues such as funding, finding a service sector receptive to the idea and finding someone with the necessary qualities. While it may not be possible to set up joint appointments in every university faculty of nursing, the philosophy of joint appointments warrants further attention and nurse educators must ensure that they do not neglect the clinical component of their role. University students must learn from mentors who take an active part in nursing care and have credibility among the clinical staff. In addition nurse educators who engage in clinical practice must be rewarded. Survival and promotion in the tertiary setting should not rest on scholarly activity alone.

The difficulties that new nursing graduates experience in making the transition from student to qualified nurse also highlights the need for more bridges between the education and service sectors. Preceptorship has gained popularity in recent years as one strategy for assisting new graduates to assume full patient care responsibilities. Preceptorship involves assigning new graduates to experienced nurses on a one to one basis so that the graduate has ready access to a role model and resource person at all times. This individualized attention is purported to lead to increased clinical efficiency and ease the transition from student to qualified nurse, however, further research is needed to substantiate these claims (Myrick 1988). Every department of nursing must look at ways of overcoming the gaps that exist between nursing services and higher education. While joint appointments and preceptorships have been found to be efficacious, solutions must be worked through in the context of each faculty's social, political, and historical situation.

Collaborative research

Clinical nurses are frequently intimidated by research yet the problem solving approach used by nurses in the nursing process and research methodology have much in common. In addition, nurses are in an ideal position to be able to suggest specific research topics and to question the rationale behind nursing actions. If the theory base of practice and the practice base of research are to be strengthened, it is important that clinical nurses undertake research and that the areas investigated by nurse researchers are seen to have relevance for practice. One way of achieving this is for clinicians and nurse researchers to undertake collaborative research. Historically, collaborative research meant that clinicians collected data for researchers who designed the project and published the results. Because nurse researchers were detached from clinical practice the integration of theory, research, and practice was often poor. Collaborative research not only brings clinicians and researchers closer together but has the additional benefit of facilitating the dissemination and implementation of research findings. Studies that are not perceived to be part of the clinical setting are less likely to influence the delivery of patient care.

Two other ways of creating links between research, theory, education, and practice are to develop nursing research liaison roles and nursing research units. The main work of the research liaison nurse comprises research and educational activities aimed at increasing research skills, research awareness, and the implementation of research findings. The research liaison nurse may work independently but preferably, he or she is part of a nursing research unit which is a centre for nursing research activity.

Every nurse must be committed to closing the practice-theory gap be it through studying nursing theory, developing personal theories, adopting or implementing existing theories, testing theory or establishing new positions such as joint appointments, preceptorships or research liaison posts. The future of nursing as a discrete discipline rests upon strong links between theory and every sphere of practice. The role of theory in clinical practice, education, and research is summarized in Figure 3.5 on page 70.

TOWARDS A DISCIPLINE OF NURSING THROUGH THEORY DEVELOPMENT

The word theory evokes many different responses among nurses—some positive, some negative. While lively discussion on the subject of nursing theory is important, it is essential that the majority of nurses value nursing theory and understand its role in the movement of nursing towards full professional status. Nursing theory defines the body of knowledge for which nursing is held accountable. As a discipline, nursing is still in the process of defining its independent functions and contributions to health care. The development of nursing theory will assist the emergence of nursing as a discipline in its own right, through increasing the autonomy of nurses in the following ways:

1. Theory based nursing practice that is specific to the discipline, will give nurses the authority to carry out independent functions because they will be valued by others as having unique and respected expertise.
2. Nursing theory clarifies, explains, and predicts nursing care and enables nurses to demonstrate that nursing care does indeed make a difference.

- Theory identifies questions or phenomena of interest
- Theory is developed and tested through research
- Theory provides a structure for analyzing research data

- Theory provides a conceptual framework to guide curriculum context
- Theory promotes creative and analytical thinking
- Theory increases recognition of nursing's contribution as a professional and scientific discipline

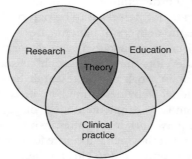

- Theory creates different ways of looking at nursing phenomena, providing a guide for assessment

- Theory interrelates concepts in such a way as to summarize existing knowledge and provides a rationale for interventions

- Theory explains how concepts are related and predicts the nature of relationships under specified circumstances, providing criteria for evaluation

- Theory stimulates creative thinking, new approaches, and behaviour

- Theory facilitates socialization into nursing by identifying the phenomena of the discipline

- Theory is developed and validated in practice

Figure 3.5 The role of theory in clinical practice, education and research

3. Nursing theory provides guidelines that allow nurses to work towards a common goal. This is important since nurses still have difficulty reaching agreement on the nature of nursing.
4. As ideas are developed and concepts are clarified and defined, nurses will build a common terminology that will facilitate communication within the profession.

The development of a scientific knowledge base will assist the emergence of nursing as a respected discipline. However, nursing theory alone will not lead to the provision of quality care. As nursing seeks increased professional autonomy through theory development, it must not lose sight of the art of nursing. While science provides a rational foundation for practice, it is the skilful blending of nursing science (theory) with the art of nursing that results in quality care and distinguishes nursing from other disciplines. Theory development must therefore encompass the art of nursing and must not unwittingly lead to the denigration of the humanistic, creative and expressive qualities in nursing. Science must not become the only respected basis for nursing practice otherwise the caring humanistic component of nursing may be undermined. To rephrase Kant's well known statement: The art of nursing without theory is blind, theory without the art of nursing is mere intellectual play.

REFERENCES

Aggleton P, Chalmers H 1986 Nursing models and the nursing process. Macmillan, London
Aggleton P, Chalmers H 1989 Next year's models. Nursing Times 85(51):24-27
Benner P 1984 From novice to expert: excellence and power in clinical nursing practice. Addison-Wesley, Menlo Park
Bronowski J 1978 The common sense of science. Harvard University Press, Cambridge
Carr W, Kemmis S 1986 Becoming critical: knowing through action research. Deakin University Press, Geelong
Chapman C M 1985 Theory of nursing practical application. Harper & Row, London
Chinn P L, Jacobs M 1983 Theory and nursing: a systematic approach. C V Mosby, St Louis
Clarke M 1986 Action and reflection: practice and theory in nursing. Journal of Advanced Nursing 11(1):3-12
Crane S 1989 Joint appointments: the Deakin experience. The Australian Journal of Advanced Nursing 6(3):21-25
Dickoff J, James P 1968 A theory of theories: a position paper. Nursing Research 17(3):197-203
Dickoff J, James P, Wiedenback E 1968 Theory in a practice discipline. Nursing Research 17(5):415-435
Duffey M, Muhlenkamp A F 1974 A framework for theory analysis. Nursing Outlook 22(9):570-574
Duffy M E 1985 Designing nursing research: the qualitative-quantitative debate. Journal of Advanced Nursing 10:225-232
Fawcett J 1984 An analaysis and evaluation of conceptual models of nursing. Davis, Philadelphia
Flew A (ed) 1979 A dictionary of philosophy. Macmillan, London
Field PA 1987 The impact of nursing theory on the clinical decision making process. Journal of Advanced Nursing 12(5):563-571
Garforth F 1971 The scope of philosophy: an introductory study book. Longman, London
Glaser B, Strauss A 1967 The discovery of grounded theory. Weiderfeld & Nicholson, London
Hardy L K 1986 Identifying the place of theoretical frameworks in an evolving discipline. Journal of Advanced Nursing 11(1):103-107
Hardy M E 1974 Theories: components, development, evaluation. Nursing Research 23(2):100-106
Henderson V 1966 The nature of nursing. Macmillan, London
Jacox A 1974 Theory construction in nursing: an overview. Nursing Research 23(1):4-12
Jennings B M 1986 Nursing science: more promise than threat. Journal of Advanced Nursing 11(5):505-512
Jennings B M 1987 Nursing theory development: successes and challenges. Journal of Advanced Nursing 12(1):63-69
Johnson D E 1980 The behavioural system model for nursing. In: Riehl J, Roy Sister C Conceptual models for nursing practice, 2nd edn. Appleton-Century-Crofts, New York

Jones J A 1988 Clinical reasoning in nursing. Journal of Advanced Nursing 13(2):185-192

King I M 1971 Toward a theory for nursing: general concepts of human behaviour. Wiley, New York

Kristjanson L J, Tamblyn R, Kuypers J A 1987 A model to guide development and application of multiple nursing theories. Journal of Advanced Nursing 12(4):523-529

Lancaster W, Lancaster J 1981 Models and model building in nursing. Advances in Nursing Science 3:31-42

McFarlane J K 1976 The role of research and the development of nursing theory. Journal of Advanced Nursing 1(6):443-451

McFarlane J K 1977 Developing a theory of nursing: the relation of theory to practice, education and research. Journal of Advanced Nursing 2:261-270

McKenna H P 1989 The selection by ward managers of an appropriate nursing model for long stay psychiatric patient care. Journal of Advanced Nursing 14(9):762-775

Meleis A I 1983 A model for theory description, analysis and critique. In: Chaska N L (ed) The nursing profession: a time to speak. McGraw Hill, New York

Meleis A I, Price M J 1988 Strategies and conditions for teaching theoretical nursing: an international perspective. Journal of Advanced Nursing 13(5):592-604

Melzack R, Wall P D 1965 The challenge of pain. Penguin, New York

Miller A 1985 The relationship between nursing theory and nursing practice. Journal of Advanced Nursing 10(5):417-424

Myrick F 1988 Preceptorship: a viable alternative teaching strategy. Journal of Advanced Nursing 13(5):588-591

Neuman B 1982 The Neuman systems model. Appleton-Century-Crofts, Norwalk

O'Hear A 1980 Karl Popper. Routledge & Kegan Paul, London

Orem D E 1971 Nursing: concepts of practice. McGraw Hill, New York

Orlando I J 1961 The dynamic nurse-patient relationship: function, process and principles. Putnams, New York

Parse R 1981 Man-living-health: theory of nursing. Wiley, New York

Pearson A, Vaughan B 1986 Nursing models for practice. Heinemann, London

Peplau H E 1952 Interpersonal relations in nursing. Putnams, New York

Polit D, Hungler B 1983 Nursing research: principles and methods, 2nd edn. Lippincott, Philadelphia

Powell J 1989 The reflective practitioner in nursing. Journal of Advanced Nursing 14(10):824-832

Hiehl J, Roy Sr C 1980 Conceptual models for nursing practice, 2nd edn. Appleton-Century-Crofts, New York

Rodgers B 1989 Concepts, analysis and the development of nursing knowledge: the evolutionary cycle. Journal of Advanced Nursing 14(4):330-335

Rogers M E 1970 An introduction to the theoretical basis of nursing. Davis, Philadelphia

Roper N, Logan W W, Tierney A J 1980 The elements of nursing. Churchill Livingstone, Edinburgh

Roy Sr C 1976 Introduction to nursing: an adaptation model. Prentice-Hall, Englewood Cliffs

Schwab J 1964 quoted in: Stevens B J 1985 Nursing theory analysis, application, evaluation. Little Brown, Boston

Stevens B J 1984 Nursing theory analysis, application, evaluation, 2nd edn. Little Brown, Boston

Thibodeau J A 1983 Nursing models: analysis and evaluation. Wadsworth, Monterey

Travelbee J 1966 Interpersonal aspects of nursing. F A Davis, Philadelphia

Weatherston L 1979 Theory of nursing: creating effective care. Journal of Advanced Nursing 4:365-375

Webb C 1989 Action research: philosophy, methods and personal experiences. Journal of Advanced Nursing 14(5):403-410

Ziegler S M, Vaughan-Wrobel B C, Erlen J A 1986 Nursing process, nursing diagnosis, nursing knowledge: avenues to autonomy. Appleton-Century-Crofts, Norwalk

4 Are we asking the right questions?

R. Lynette Russell

It was so easy to say what I had to say. To say it. But not to write it. How to put down on paper...the eloquent signs of the body and face which go with the spoken word, the silences, the tone and the music of the voice, the look so filled with unwritten words, but nevertheless comprehensible, the hands, like plates of fruit, filled with unspoken sentences; in sum, everything which gives words the precise meaning which one wants to give them (Colliere 1988).

INTRODUCTION

A question that has consumed the energy of many nurses is one which appears, on the surface at least, to be an easy question that any nurse could, in fact should, be able to answer. It is a question to which many nurses, from all branches of the profession throughout the world, have devoted a great deal of time in attempting to answer. In addition the nursing literature is replete with learned attempts to answer this same question. It is a question that, almost inevitably, forms the subject of addresses at nursing conferences or seminars. If it does not form the subject of an address at such forums it usually comes up as a comment or question during the discussion periods. I still remember, quite clearly, one such incident at a conference when a nurse said, '...but we do not even know what nursing is!'. This comment was made by a registered nurse who had been in practice for a number of years. The question that is asked so frequently, both by members of the nursing profession and by those from outside the profession, is, 'What is nursing?'

It will be argued that the time has come to stop devoting so much energy in trying to find the definitive answer to this, or similar questions. Enough of the energy of the nursing profession has already been used in such attempts. To provide support for this contention an overview of the ways in which we have defined, described, discussed, examined, and evaluated nursing and nursing practice will be given. The purpose of this overview is to demonstrate, quite clearly, that we have already exhaustively defined and described nursing. That is, we can answer the perennial question of 'What is nursing?'. These attempts to develop a definitive definition of nursing have the added problem of being retrospective in nature. That is, we often define what nursing was, not what it is now, or what it will be in the future. Nursing as

73

a dynamic and changing discipline is disadvantaged by such retrospective definitions. The major disadvantage, however, of our present and past efforts to definitively define nursing is that it has caused the intellectual and emotional energy of the profession to remain concentrated in an area which is now inappropriate. This intellectual and emotional energy would be better utilized in defining and refining the knowledge base that is unique to nursing, that is, in developing the discipline of nursing itself. Although much has already been accomplished in this vital endeavour, much more remains to be done. To contribute to this endeavour we, the members of the nursing profession, need to ask and seek answers to new questions, for example, 'What do we want nursing to be?', 'How do we want to practise nursing in the future?', 'Where do we want to practise nursing?', and last, but not least, 'How can we achieve changes in nursing and in nursing practice that we, the nursing profession, see as necessary?'. It is by asking such questions that we will be able to determine the future of nursing whilst, at the same time, continue to develop the unique discipline that is nursing.

THE WRONG QUESTION

What is nursing?

At first glance it appears difficult to understand why nurses continue to spend so much time in attempting to answer the question of what is nursing. Even a cursory look at introductory nursing textbooks demonstrates that considerable space is devoted in these texts to what appears to be clear, easily understood answers to this question (Taylor et al 1989). Many of these texts commence, for example, with a discussion on what nursing is by defining the word 'nurse' as originating from the Latin word 'nutrire', that is, 'to nourish' (Taylor et al 1989). A number of different definitions of nursing, such as those accepted by the International Council of Nurses, the American Nurses' Association, and the Canadian Nurses Association, are then presented.

It is usually at this stage that some form of qualifying statement is made that a satisfactory definition of nursing still remains elusive. Nurses themselves, it appears, often disagree over the most appropriate definition. It may be, therefore, that it will not be possible to arrive at a definition which is universally acceptable to all members of the nursing profession (Wolff et al 1983). Perhaps part of the answer to this problem of arriving at a satisfactory definition of nursing is suggested by the following which states that 'nursing has never existed in isolation. From the beginning of time, the role of the nurse has been defined by the groups and social structure in which people were living' (Taylor et al 1989).

These introductory nursing textbooks then provide fairly detailed descriptions of the roles of the nurse in today's society (Wolff et al 1983). It is interesting to note that, unlike the definitions of nursing, the roles of the nurse are confidently given without any qualifying statements. For example, one authority (Wolff et al 1983) gives the roles of the nurse as caregiver, patient advocate, teacher, counsellor, co-ordinator, leader, role model, and administrator. Another prefers to describe four main aims of nursing which are: promoting wellness, preventing illness, restoring health, and facilitating coping (Taylor et al 1989).

Textbooks then describe, often in quite minute detail, the settings in which nurses work (Wolff et al 1983, Kozier & Erb 1987, Taylor et al 1989). In addition these texts also include descriptions of expanding career roles and functions of nurses (Kozier & Erb 1987, Taylor et al 1989). It is when thinking about this variety of settings in which nurses work, that the difficulties being experienced by the profession in arriving at a clear, concise definition of nursing that is acceptable to all practitioners becomes much easier to understand. Will it ever really be possible to develop a definition of nursing that encompasses such diverse areas of clinical practice as intensive care, community health, psychiatric nursing, general medical and surgical nursing, geriatric nursing, and midwifery, whilst at the same time being applicable to nurse researchers, managers, and academics?

No attempt has been made to do an exhaustive search of the nursing literature in this area. Even a cursory examination of readily available current nursing textbooks demonstrates that there is a wide range—in addition to the introductory nursing texts—which are devoted to: describing and discussing the various definitions of nursing that have been advanced; examining the roles of nurses as proposed in the literature; and discussing developments in isolating a body of knowledge which is specific to the discipline of nursing. One of these looks, for example, at the various definitions of nursing, and at theory development in nursing amongst other issues (Moloney 1986). Another also examines definitions of nursing, then looks at the work of nurse theorists and the roles of the nurse (Meleis 1985). A final example examines the definitions of nursing and then looks at the foundations and framework of the discipline of nursing. This is then followed by a detailed examination of the role of the nurse (Doheny et al 1987). And still we can say we are unable to answer the question 'What is nursing?'. Perhaps the following comment, made in the context of a discussion about our current obsession with the idea of professionalism and our preoccupation with gaining professional status for nursing, may provide part of the answer to our continuing difficulty in finding a satisfactory answer to the question of what is nursing: '...there has been a transition in nursing from self-confidence to obsessive self-scrutiny' (Jolley & Allan 1989). The writer then goes on to say that in accepting the standards of other professions '...nursing has thereby deprived itself of its own unique identity' (Jolley & Allan 1989).

Definitions of nursing

It may be of value to pause for a while and look briefly at some of the definitions of nursing that have been advanced. These definitions have been forthcoming by numerous groups of nursing practitioners, doctors, political scientists, legislators, educators, the general public, and others since Florence Nightingale's era (Brooks & Kleine-Dracht 1983, Moloney 1986). The first definition that is commonly cited is that of Florence Nightingale who, in the mid-1800s, defined nursing as a process to put 'the patient in the best condition for nature to act upon him' (Nightingale 1860). It was also Miss Nightingale who first described nursing as both a science and an art (Miller 1989). Important definitions of nursing, or descriptions in some instances, were also proposed by Hildegard Peplau (1952), Ernestine Wiedenbach (1960), Faye Abdellah (1960) and Ida Orlando (1961), (Kozier & Erb 1987, Doheny et al 1987).

It was during this period that the definition that has perhaps gained the widest acceptance by the nursing profession was developed by Virginia Henderson in 1960 (Henderson 1966). The concepts within this definition were further developed and defined in her nursing textbook (Henderson 1966). The definition developed by Henderson was adopted by the International Council of Nurses in 1972 (Taylor et al 1989). Prior to this, however, Henderson had developed a statement for the International Council of Nurses in which the activities which comprise basic nursing were outlined (International Council of Nurses 1960, Henderson 1966). It is perhaps worthwhile to quote the definition developed by Henderson in 1960 once again:

The unique function of the nurse is to assist the individual, sick or well, in the performance of those activities contributing to health or its recovery (or to a peaceful death) that he would perform unaided if he had the necessary strength, will, or knowledge. And to do this in such a way as to help him gain independence as rapidly as possible (Henderson 1966).

It is not difficult to understand why such a definition of nursing has gained such a wide acceptance. It has the beauty of being clearly stated and of being readily accessible to all members of the profession. It also can be seen as applicable to the wide range of settings in which nurses practise.

It is of interest to note that in the years prior to the development of this definition there had been an explosion of activity on the part of American nursing to develop an acceptable definition. In 1950 the American Nurses' Association, for example, embarked on a five year investigation of the functions of the nurse. This was followed, in 1955, by the development of an approved definition of nursing practice designed for inclusion in nurse practice acts. This definition was strongly criticized as being very general and applicable to groups other than nursing. It did, however, suggest that nurses observed, cared for, and counselled patients; were responsible for supervising other health personnel without supervision by a physician; and gave medications and treatments as prescribed by the physician (Henderson 1966). In addition to Henderson, definitions of nursing were developed by Dorothy Johnson (1960–1980), Imogene King (1968–1980), Dorothea Orem (1969–1980), Myra Levine (1973), Sister Callista Roy (1976–1984),

Martha Rogers (1970–1980), Bette Neuman (1982), and Madeleine Leininger (1984) (Doheny et al 1987, Kozier & Erb 1987).

These efforts to develop a definition of nursing, one that will answer the oft put question of 'What is nursing?' to the satisfaction of the majority of nurses, has not been confined to other countries. Many attempts have also been made within Australia to develop a clear, acceptable answer to this question (Ramsay 1970, Saint 1971, White 1972, Royal Australian Nursing Federation (RANF) 1983, Australasian Nurse Registering Authorities Conference (ANRAC) 1990). The simplest of these is that 'a nurse is a person, who having completed an approved program of nurse education, is licensed by a nurse registering authority to practise as a nurse', (Australian Nursing Federation (ANF) 1989). This type of definition of a nurse has been accepted in Australia for some time. For example, a major project was conducted by the National Health and Medical Research Council (Nursing Committee) in 1972. The purpose of this study was to define and identify the present and future roles of the nurse in Australia (White 1972). This study accepted the International Council of Nurses definition of a nurse which is very similar to that given above (World Health Organization 1960, White 1972). This definition had also been adopted in Victoria (Ramsay 1970).

When such definitions of a nurse are adopted, the need to ensure that the content of basic nursing programs is acceptable to the profession is obvious. Equally as obvious is the need to ensure that those who have the power to license these programs and register their graduates support a concept of nursing which is acceptable to the profession as a whole.

Role statements

Attempts in Australia to clearly define what nursing is have included the development of statements about the roles and functions of the registered nurse. One example is the statement of the functions of the registered nurse developed following widespread consultation, by the Nurses Education Board of New South Wales (NEB) which gives an exhaustive list of nursing tasks under seven functional areas. These functional areas are: professional responsibility, basic nursing care, specific nursing procedures, observation and action, human relations, administration, and education (NEB 1977). This statement provides, therefore, an excellent summary of what was perceived to be the functions of a registered nurse at the time. A second example, developed by Australian nursing organisations, lists the roles of the nurse to include the promotion of health; the prevention of health breakdown; the care of the physically and mentally ill, and disabled and dying people of all ages in all health care settings; and the facilitation of spiritual integrity. Nurses, it is argued, work with people who are healthy as well as those with some manifestation of health breakdown (ANF 1989). A third example, a more recently released document developed by ANRAC, states that the role of the registered nurse is composed of a number of integrated components which include clinician, care coordinator, counsellor, health teacher, client advocate, change agent, and clinical teacher/supervisor (ANRAC 1990). Again this document was developed following widespread consultation with the nursing profession. These and similar documents (Saint 1971, Sax 1978, RANF 1983), as they give what were seen to be the functions and roles of the registered in the Australian setting, can help to provide a partial answer to the question 'What is nursing?'.

An Australian study of the perceptions of the functions of nurses, as held by university students of nursing, provides a further interesting perspective on this question of 'What is nursing?'. The most frequently cited functions of nurses, as perceived by the students in this study, were caring, communicating, promoting health, intervening and educating (Pelletier et al 1989). The authors argue that the research findings suggest that the students' perceptions of nursing functions reflect media impressions (Pelletier et al 1989). They go on to say that it seems that the students in all three groups maintained the established societal belief that nurses are essentially care providers (Pelletier et al 1989).

Descriptions of nursing

Unlike the early definitions by Nightingale and Henderson, later definitions of nursing within the nursing literature become increasingly difficult to use or quote as clear, concise, stand alone statements. One example of these later definitions is that developed by Martha Rogers. Rogers developed a broad, holistic definition of nursing in which the person was perceived as central to nursing's purpose. A systems perspective was used to describe nursing as a humanistic science that could explain and predict the nature and development of individuals (Doheny et al 1987). Rogers saw nursing as being concerned with maintaining and promoting health, preventing illness, and caring for and rehabilitating the sick and disabled. Nursing, according to Rogers, seeks to promote symphonic interaction between the environment and person, to strengthen the coherence and integrity of the human being, and to direct and redirect patterns of interaction between people and environment so that maximum health potential can be realized (Kozier & Erb 1987). Nursing, according to Rogers, is both a science and an art (Doheny et al 1987).

Perhaps a more 'user friendly' definition or description of nursing than Rogers's is that of Dorothea Orem. Orem sees nursing as a helping or assisting service to persons who are wholly or partly dependent, and as a creative effort by one human being to help another human being. Nursing is seen as a deliberate action, a function of the practical intelligence of nurses, an action to bring about humanely desirable conditions in persons and their environments. Orem sees nursing as distinguished from other human services and other forms of care by its focus on human beings (Doheny et al 1987, Kozier & Erb 1987).

It would be remiss not to mention, even if it is in passing, the work done by Patricia Benner in describing what nurses do. Benner undertook descriptive research, what she terms 'a dialogue with nurses and nursing' (Benner 1984) and identified five levels of competency in clinical nursing practice. These levels were novice, advanced beginner, competent, proficient, and expert. This research was undertaken with nurses, who were interviewed and observed either individually or in small groups, using patient care situations. As a result of this research a number of domains of nursing practice were isolated including the helping role; the teaching-coaching function; the diagnostic and patient-monitoring function; effective management of rapidly changing situations; administering and monitoring therapeutic interventions and regimens; monitoring and ensuring the quality of health care practices; and organizational and work-role competencies. For each of these domains of nursing practice Benner gives examples, or exemplars, based on actual episodes experienced by nurses during their nursing practice. In this and later work Benner developed the thesis that caring is central to human expertise, to curing, and to healing. Nursing was viewed as a caring practice whose science is guided by the moral art and ethics of care and responsibility. Additionally, she argues that caring as a moral art is primary for any health care practice (Benner & Wrubel 1989). The insights into nursing and nursing practice that are the outcomes of this, and other similar research, are enlightening and contribute to our understanding of what nursing is.

Another nurse leader who has provoked some valuable discussion about what is nursing is Margretta Styles (1982). In the introduction to this work Styles invites nurses to search with her for a total view of nursing and for our personal meaning as nurses. Such a pilgrimage, according to Styles, would take us 'first through the general field of professionalism...Then, we will open up our own frontiers with the assertion of an ideology and directional model—a manifesto or social contract—for nursing; exploration of the nature of nursing and the conditions under which it is practised; professional, academic, socialization, and governance models to enlarge our capacities and social legacy; and, most deeply, contemplation of those personal qualities that are passages to professionhood' (1982).

Styles' work, like that of Benner, proves to be a fascinating examination of nursing which can provide us with many valuable insights into the profession.

Theories and models of nursing

It is at this stage, however, that the water becomes cloudy, as these definitions and descriptions of nursing slowly become transformed into theories or models of nursing. In fact, in many of the later nursing textbooks, definitions of nursing such as Henderson's are so described (Meleis 1985, Kozier & Erb 1987). It may be useful, at this stage, to quote the explanation of a theory.

Theory involves intellectual operations and is comprised of facts, principles, and concepts that are arranged to show their interrelatedness. A theory describes something, a happening or a phenomenon. In more common terms, a theory is used to explain phenomena and organize ideas and knowledge. Theory development enables one to describe, explain, predict, control and/or prescribe phenomena of interest (Doheny et al 1987).

The difficulty with later definitions of nursing, or theories as they are now described, is their inaccessibility to the general nursing community. It has now become necessary for nurses to take courses, at undergraduate and postgraduate level, to study current nursing theories and to develop an understanding of what they are. In addition it can be argued that many in the general nursing community do not see nursing theories and models as relevant to their day to day practice in the clinical setting (Miller 1989). It is difficult to imagine, therefore, that something that is seen as not relevant to clinical practice, that is, nursing theories or models, will become acceptable to the majority of the nursing profession as the one true definition or explanation of what nursing is. It has been argued by a number of authorities that there is a 'widespread belief in nursing, that experience is superior to thought in every way...' and that this is '...one aspect of a certain anti-intellectual bias that is also evidenced in the resistance to identify, test, and validate nursing practices within an appropriate theoretical framework' (Smith 1981). The development of nursing theories and models has not, therefore, made it any easier for the nursing community to formulate a clear, acceptable, answer to that perennial question 'What is nursing?'.

Task analysis and costing nursing

At the same time as attempts were being made by the American Nurses' Association to develop a definition of nursing, thousands of American nurses were participating in the development of statements on functions, standards, and qualifications for practice in the various fields of nursing (Henderson 1966). Henderson, in summarizing these efforts at the time stated that 'major efforts have been made by individuals, small groups, and organized nursing to formulate a statement of its functions, but we must conclude that this is still unfinished business. This leads into a further area where nursing has been subjected to some very detailed analysis, the area of 'task analysis'or 'job analysis'. Job analysis has been defined as 'a method used to discover the component elements of a job by observation, study, and recording pertinent information relating to the nature of a specific job' (Morlan 1956).

In these types of studies the actual activities carried out by nurses whilst performing their job have been studied in some detail (Morlan 1956). Within the Australian setting an interesting example of this type of study was carried out on behalf of the Nurses' Education Board of New South Wales (1984). The aims of this study were to identify nursing care activities; to document and analyze cognitive processes associated with nursing decisions and patient care; and to develop a methodology and instrument for analyzing decision-making and problem-solving by nurses in relation to patient care (NEB 1984). This study formulated six major nursing intervention categories; observational, supporting/assisting, preventive, educative, rehabilitative, and administrative. All nursing interventions were then grouped under these categories. For each of these six categories detailed listings of nursing interventions were then developed. Studies such as this provide insights into and valuable research data about what nurses do. It is somewhat puzzling, however, that such little use has been made of the findings from this study or ones that are similar in nature.

In addition to task or job analysis studies, extensive efforts have also been made to analyze the cost of providing nursing services and to determine the effectiveness of these services (Bulechek & McCloskey 1990, RANF 1983, 1984, 1985, Leininger 1984). Such studies also provide many invaluable insights into nursing. It is difficult to imagine, for example, that nursing services can be costed adequately or that the effectiveness of these services can be evaluated if they are not, firstly, described or defined in some meaningful way. These studies can, therefore, also contribute to the development of an acceptable definition or theory(s) of nursing as they further increase our understanding of what is nursing and nursing work.

A further area in which nursing activities have been subjected to detailed scrutiny is the research into patient classification systems. These systems attempt to quantify the amount of nursing care required by a client and are in widespread use for the allocation of nursing resources both in Australia and overseas. An example of these tools is the Rush-Medicus Classification Instrument (Bulechek & McCloskey 1990). Although a number of these tools were originally developed to predict staffing needs, they have been recently used to determine the cost of nursing care. Again, it is difficult to believe that systems which we use to determine how much nursing care is required by a client and the cost of this care have been developed by a profession which argues that there is no clear and acceptable answer to the question 'What is nursing?'(Bulechek & McCloskey 1990).

Regulation of nursing—legislation, competencies, and standards

A further area that is worth some examination when attempting to answer the question 'what is nursing?' is government legislation which directly affects the nursing profession. In Australia, legislation to establish registration authorities was first introduced in South Australia in 1920, Western

Australia in 1922, Victoria in 1924, New South Wales in 1925, Tasmania in 1927, Queensland in 1928, and the Australian Capital Territory in 1933. The Council of the Australasian Trained Nurses Association, a professional nursing organization which had been responsible for establishing a register of trained nurses and for prescribing standards for nurse training, saw these registration acts as a mechanism that would protect its members and provide them with official recognition (Russell 1990).

Although the powers of the boards established by legislation varied from state to state, their primary responsibilities were similar. These were to maintain a register of trained nurses; recognize hospitals as training schools; and conduct examinations to admit nurses to the register. It should also be noted that in maintaining a register of trained nurses these authorities were also given disciplinary powers and could remove names from the register. The boards also assumed responsibility for the education of nurses (Russell 1990).

The responsibility for the education of nurses was, prior to the transfer of nurse education into the tertiary sector, carried out by prescribing minimum standards for both the theoretical and clinical components of nurse training; by setting the age of entry, the educational standards of entrants, and the period of training; and by accrediting training schools for nurses (Russell 1990).

The registration authorities developed 'minimum standard' syllabi which those conducting preregistration programs were to adhere to. Using New South Wales as an example, the last syllabus prior to the transfer to the tertiary sector, consisted of one thousand hours of theory (Nurses'Registration Act 1953). This theory was divided into three main headings: the biological and physical sciences, behavioural and social sciences, and health sciences. There was also a fourth untitled section which contained two subjects: the principles of unit management and the principles of education. By examining the content of these syllabi, over time, an interesting insight into developments in nursing and nursing practice can be gained. There was, for example, a gradual increase in the content in the biological and physical sciences and the behavioural and social sciences within these syllabi. There was also an increase in the number of speciality areas in the health science or nursing component of the syllabi, with a concomitant prescription by the Board for students to gain practice in these speciality areas during the courses (Russell 1979, 1990). A similar pattern can be isolated in each state. These powerful statutory government bodies had, therefore, a major effect on the education of nurses in each state.

Little of this has changed following the decision to transfer nurse education into the tertiary sector throughout Australia. There has been, however, a move by nurse registration or regulation authorities towards the introduction of broadly based competencies and away from the prescription of a minimum standards syllabus or curriculum for nursing programs. A competency has been defined as 'the ability to apply knowledge and skills with understanding and the appropriate attitude to specific activities and responsibilities (Allan 1989). Institutions conducting pre-registration programs are required to demonstrate, to the satisfaction of the registration or regulatory authority, that their programs meet these competencies in order to ensure that their graduates can gain registration on completion of a course. Again, these competencies were developed following widespread consultation with the nursing profession. It could be argued, therefore, that they reflect the profession's current understanding of what constitutes nursing.

In New South Wales, for example, the Nurses Registration Board (NRB) developed a set of guidelines and competencies for courses leading to registration as a nurse (1988a). The guidelines make it clear that although the registration authority no longer carries out its responsibility for the education of nurses by, for example, setting the age and educational standard for entrants, it still determines many aspects of that education.

The competencies which the Board expects to be achieved by graduates of nursing programs leading to registration are given under seven broad headings. These broad headings are: assessment, planning and intervention, safety, health promotion, habilitation and rehabilitation, communication and interpersonal skills, and management of professional practice (NRB 1988b). Under each of these seven broad headings there are specific objectives which give further details of what each competency means, for example, under Competency 1, Assessment, it states that 'the graduate nurse should be able to assess and monitor the physiological, psychological and social condition of the individual, the family or group with a health or illness problem, according to age, disability, socio-cultural background and environment' (NRB 1988b). The following objectives are then given '...in developing this competency the nursing student should be able to: apply principles of nursing and related sciences to the process of assessment and monitoring; use an analytical approach in assessment and monitoring; identify the health needs of individuals, families and groups; recognise changes to health status following initial assessment' (NRB 1988b). These competencies are, therefore, quite specific. In addition the Board states its philosophy for a basic nursing program. It is reasonable to assume, therefore, that the nurse registration authority in New South Wales has a clear view on what is nursing and what is nursing work in order to be able to set such guidelines and to develop appropriate competencies for basic pre-registration nursing programs.

The Australasian Nurse Registering Authorities Conference (ANRAC), at which are represented all Australian state and territory nurse registering authorities, has recently completed an exciting project in which national competencies for the registration and enrolment of nurses were formulated, validated, and refined. Again this process was done through wide consultation with members of the nursing profession. In addition assessment technology being developed can be used to determine if these competencies have been met (ANRAC 1990). The preamble to these competencies states that 'in preparing the statements of competencies it was necessary to identify the beliefs about nursing and its practice that underpinned them, and to describe the role of the registered and enrolled nurse'.

The role of the registered nurse is seen as being composed of a number of components and, in addition, as including a responsibility to examine nursing practice critically. The individual registered nurse should also incorporate the results of personal action research or the research findings of others when carrying out the role. It is stated that the registered nurse has a responsibility to understand the role and function of enrolled nurses and to determine, on the basis of client needs, whether nursing will be given by a registered nurse or an enrolled nurse (ANRAC 1990).

Eighteen competencies, with a number of subsets, are then given as essential for those persons seeking registration in Australia. Two examples of these competencies are: to maintain a physical and psychosocial environment which promotes safety, security, and optimal health; and to formulate a plan of care in consultation with individuals/groups taking into account the therapeutic regimes of other members of the health care team (ANRAC 1990). This document provides very clear answers to the question of 'What is a registered nurse?' as perceived by the registration authorities in Australia.

Australia is not alone in taking the approach of setting competencies to be met by preregistration nursing programs. In the United Kingdom, for example, the competencies approach has also been adopted by the nurse regulation authorities with work on identifying nursing competencies beginning as early as 1970. This work has continued up until the present and the new scheme for the education of registered nurses, called Project 2000, has been based on the use of competencies (Allan 1989).

To return to Australia, each of the separate state registration or regulation authorities sets the standards to be met by those wishing to be admitted to the register as a nurse. This, in turn, affects the type of educational programs that are offered. These registration authorities also have disciplinary powers which can include removing names from the register. These statutory authorities have, therefore, played a major role in determining standards for the nursing profession and will continue to do so. It is equally as obvious that they have, and will continue to have, a major effect on determining what a nurse is and what nursing is by the criteria, as given in the competencies, that are set for admission to each register.

To emphasize this point, let us return for a moment to a previously cited definition of a nurse as accepted by a major Australian nursing organization, the Australian Nursing Federation. This definition states that 'a nurse is a person who has completed an approved program of nurse education and is licensed by a nurse registering authority to practice as a nurse' (ANF 1989). The importance of these state registration authorities in determining what a person needs to know or be able to do before being granted registration as a nurse, (that is in determining what a nurse is and in turn what nursing is), should not be underestimated. It is equally as obvious that these authorities must be open to a wide range of inputs from the nursing profession as a whole to ensure that what they prescribe accurately reflects the views of the nursing profession itself.

Countries outside of Australia have also, in many instances, established similar government authorities (Grippando 1986, Taylor et al 1989, Russell 1990). In the United States of America, for example, each state has a nurse practice act which regulates nursing and within these acts is a legal definition of nursing (Grippando 1986). The definitions from the various nurse practice acts in America also provide a very clear answer to the perennial question 'What is nursing?' At the very least, they provide a clear answer to what is seen as the current activities of those designated as registered nurses within the work environment.

In each state in America the nurse practice acts are administered through a board of nursing or similar body (Grippando 1986). There is also, as in Australia, a National Council of State Board of Nursing Inc., which consists of representatives from all state boards of nursing. As in Australia, agencies such as these have a tremendous influence on what is recognized as appropriate activities for those to be accepted, under the licensure laws, as registered nurses.

In addition to nurse practice acts in the USA many efforts have been made to develop acceptable standards of nursing practice. Standards have been developed for many areas of nursing practice, by the American Nurses' Association, and are made widely available. As these standards have been designed to support and assist individual nurses in the performance of their professional roles they provide a further excellent illustration of what nurses do (Grippando 1986).

Standards for nursing practice have also been developed in Australia by the National Professional Development Committee of the then Royal Australian Nursing Federation (RANF). These standards were developed following an extensive consultative process with many Australian nurses. Draft standards were published for comment, revised, and then republished twice in response to such comments. Groups of nurses, including committees at branch and local levels, and the National Conference held in Melbourne in October 1982, all contributed to the development of these standards (RANF 1983). As a brief example of these standards, Standard One is that 'the registered nurse fulfils the obligations of the professional role'. For this standard a number of nursing behaviours are then isolated, for example, 'the registered nurse in any practice setting complies with the profession's code of ethics; functions in accordance with legislation affecting nursing practice; and maintains the rights and safety of the patient'. Again, these standards present a clear picture of what a nurse is and what nursing practice is. The standards also form the invaluable basis for the evaluation of nursing practice and the performance of the individual nurse.

Whither nursing?

It should now be obvious that we have attempted to define, describe, examine, discuss, and evaluate nursing exhaustively in a relentless pursuit of an answer to the question 'What is nursing?'. A factor which will always contribute to our inability to answer this question is the diversity of speciality areas in which nurses practice and the equally diverse settings in which this practice occurs. It may never be possible to develop a clear, precise definition of nursing that will satisfy clinical practitioners in such diverse areas as intensive care, community health, psychiatric nursing, general medical and surgical nursing, geriatric nursing, and midwifery and which will also be acceptable to, and applicable to, nurse researchers, managers, and academics. We could, of course, continue to subscribe to the view that the only real nurses are those who work in clinical settings. This approach simplifies the task of developing an acceptable answer to the question 'What is nursing?'. It is, however, essential that the nursing profession recognizes and accepts those who do not work in the clinical setting as vital members of the nursing profession. Therefore, it is necessary that any definition or explanation of what nursing is includes those who practise as nurse clinicians, nurse managers, nurse academics, and nurse researchers.

Given the very real threats to the continuation of nursing practice as we understand it today, and to the nurse's place as an essential member of the health care team (Pilkington 1989), it would appear vital that we clearly state what we want nursing to be and where we see that nursing, as we perceive it, should be practised. To do this we need to move away from these continuing attempts to define precisely what nursing has been or is at the present. A further urgency is added to this need by the rapid changes that are occurring in all areas of the health care sector, changes which are stimulated by rapid advances in knowledge and the associated changes in technology, coupled with the changes occurring within society itself. It would seem vital, at this particular stage of the development of the nursing profession, that we 'stake our claim' to what we see as the territory of nursing. If we fail to do this before the very near future, other aspiring groups of health or health related groups will. We may find, therefore, that the territory that we see as nursing has become the exclusive territory of another health or health related discipline.

THE RIGHT QUESTIONS

What do we want nursing to be?

Increasingly the approach being taken in the nursing literature is to concentrate on what differentiates nursing from other health professionals rather than on attempting to develop a definition of what nursing is. An example of this approach is that of Webster (1990) who states that nursing is distinguished from other professions by the nature of that which it wishes to create, that is, the enhancement of the health of the individual and community.

This leads to attempts to determine what is the unique focus or essence of nursing, a focus which also differentiates nursing from other helping professionals. The focus that has been the subject of increasing attention, by Benner (1984) and others (Leininger 1984, Watson 1988) is that of caring. These attempts to determine what differentiates nursing and nursing practice from other helping professionals may, in the long term, prove more fruitful than those which have surrounded the attempts to define nursing.

As a concomitant to these attempts to determine what differentiates nursing from other helping professions, there has been a steady progress towards isolating a body of nursing knowledge (Meleis 1985, Moloney 1986, Doheny et al 1987, Bulecek & McCloskey 1990, McCloskey & Grace 1990,). This knowledge will be unique, in many ways, to nursing and will also help to differentiate nursing from other helping professionals.

All of these activities will, therefore, provide a contribution to the continuing debate on what nursing is. It may be time, however, for the profession to accept that 'the glorious thing about nursing is that it cannot be defined. The irony is that we never give up trying' (Brooks & Kleine-Dracht 1983).

The nursing literature, however, contains many examples of emerging new directions for nursing that can help us to answer the question of 'What do we want nursing to be?'. One of these new directions is a change in focus from the traditional cure concept of caring for the ill individuals, to a concept that includes the prevention of illness, health promotion, and maintenance in caring for individuals, their families, and society (Doheny et al 1987). This theme is picked up by many others who argue that nursing is broadening its evolving role in health care to include health promotion, the prevention of illness, and the provision of health education and interventions that can change behavioural patterns and thus reduce the risks of serious illness (Moloney 1986, Rafferty 1987-88).

This change in focus is well demonstrated, for example, in the competencies developed by the New South Wales Nurses Registration Board (NRB 1988) and the Australasian Nurse Registering Authorities Conference (ANRAC 1990). This change in focus has been reflected, therefore, in the curricula developed for undergraduate preregistration nursing programs offered by the higher education sector throughout Australia.

The need for the profession to either embrace this change in focus wholeheartedly or to modify or reject such a change should be obvious. At the same time the need for the profession to determine if it wishes to retain the well defined nursing role of caring for the sick, that is the 'traditional cure concept' of nursing, is equally as pressing.

How do we want to practise nursing in the future?

The time has come for the nursing profession to answer this vital question, that is 'How do we want to practise nursing in the future?' There has been, for example, a rapid expansion of the traditional role of the nurse—that of caring for the sick—a role that is, normally, carried out within an institutional setting. This expanding role of the nurse, often as a result of rapidly changing technology, is most clearly seen in high dependency areas such as intensive care, renal dialysis, neonatal intensive care, and so on (White 1972, Sax 1978, Marles 1988). This expanded role has, too often, been dependent on ad hoc delegation by medical officers, a process in which nurses are typically acquiescent (White 1972, Marles 1988).

In addition there has been the development of new roles for nurses. Of these, clinical specialists, nurse practitioners, and nurses as primary health care workers are of particular interest. A number of these new roles, unlike the traditional role of the nurse, can be practised in non-institutional settings.

The clinical nurse specialist's role was first developed in America and was conceptualized as a nurse who would serve as a role model in the delivery of high-quality nursing care to patients (deYoung 1985, Moloney 1986). This role appears to be, however, more an extension of the traditional role of the nurse than a new role.

The nurse practitioner, however, is a totally new role which was defined, by the American Nurses' Association in 1973, as a registered nurse who had received additional preparation in a specialized education program, normally at Master's degree level (Moloney 1986). Nurse practitioners can practise in individual practice, or in group practices or private hospitals, or within a group medical practice (Barham & Steiger 1982, Moloney 1986, Andersen 1990). The evolution of this role is interesting as it developed, at least in part, from a shortage of doctors in the paediatric area. An interesting parallel can be drawn between this shortage and the looming shortage of resident medical officers in New South Wales. As a result of this shortage registered nurses are to undertake special programs to develop extended skills in order to carry out some parts, at least, of the resident medical officers' normal role. Other factors that were important in the development of the new role of nurse practitioner included an increasing demand by nurses for autonomous and independent practice. There is some concern, however, that this practitioner role actually represents an identification with the practice of medicine rather than the practice of nursing (Moloney 1986). A similar concern can also be voiced about the role being undertaken by clinical nurse specialists in the high technology areas.

A further developing role for the nurse is that of primary health care worker (Donahue 1986, Kinross 1986, Moloney 1986). In an interesting study, which included the perceptions of their future by Victorian nurses, it was found that nurses were becoming more involved in primary health care

(Marles 1988). It has been argued, however, that the role of the remote area nurse in Australia already encompasses much of this role (Kirke 1986). Primary health care is, however, an area that is worthy of further investigation as a practice setting for nurses.

Where do we want to practise nursing?

It is difficult, however, to argue that changes in the focus of nursing, that is a change from the traditional cure concept of caring for ill individuals to a concept that includes the prevention of illness, health promotion, and maintenance in caring for individuals, their families, and society (Doheny et al 1987), actually reflects the realities of the workplace. Between March and July 1989 there were some 332 900 qualified people registered as nurses throughout Australia. Of these, some 57%, that is, approximately 189 753, were working within the nursing profession. Over 60% of qualified nurses working in nursing stated that they were located solely at hospitals. Of these registered nurses working in hospitals, estimated at 145 800, 48% (69 984) were working in the general clinical field; 32% (46 656) in specialist clinical fields; and 10% (14 580) in administrative/supportive positions (Australian Bureau of Statistics 1990).

It could be argued, therefore, that although these nurses would be involved in some health education interventions, the majority of their activities would still be centred around the care of individuals with physical or psychological disturbances. That is, the majority of current nursing practice still revolves around providing nursing care for the sick. It can also be argued that there has been little change to the venue, that is from an institutional setting to a non-institutional setting, in which the majority of nurses practise. Additionally it would appear that there has been little opportunity for the nurses to develop as independent, rather than as interdependent or dependent, practitioners within these institutional settings.

How can we achieve change in nursing?

It can be argued that much of the change that has occurred in nursing has been 'change by drift', that is, changes that have just happened rather than changes that have been the result of planning. On the whole we have allowed our profession and the environment in which that profession works to change without our involvement, almost without our noticing it (Brooten et al 1988). It is not, nor should it be, the prerogative of the medical profession, or any of the other health professionals, to decide what nurses should do (White 1972, Nuckolls 1990). We, that is the nursing profession itself, should seek to reshape our own place in the health care sector. One of the ways in which we could do this is by allying ourselves more closely with the self-stated needs of the patients, as articulated through the consumer health care movement (Jolley 1989). Another is to develop new perspectives as nursing's transition from an illness-care orientation to health promotion and health maintenance increases, and as future health needs of society begin to surface. In addition a changing health care system requires that nurses reorientate nursing to meet an evolving, rather than a static, role in health care (Jolley 1989).

As the 21st century approaches there are many opportunities for the members of the nursing profession to redefine its position, opportunities that we must grasp. It is still true that the public appreciates the field of medicine more than that of nursing although both services require a great deal of knowledge and skill on the part of practitioners. Yet the privileges and rewards expected by the medical profession, and afforded to them by society, are in sharp contrast to those generally expected by nurses and accorded to them by those they serve (Moloney 1986). The same can be said of many of the other health care professions.

In order to grasp these opportunities all members of the nursing profession need to participate in planned change. Becoming involved in planning change will demand a heavy investment of individual and collective time and energy. The rewards to the nursing profession, however, would be commensurate (Brooten et al 1988). It should also be noted, that planning change can have a unifying effect upon the nursing profession rather than a divisive effect. Applied within nursing, it can help the profession clarify its goals and increase its effectiveness in seeking to improve its own status and to create a better healthcare system for people (Brooten et al 1988).

CONCLUSION

It has been argued that it is time we stopped trying to find a definitive answer to the question 'What is nursing?'. This is a question that has successfully defied answers, even despite the considerable collective energy devoted to it by the nursing profession. The time for such detailed and definitive definitions is past. Definitions of nursing can have the effect of limiting the scope of nursing practice rather than of allowing this practice to expand into new horizons. The same can be said for continuing attempts to develop definitive role statements or to describe nursing by the use of a task or job analysis approach. Rather we should move forward, with confidence, into the future whilst stating clearly what we, the nursing profession, see as the future role of the nurse both within and outside the health care setting in Australia: a future role that may be quite different from that role of the nurse that we know today. There is much in the nursing literature that will help us in this endeavour and some of this will be found in the work that has already been done on defining and describing nursing. The continuing efforts to expand and develop the body of nursing knowledge, that is the discipline of nursing, will also contribute to this endeavour. In addition, we need to seek the answer to a number of questions. These questions should be: 'What do we want nursing to be?', 'How do we want to practise nursing in the future?', 'Where do we want to practise nursing?' and, 'How can we achieve changes in nursing and in nursing practice that we, the nursing profession, see as necessary?' In seeking the answers to these questions we should strive to develop our own strategies for change so that the practice of nursing becomes what we, the members of that profession, want it to be. Such change may mean that nursing practice, as we understand it today will change quite dramatically. It will also mean that the form this change will take, rather than being imposed or resulting from change by drift, will be determined by the nursing profession itself. Only then can it be said that we are making progress.

REFERENCES

Allan P 1989 Nursing education: A luxury or necessity? In: Jolley M, Allan P (eds) Current issues in nursing. Chapman & Hall, London
Andersen B 1990 The practitioner role: In search of definition and sustainable development. 38th Annual Oration, The New South Wales College of Nursing, Glebe
ANRAC 1990 National competencies for the registration and enrolment of nurses in Australia. Australasian Nurse Registering Authorities Conference, North Adelaide
Australian Bureau of Statistics 1990 Career paths of qualified nurses. Commonwealth Government Printer, Canberra
Australian Nursing Federation 1989 Nursing in Australia: a national statement. ANF, South Melbourne
Barham V, Steiger N 1982 Health maintenance organizations and nurse practitioners: the Kaiser experience. In: Aiden L (ed) Nursing in the 1980s: Crises: Opportunities: Challenges. Lippincott, Philadelphia
Benner P 1984 From novice to expert. Addison-Wesley, Menlo Park
Benner P, Wrubel J 1989 The primacy of caring. Addison-Wesley, Menlo Park
Brooks J, Kleine-Dracht A 1983 Evolution of a definition of nursing. Advances in Nursing Science 5(4):51-78
Brooten D, Hayman L, Naylor M 1988 Leadership for change: an action guide for nurses, 2nd edn. Lippincott, Philadelphia
Bulechek G, Mc Closkey J 1990 Nursing intervention taxonomy development. In: McCloskey J, Grace H (eds) Current issues in nursing. 3rd edn., CV Mosby, St Louis
Colliere M 1988 Nursing: Thoughts on nursing service and identification of the service offered. International Nursing Review 27(2):49-52, 27(3):79-87, 27(11):114-110
de Young L 1985 Dynamics of nursing. 5th edn., CV Mosby, St Louis
Doheny M, Cook C, Stopper Sr M 1987 The discipline of nursing, 2nd edn. Appleton & Lange, East Norwich
Donaghue S 1986 Transition to primary health care—an Australian perspective. Nursing in Transition. 8th National Conference, College of Nursing, Australia, Darwin
Grippando G 1986 Nursing perspectives and issues, 3rd edn. Delmar, New York
Henderson V 1966 The nature of nursing: A definition and its implications for practice, research, and education. Macmillan, New York
International Council of Nurses 1960 Basic principles of nursing care. Devonshire Press, Torquay
Jolley M 1989 The professionalization of nursing: the uncertain path. In: Jolley M, Allan P (eds) Current issues in nursing. Chapman & Hall, London
Jolley M, Allan P (eds) 1989 Current issues in nursing. Chapman & Hall, London
Kinross N 1986 Nurses and primary health care: An international perspective. Nurses in Transition. 8th National Conference, College of Nursing, Australia, Darwin

Kirke B 1986 Primary health care—a Territory remote area perspective. Nurses in
    Transition. 8th National Conference, College of Nursing, Australia, Darwin
Kozier B, Erb G 1987 Fundamentals of nursing: concepts and procedures, 3rd edn.
    Addison-Wesley, Menlo Park
Leininger M 1984 Care: the essence of nursing and health. Slack, Thorofare
McCloskey J, Grace H (eds) 1990 Current issues in nursing, 3rd edn. CV Mosby, St Louis
Marles F (Chairperson) 1988 Report of the study of professional issues in nursing.
    Government Printer, Melbourne
Meleis A 1985 Theoretical nursing: development & progress. Lippincott, Philadelphia
Miller A 1989 Theory to practice: implementation in the clinical setting. In: Jolley M, Allan
    P (eds) Current issues in nursing. Chapman & Hall, London
Moloney M 1986 Professionalization of nursing: urrent issues and trends. Lippincott,
    Philadelphia
Morlan V 1956 Job analysis—what and why. American Journal of Nursing 56(10):1285-
    1287
New South Wales Nurses' Registration Board,1988a Competencies. Sydney
New South Wales Nurses' Registration Board, 1988b Guidelines and competencies for
    courses leading to registration, Sydney
Nightingale F 1860 Notes on nursing: What it is and what it is not. Harrison, London
Nuckolls K 1990 Who decides what the nurse can do? Nursing Outlook 20(3):31-37
Nurses' Education Board of NSW 1977 The functions of a registered nurse. The Lamp
    34(1):19-21
Nurses' Education Board of NSW 1984 An analysis of patient care provided by nursing
    personnel, Volumes 1 & 2. Government Printer, Sydney
Nurses Registration Act,1953, as amended, 1978 Regulation 4(1) (a) Schedule A, General
    Student Nurses. Government Printer, Sydney
Pelletier D, Adams A, Donoghue J, Duffield C 1989 The functions of a nurse: perceptions
    held by university students of nursing. Australian Health Review 12(3):43-55
Pilkington P 1989 Reclaim the role. The Lamp 46(8):22-28
Rafferty C 1987/88 An apologist's theories for the nursing profession: adaptation and art.
    Nursing Forum XXIII(4):124-126
Ramsay Dr A H (Chair) 1970 Report of the committee of enquiry into nursing in Victoria.
    Government Printer, Melbourne
Royal Australian Nursing Federation 1983 Standards for nursing practice. RANF, South
    Melbourne
Royal Australian Nursing Federation 1984 Nurse staffing methodologies : An exploration of
    the issues. RANF, South Melbourne
Royal Australian Nursing Federation 1985 Costing nursing care: budget planning,
    management and justification. RANF, South Melbourne
Russell R L 1979 General nurse training in New South Wales 1925-1973. BA (Hons) thesis.
    University of Newcastle, Newcastle
Russell R L 1990 From Nightingale to now: Nurse education in Australia. Harcourt Brace
    Jovanovich, Sydney
Saint Prof E (Chair) Report of the committee of inquiry into nursing. Nursing in Queens-
    land. Royal Australian Nursing Federation, Brisbane
Sax Dr S (Chairman) 1978 Report of the committee of inquiry into nurse education and
    training to the Tertiary Education Commission. Nurse education and training. Austral-
    ian Government Publishing Service, Canberra
Smith J 1981 Nursing science in nursing practice. Butterworths, London
Styles M 1982 On nursing: Toward a new endowment. CV Mosby, St Louis
Taylor C, Lillis C, LeMone P 1989 Fundamentals of nursing. Lippincott, Philadelphia
Watson J 1988 New dimensions of human caring theory. Nursing Science Quarterly
    1(4):175-181
Webster G 1990 Nursing and the philosophy of science. In: McCloskey J, Grace H (eds)
    Current issues in nursing, 3rd edn. CV Mosby, St Louis
White R 1972 The role of the nurse in Australia. TERC, Univervisity of New South Wales,
    Kensington
Wolff L, Weitzel M, Zornow R, Zsohar H 1983 Fundamentals of nursing, 7th edn.
    Lippincott, Philadelphia
World Health Organization 1960 Expert committee on nursing, fifth report. Technical
    Report Series.347, Geneva

FURTHER READINGS

Aiken L, Gartner S (eds) 1982 Nursing in the 1980's: Crises, opportunities, challenges. Lippincott, Philadelphia

Australian Institute of Health 1988 Health workforce information bulletin No 13: Nurse workforce 1986. AGPS, Canberra

Cohen H 1981 The nurse's quest for a professional identity. Addison-Wesley, Menlo Park

College of Nursing Australia 1986 Nurses in transition. 8th National Conference, Darwin Institute of Technology, Darwin

Congalton A 1962 The public image of nursing. NSW College of Nursing, Sydney

Daniels K (Chairperson) 1986 Committee to review Australian studies in tertiary education: Nurse education and Australian studies. Canberra

Emden C, Young W 1987 Theory development in nursing: a Delphi study in innovations in nursing. 9th National Conference College of Nursing, Australia, Hobart

Friss L 1977 What do nurses do? Journal of Nursing Administration VII(8):24-28

Garratt S A 1987 Practice—A challenge. In: Innovations in nursing. 9th National Conference, College of Nursing, Australia, Hobart

Henderson V, Nite G 1978 Principles and practice of nursing, 6th edn. Macmillan, New York

Katz F, Mathew K, Pepe T, White R 1976 Stepping out: nurses and their new roles. University of New South Wales Press, Kensington

Keane B 1987 Nurse consultancy—the mega trendy option. In: Innovations in nursing, 9th National Conference, College of Nursing, Australia, Hobart

Lindner C 1989 Work measurement and nursing time standards. Nursing Management 20(10):44-49

McCue H, White R 1983 Innovation in nursing curricula: a survey of developments in Australia. Research and Development Monograph No. 2. University of New South Wales Press, Kensington

Minehan P 1977 Nurse role conception. Nursing Research 26(5):374-379

National Health and Medical Research Council 1974 The role of the nurse in Australia. Australian Government Publishing Service, Canberra

Nurses Registration Act 1953 As amended. Goverment Printer, Sydney

Nurses Registration Act, 1953, Regulations, as amended. Government Printer, Sydney

Olade R 1989 Perception of nurses in expanded role. International Journal of Nursing Studies 26(1):15-25

Parker J 1986 Changing perspectives upon nursing. In: D'Cruz J V, Bottorf J L (eds) The renewal of nursing education. La Trobe University Health Service, Melbourne

Royal Australian Nursing Federation 1975 Report of a working party of nominees of the RANF, College of Nursing, Australia, the National Florence Nightingale Committee of Australia, and the New South Wales College of Nursing. Goals in nursing education: Part II. Melbourne

Royal Australian Nursing Federation 1983 Standards for nursing divisions. RANF, South Melbourne

Stevens B 1974 New York state definition of the practice of nursing : Implications for nursing education. Journal of Nursing Administration IV(3):37-41

Wright S 1989 Changing nursing practice. Arnold, London

5. Mapping the terrain of the discipline

Betty M. Andersen

Frequent reference is made to the discipline of nursing. Indeed the title of this book focuses attention on the application of the concept of discipline to nursing and the title of this chapter implies a process of identifying what the parameters of such an application are. Both the title of the book and the chapter however should lead the reader to conclude that the process of discipline exploration in nursing in Australia is at an early and unsophisticated stage of development.

Donaldson & Crowley (1978), in reviewing the discipline of nursing, conclude that most nursing authors tend to emphasize theoretical reflections which lead to an understanding of the nature of nursing rather than 'explicating the structure of the body of knowledge which constitutes the discipline of nursing'. It is the belief of this writer that both processes are essential to an understanding of how conceptualizations about nursing can satisfy the characteristics of a discipline. Schwab (1964) recognises levels of understanding and development of a discipline by using two metaphors in introducing the difficult subject of the meanings and significances of the structure of a discipline. He talks first about 'mapping the terrain' then the need to follow up by 'exploring [in more detail] the land' itself.

This chapter will outline the processes adopted in 'mapping the terrain' and in beginning to 'explore the land' of nursing in some detail. It does this in an attempt to make sense of the practice of nursing and to allow a structure of the discipline to emerge. Further it will relate the processes resulting in this theory development to theoretical considerations of the structure of disciplines.

The location of nursing education within the tertiary sector reinforces the need to understand what is meant by the concept of a discipline and how to justify the profession's claim to discipline status. Not only is clarity in this development essential to the educational process but also to enable the profession to monitor, manage, and research practice itself. Recognizing these facts should consolidate the process of achieving strong links between practice, theory development, research, and education.

Donaldson & Crowley (1978) suggest that there is an urgent need for a clear explication of the structure of the discipline which is made more explicit than it is at present. Apart from its significance in the justification of doctoral programmes they suggest that the very survival of the profession is at risk unless the discipline is defined. In making this claim they quote Armiger (1974) who noted, 'There exists to-day an unprecedented need for identification of the uniqueness of nursing science and practice, lest overriding forces in contemporary society lead to disintegration of nursing as a distinct profession'. Sixteen years later the need is even greater, not only because of the mushrooming growth of health-related therapies taking over aspects of nursing function but because territorial attitudes of some specialist nursing groups deny the existence of a generic entity. It is this generic entity which is at the heart of the structure of nursing's discipline.

THE APPLICATION OF DISCIPLINE THEORY TO NURSING

What then is meant by theorists using the term discipline? Do different types of discipline exist? What determines membership of one discipline rather than another? It is not the purpose of this chapter to address these questions but rather to address characteristics, structural, and organizational issues. There is no single accepted organization, even among well-established disciplines. This problem arises according to Schwab (1964) because the problem of organisation is a problem of classification primarily, and in classifying groups of complex things, different bases can be justified. However Schwab continues the discussion by suggesting four recognized organizational bases, namely:

1. The subject matter, what is aimed at in investigation, or in work on
2. The practitioners, what competencies and habits are required to carry on their work
3. The methods (syntax), and modes of enquiry by which the subject matter is addressed
4. The ends, the kinds of knowledge or other outcomes at which they aim.

Certain disciplines may satisfy inclusion more readily on one or two bases than others, for example, physics, history. Nursing's uniqueness is not generally considered to be its subject matter nor its methods of enquiry but rather, according to Donaldson & Crowley (1978), its special 'perspective' more likely to equate with Schwab's fourth basis and to some degree to the second basis.

Understanding what is inherent in the construct, discipline, involves more than clarifying or justifying a classification basis. It entails an understanding of the structure of a discipline. Schwab (1964) distinguishes two interrelated elements when describing the structure of disciplines, namely, the substantive structure and the syntactical structure. What is meant by the substantive structure has been variously explained in terms of subject matter (Kim 1983), themes, boundaries (Donaldson & Crowley 1978), that which is of interest to the discipline. Patel et al (1989) describe structure in terms of the organization of concepts in relation to each other. In so doing they take up Schwab's identification of conceptualizations and networks of conceptualizations or structures. He further suggests these conceptualizations may initially be borrowed (from other disciplines), or invented then tested out, resulting in tentative theory development which leads to further clarification of the initial conceptualisations and allows the development of concept networks.

Again according to Schwab (1964), the identification of these conceptual structures is critical to any discipline. This is so because these structures direct enquiry by generating 'telling' questions, allowing the researcher to know what data to collect, how to interpret the findings and how to incorporate them into the discipline's body of knowledge. Therefore the first challenge to a professional group embarking on the process of developing its discipline base is to identify what are its conceptual structures and what are the powers and limitations of enquiry generated by these structures.

Already reference has been made to the process and products of enquiry. The syntactical structure of a discipline is concerned with just this; with the way a discipline pursues knowledge—the research methodologies or the procedures for conducting enquiry—and the ways it verifies knowledge, or the criteria by which it allows the acceptance of statements as true within the discipline.

It is against this background summary that the process and products of enquiry about to be described need to be evaluated. What is to be recorded here had its formal beginnings sixteen years ago in response to a challenge issued by the School of Nursing, Cumberland College of Health Sciences, to provide a research basis for a tertiary level nursing education programme. No Australian conceptual framework was available out of which the research could emerge. The process of developing such a framework was set in train by asking a simple question, 'what is the nature of nursing?' No simple answer resulted, rather an ongoing process (syntax) was set in train which ultimately resulted in a series of interrelated theoretical models. The products were important because they provided the basis for research, the conceptual framework for nursing curricula, and the claim that a structure of the discipline and an identifiable knowledge base for nursing was emerging. However, the processes and underlying assumptions provide valuable insights into the earliest attempts to formulate nursing theories in the absence of an identified discipline structure. These theories were grounded in practice because of the belief that practice should drive theory, research, and education. Can theories derived in this way be taken seriously?

THEORY FROM PRACTICE

The validity of theory derived from practice has long been debated. The more traditional western view of epistemology denies the validity of the methods and products of thinking out of action-taking. Some notable exceptions to this position have been developed. According to Benne (1985), Dewey, an American pragmatist, and others of like persuasion sought to shift the definition of knowing from the products to the process and methods of knowing. Inherent in the case against knowing from doing is the argument that thinking and doing, theory, and practice are antithetical. However, judgment theory according to Dewey (1933) and Peel (1971) establishes a clear relationship between thought, judgment and action. As clinical judgment is central to professional nursing practice, this writer would argue there is no case to divorce thinking (and knowing) from doing. Indeed nurses as action-based thinkers do confront the problematic in patient situations, circumstances and/or status and in practice protocols and goals. The result, if conceptualized, can provide explanations, prediction, clarity and direction to practice, research, and education.

Kant (1781) suggests that in respect of time, no knowledge of ours is antecedent to experience but begins with it. We are indeed caused to think by objects affecting our senses, to compare, to connect, or to separate our impressions. He goes on to describe knowing from experience as a compound, a combination of knowing emerging from direct, concrete experience and knowing supplied by cognitive activities, set in train by the experience but independent of it. He also suggests it is difficult to distinguish the one form of knowing from the other till long practice has made us attentive to and skilful in separating it.

With these arguments in mind, it seems acceptable to use practice as the starting point to identify a conceptual structure, to ask questions, collect data and to interpret findings. The paradigm which drove the project can best be represented as *practice-theory-practice*. This paradigm was to undergo further change as a result of reflection on the continuing process. The nature of the change will be discussed later. The importance of the conceptual structure has been highlighted because it both informs the enquiry process (the syntactical structure) and is in turn informed by it. Any pioneer researcher, however, faces something of a dilemma when no clear boundaries or conceptual structures of a discipline exist. Schwab (1964) suggests that, at this stage of development, enquiry begins in virtual ignorance. However, he points out that ignorance can't initiate an enquiry, and any subject complex enough to need enquiry will need a framework to guide decisions of what is relevant or irrelevant, important or unimportant. In his words this guide is achieved initially by borrowing or inventing a conception.

It was realized at the outset of this writer's enquiry activity that the phenomenon (nursing) was complex and to achieve an effective outcome, a structure was needed to prescribe the scope and allow superordinate organisers to emerge. Now, with hindsight, it is easy to associate the steps taken and the outcomes of the extended enquiry process with an exploration of the structure of the discipline as outlined by Schwab. However, at the outset of the research there were different more limited stimuli driving the enquiry and different specific ends being pursued.

Already the starting point has been identified as practice. In actual fact the concept of practice was narrowed to an initial consideration of what a practitioner did in carrying out the roles and functions of a professional nurse. This locus of enquiry, acting as the initial conception, equates to the second basis for the classification of a discipline as identified by Schwab (1964). A second, but 'borrowed' conceptualization, problem-solving, emerged from the analysis of the practitioner function providing a perspective through which to view the activity of nursing. Moreover this borrowed conceptualization generated the need to explore the relationships among thought, judgment and action-taking; the behaviours inherent in each; and their relevance to the nursing activity. One by one additional key concepts continued to emerge as a result of asking the initial question, 'what is the nature of nursing?' and of analysing it in terms of what the practitioner did.

Very significant among these emerging concepts was the *goal*-oriented nature of practice which had to relate to concerns about *people*; in particular about their *health needs and problems* when significant changes to their health status occurred. Inherent in the concept of goal-oriented behaviour, in which the nurse takes action to bring about change in a person's situation, is the concept of *intervention*. Intervention in this action context may be direct, in the form of *care-giving*, or may be more indirect as a *care-facilitator* when the person with the problem is caused to develop self-care skills or initiatives. This perspective highlights another significant concept, namely the *relationship* between the recipient and initiator of care. One final concept, *context*, emerged at this time as exerting an influence on all of the other conceptual structures.

The two initial concepts, therefore, even at the earliest stage of the investigation, led to a system or network of concepts emerging as crucial if a comprehensive understanding of the practice were to be achieved. Schwab (1964) places considerable emphasis on the role of conceptual structures in giving a discipline its special knowledge base. Not only do these structures guide the enquiry process for the discipline and form the reference point around which the discipline's knowledge is formulated but the network of interrelated schemas ensures cohesion and internal consistency. The parts of the structure which give rise to subject matter are important, but so too is the relatedness among the parts. The nature and scope of this relatedness may well contribute to the uniqueness of nursing as a professional discipline.

The primitive conceptual network resulting from the first question 'what is the nature of practice?' and the two basic concepts, practitioner functions and problem-solving, generated the following additional questions:

- What is the nature of the goal/s to which the practice is directed?
- What is the nature of people—the person who is the recipient and the person who is the initiator of care?
- What is the nature of the relationship between the initiator and the recipient of care?

• What is the nature of the context within which the activity takes place?

These 'telling' questions define the parameters of the enquiry which forms the basis of this chapter. They suggest that a series of interactive conceptualizations is more likely to provide nursing with a discipline structure than would a single model. Further, these parameters may be equated with Kim's (1983) boundaries which she suggests are based on the major phenomena or subject matter with which the profession deals. There is, however, a need for elasticity in identifying these boundaries (Kim 1983) which, it would seem, closely relate to Schwab's (1964) conceptual structures. She cites Fawcett (1978) as categorizing the concern of nursing in terms of man; health; environment; and nursing. Donaldson and Crowley (1978) suggest there is evidence of a remarkable consistency among nurse scholars about what they conceive to be the essence of nursing with three general themes emerging as the basis of their enquiry, namely, concern with:

1. 'The principles and laws which govern the life processes, well being, and optimum functioning of human beings—sick or well.'
2. 'The patterning of human behaviour in interaction with the environment in critical life situations.'
3. 'The processes by which positive changes in health status are affected.'

Some areas of overlap between the themes of the American theorists and this writer can be recognized.

THE PROCESS OF CONCEPTUALIZING PRACTICE

As has been stated, the process began with the simple question, 'what is the nature of nursing?' This question had no simple answer, rather it generated many answers and more questions which took the enquiry down branching pathways in which a number of ideas and steps were explored or carried out simultaneously. The difficult part of the process was not in the generation of ideas and answers; this was achieved by means of a direct appeal to, and reflection on, actual practice. Nor was the problem in the identification of factors which influenced practice, but rather in the establishment of relationships among sometimes apparently disparate parts. Many answers and undisciplined ideas needed to be organized in order to test the validity of the perceived relationships. This organizational task was approached by adopting different strategies, for instance, a central or focal concept or theme was sought among the answers to each of the initial five questions. This identification was followed by the development of schematic models and/or frameworks. These schemata and frameworks served not only to reduce large quantities of ideas, but to organize systematically the relationships among the key elements or concepts or ideas and to identify gaps within the emerging conceptual systems. The final step in the initial phase of the task was the elaboration of the key concepts and the nature of their interactiveness by a series of propositional statements sequentially organised as core ideas. Other theorists no doubt may well reverse the process by starting with prose.

The outcome of this series of activities, which centred on reflecting, asking questions, gaining answers, selecting focal concepts, and representing relationships, was a series of interactive schematic models and accompanying core ideas first published in Andersen (1976) and again in 1978 and 1984. Those currently in use have undergone further refinement and/or elaboration both by this writer and faculty of the School of Nursing and Health Studies, University of Western Sydney, Macarthur. The latest revision was carried out for the purpose of course documentation and reaccreditation in 1989.

The finished product may convey to the reader a false sense of the ease with which the structural elements were identified and articulated to achieve the interactive framework about to be discussed. Indeed the process has been a long one, characterized by reflection, enquiry, a frequent revisiting of concepts and their relationships with other concepts, and revisions of the schematic representations in terms of their fit or relevance to the real world of practice. There is no doubt that the process will continue, indeed must do so as insights gained along the way, in response to changes in practice and to reflecting on their impact, further inform and illuminate the profession's understanding of its discipline.

THE PRODUCT OF REFLECTION AND ENQUIRY

In order to provide the reader with a broad sweep of the theoretical terrain explored by this writer, it is intended to begin with the end product. This will allow the reader, with the assistance of a schematic representation, to consider the relationships among some key structural elements of practice. It is then intended to return to examine in more detail each of the constituent parts, to apply the zoom lens, as it were, to these various key reference points. Any simplistic representation of a complex activity runs the risk of appearing to do an injustice to the activity. In presenting this abridged version before the details, it is intended to provide the reader with a summarized statement, a series of reference points and a framework into which the details can be placed.

Summarised statement

Nursing is a dynamic, interactive and goal-oriented activity in which enquiry processes guide intervention. Intervention processes are seen to be necessary in response to actual or possible changes to the desired state of being (health) which interfere with, or have a potential to interfere with, a person's or group of people's ability to engage in activities of daily living. Both the nature and goals of intervention, whether direct or indirect, are determined by a number

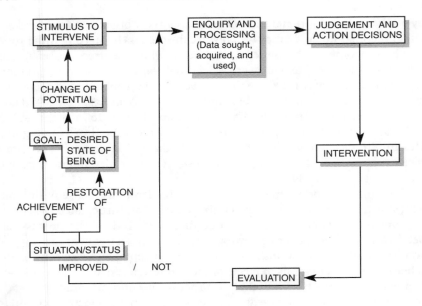

Fig. 5.1 Abridged nursing activity model.

of factors, not the least of which is the nature of the health need and the extent of health breakdown. Their determination is supported by enquiry and they are influenced in turn by the quality of judgment brought to bear on the patients'/clients' situation(s) (Fig. 5.1).

As a result of the first set of core ideas, which amplified the nature of the nursing activity there was need to extend the enquiry further to consider the following:

1. The nature of, and relationship between 'health' and 'health break-down'. This was necessary because they are both significant variables in determining the quality of life people lead, which may in turn be reflected in the extent to which people are able to engage in the activities of daily living in an integrated way. The outcome of this exploration is relevant also because it clarifies the goal(s) to which the practice is directed and the nature of intervention in general terms, including the modes of care.
2. The meaning, scope and parameters of the concept of 'intervention'. It is the process whereby action decisions are translated into action taking, whether that action involves direct care giving, facilitation of care and/or strategies which pre-empt the need for care. Its purpose is to achieve the goal of patient/client situation improvement (formerly expressed as 'problem solution').

The more detailed analysis of the concept of intervention, as it applies to nursing across all types of specialist practice, convinced this writer that common roles and functions could be identified. This commonality provides the justification of the claim that a generic basis to all nursing practice exists. Without such a basis it is difficult to sustain an argument that *a* discipline of nursing exists and that comprehensive nursing education programmes are valid. Though, it is claimed, the roles and functions are identified as common to all types of nursing, changes in frequency of performance, dominance and/or complexity may occur. This is true even within one field of nursing practice, for example 'medical' nursing, depending on the nature of the breakdown, chronicity, and response to treatment, and so on.

Because there was need to explore these variations and to test the generalizable nature of roles and functions, a framework evolved, known as the Care Activity Framework. It allows the application of the generic roles and functions model to any specific care activity. It should be noted that the choice of term 'care activity' is deliberate and does not equate to a procedure or a task. It embodies a cluster of activities which collectively contribute to care and require that the nurse carry out a number of functions and indeed play various roles. The completion of the care activity analysis provides further elaboration as it requires the identification of skills, behaviours, principles, and concepts, all of which are essential to effective care giving or facilitating involved in that example of care.

In the process of the identification and definition of roles and functions and the analyzes involved in clarifying the concept of care activity, two primary roles, care-giver and care-facilitator emerged. Further elaboration of these concepts focused attention on yet another key conceptual element, namely the role relationships between the initiator of care and the recipient. (In later deliberations the inclusion of family and/or significant others extended the scope of the role relationships needing to be considered.) The concepts of dependence and independence allowed such relationships to be explored and the need for changes in function emphasis to be identified.

Thus the network of conceptualizations was extended by the development of three more interrelated models or frameworks which emerged from the analysis of the concept of intervention. These models are known as, Roles and Functions, Care Activity Framework and Role Relationships. The interactive nature of the ideas, functions and practices, represented by the models, is clearly illustrated by their collective influence on the determination of intervention goals and modes or focus of care. Similarly these goals and modes of care are influenced by the stimuli to intervention which are generated by the nature of the health needs or health breakdown problems and other circumstances involved.

Schematic relationships of key structural elements

Figure 5.2 represents schematically and again in summary form the relationships among the key conceptualizations presented ultimately as models—

conceptualizations which resulted from addressing the first four of the original five questions by means of the process previously outlined briefly. Though it is desirable to organize these individual conceptual structures within a superordinate structure, as represented by Figure 5.2, they have been separated out in the process of amplification in order to recognize their significance in the elaboration of the concept intervention, and to begin the more detailed process of 'exploring the land'. This exploration in turn allows the identification of the knowledge base to be incorporated into the structure of the discipline.

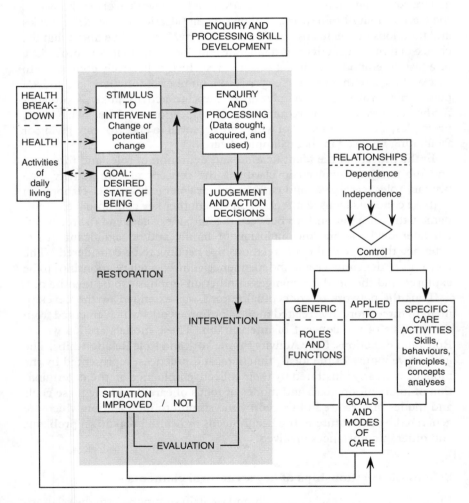

Fig. 5.2 Schematic relationships of key structural elements.

The conceptual network

It is time to examine one by one the individual models which collectively form an example of a network of conceptualizations referred to by Schwab (1964). It is from this network that more detailed analysis can be carried out, resulting in better understanding of the substantive structure of the discipline of nursing.

The nursing activity model

The Nursing Activity Model (Fig. 5.3 on page 106) was the first product of the process previously described which evolved directly from an analysis of actual practice. It can be described as a representation of the process of enquiry as it applies to and shapes nursing intervention, in that it establishes a clear relationship between thinking, judgment, and action-taking. This action-taking or intervention has as its goal, situation improvement (initially described as problem solution) and thereby the maintenance and/or restoration of a desired state of being. The activity is more than the sum of its parts or elements. Change to the nature or performance of any of the elements will have consequences for performance in other elements and in particular for the care being provided.

This model, currently in use, has undergone review on two occasions since it was first published in 1976, as a result of its application in various fields of clinical practice and of extensive experience with the problem-solving process in nursing. There was no significant change to the essence of the model; however the phrase 'situation in need of improvement' was substituted for the term 'perceived problem'. A second addition resulted from recognition being given to the fact that when exploring a problem or situation, an enquirer may need to acquire new theoretical knowledge as well as recall prior knowledge and use current client information.

There were decided advantages in not focusing on the phrases 'problem-solving' or 'problem identification'. In the realities of practice, nurses encounter people in situations which are often complex, and who have needs as well as problems, many of which cannot be solved but may be improved. To focus on a problem or a diagnosis may result in the opposite outcome to the holistic care claimed as characteristic of nursing. Focusing on single problems also tends to cut short the process of enquiry which in turn affects the quality of judgment and consequently the actions taken or proposed.

The model represents an activity called into being in response to a change in a person's situation (desired state of being) in which health need/s or health-breakdown problem/s have already interfered, or have the potential to interfere, with the person's ability to engage in the activities of daily living. The enquiry process is stimulated, resulting in the gathering of patient/situation related information from a variety of relevant sources by direct and indirect means including observations, investigations, interviewing. What

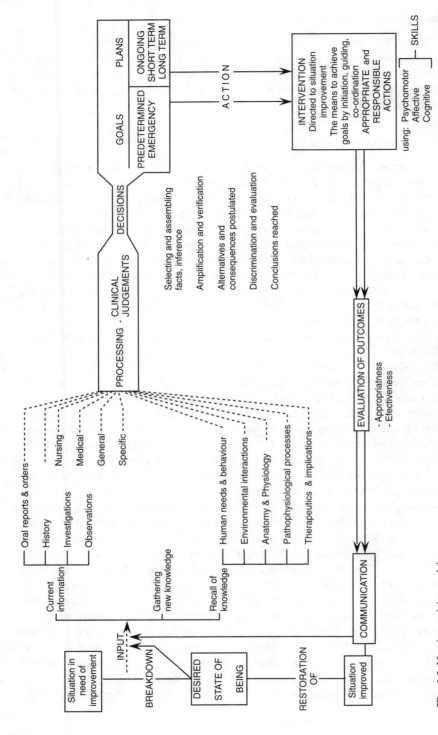

Fig. 5.3 Nursing activity model.

and how to observe, investigate, and ask about may well be influenced by concurrent recall of prior knowledge about human needs and behaviour; environmental interactions; anatomy and physiology; pathophysiological and psychopathological processes; and therapeutics and their implications. When this recall is insufficient to guide the assembling of data, the need to acquire new or further knowledge is acted on, often by recourse to texts, journals or to other personnel with more specialized knowledge.

The result of the acquisition of information and knowledge recall has to be processed in order that judgments may be made and actions set in train. A number of skills are used in reaching the judgment stage which may be being applied simultaneously, very speedily and without the user being conscious of the processes being invoked. Often the duration of the process is more protracted for a variety of reasons. However, in other instances the response may appear to be more of a reflex action, for example in certain emergency situations where predetermined protocols provide a framework for initial action-taking. These protocols, however, are also the product of a systematic decision making process.

Goal definition, sometimes more formal than at other times, facilitates the planning and coordinating of care to meet ongoing needs both in the short and long-term, according to determined priorities and inclusive of prescribed treatments. The concept of intervention has been adopted to describe the processes which transform the judgments and action decisions into appropriate and responsible activity with, or on behalf of, the patient or client and/or family or significant others.

This conceptual label was chosen to provide a superordinate organizer for what in reality represents a multi-faceted set of performances or phenomena and to allow empirical explanation to unfold. Other labels of equal generalizability could be used. The outcome of intervention should be an improvement in the situation, a meeting of needs and sometimes a contribution to the solution of problems. Both the intervention process including the nurse's performance, and the patient/client outcome are evaluated and reported, in terms of effectiveness and appropriateness.

Because the concept of intervention is so central to the activity, the zoom lens was applied and a more detailed analysis undertaken. A series of propositional statements resulted. They have in turn generated further enquiry by faculty of the School of Nursing and Health Studies, University of Western Sydney, Macarthur.

Intervention:

- Transforms deliberate action decisions into activity in an effort to improve situations, solve or prevent problems, and establish or maintain a desired state of being;
- Is concerned with assisting the individual and/or groups of people to carry out the activities of daily living in as integrated a way as possible and to meet any deficiencies which may occur;

- Involves the assumption of two primary roles, health care giver, and health-(self) care facilitator;
- Based on these primary and related sub-roles, may entail performance of any or all of seven distinct function categories, namely: assessment; structuring the environment; physical and behavioural care initiatives; management; communication, research and education/facilitation;
- Activities, though involving the performance of functions, can further be classified in terms of modes of care, namely: therapeutic, habilitative, rehabilitative, palliative and/or preventive;
- Initiation and implementation are influenced by the quality of: judgment brought to bear on the patient/client situation; competence in technical, basic, and interpersonal relationship skills; and communication ability;
- Processes in respect of individuals are influenced by the context of care, the nature of the health needs, health-breakdown problems, consequences and/or outcomes and in general terms by political, economic, legal, and ethical constraints/controls and by cultural values.

The intervention goal, situation improvement, and therefore the maintenance or restoration of the desired state of being, can best be understood when a detailed examination of the concept of health and its relationship to health breakdown is undertaken.

Health: health-breakdown and intervention relationships

Chronologically the second conceptual framework addressing the many relationships (Figs 5.4 and 5.5) developed as a result of the question, 'What is the nature of the goal to which the activity of nursing is directed?'. There is no doubt that concern with health needs, health breakdown problems, consequences and outcomes is central to generic nursing practice. Traditionally health and disease were described as being on a continuum. In the initial research conducted by this writer, the concept of a continuum was abandoned and a circular representation of the relationships developed. However a subsequent major change was made at the time of the first revision in 1983-84. The concept of disease was found to be too restrictive and not representative of all care problems/situations encountered by nurses, and therefore was not generalizable to all fields of practice. The term disease was replaced by the phrase health-breakdown, in which disease processes, pathophysiological or psychopathological, were regarded as one example of breakdown.

The new model 'Integrated Health/Breakdown and Intervention Model' improves the former Health/ Disease Relationship model in three ways. Firstly it incorporates the concepts of impairment, disability, and handicap as consequences of breakdown. These consequences may occur concurrently with a disease process or become apparent subsequently, that is

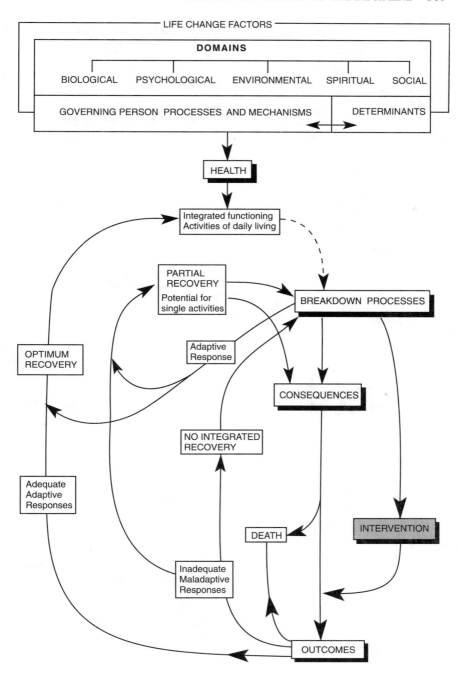

Fig. 5.4 Simplified integrated health/breakdown and intervention model. The components are shown in more detail in Figs 5.5 and 5.6.

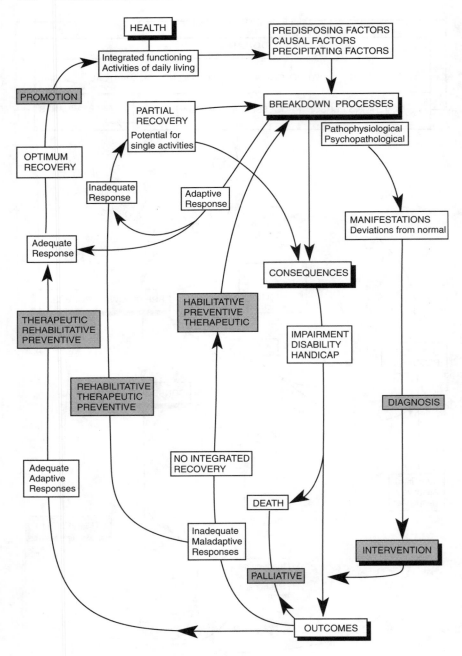

Fig. 5.5 The breakdown and intervention phases of the integrated model in detail.

beyond the time when the original disease or health breakdown process has passed. Further these consequences may themselves precipitate additional breakdown, all of which interfere with an individual's ability to engage in the activities of daily living.

The second improvement is brought about by identifying the modes of care— therapeutic, rehabilitative, habilitative, palliative, and preventive and how they are influenced by the potential nature of patient response. The nature, focus, and range of intervention activities is shown to be influenced by the time, relative to breakdown, at which intervention occurs. Similarly these considerations will determine which roles, role-relationships, functions, and skills will be needed and which will be dominant. Thus the model not only sets out to extend the framework already developed, by exploring health and its relationship to health breakdown, but it incorporates or transfers key concepts from the first model or framework. In this way interactiveness of the models is demonstrated and an internally consistent network of conceptualizations, or structures as proposed by Schwab (1964) is ensured.

A concept of health

The third aspect of improved development came about as a result of exploring the concept of health more fully. Originally it was represented simply by a consideration of the factors seen to be essential to health development, maintenance, and restoration. They were classified as belonging to the physical, psychosocial, environmental, and spiritual domains. Needs in these domains were seen to be relative in terms of the age continuum and whilst basic needs were known to be common, other needs varied not only in terms of age but of developmental stage, culture and technological evolution. Health was regarded as essential to survival, with coping and adaptation processes developing either as innate or acquired mechanisms.

The new amplified Health model (Fig. 5.6), though retaining many of these concepts, goes further in that it describes health as both a state and a process. As a state it is relative and is reflected in an individual's capacity to engage in the activities of daily living in an integrated way, which in turn contribute to survival and fulfilment as a human being. As a process, health is dynamic and is characterized by adaptive and maladaptive responses which may or may not help maintain the desired state of equilibrium necessary to sustain a high level of wellness in each of the major domains, biological, psychological, spiritual, environmental, and social. There are numerous person-centred processes and mechanisms and intrinsic and extrinsic determinants which need to be established and developed to allow essential life needs to be met. Variations in any of these processes or mechanisms may be reflected in variations in the level of wellness and/or in

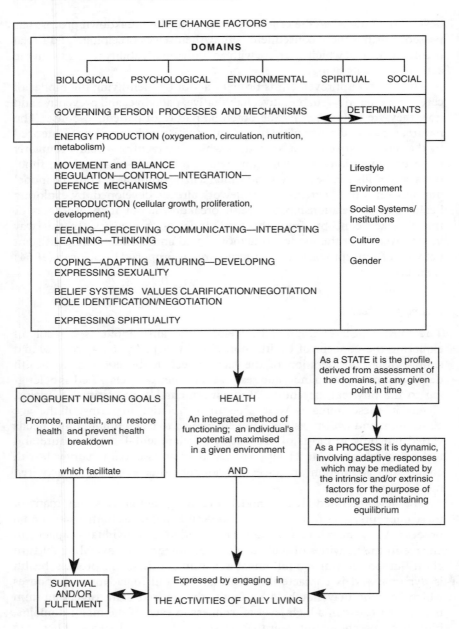

Fig. 5.6 A model of the concept of health and its components.

health breakdown. The relationships among these concepts and the goals of nursing intervention are clarified in the Concept of Health and its Components Model (Fig. 5.6).

Changes of sufficient magnitude to the desired state of being, which are not compensated for, lead to health breakdown (Figs 5.4 and 5.5) which may be due to certain predisposing, precipitating, and/or causal factors. Identification of these factors and an understanding of their role, provides nursing with two important foci for goals and modes of care, namely, health promotion and prevention of breakdown or disease processes.

When breakdown processes are set in train and adaptive responses are inadequate, *pathophysiological* and *psychopathological* processes may result in manifestations of deviation from 'normal' which need to be recognized. Similarly the *consequences* of breakdown processes (of whatever origin), impairment, disability, and handicap, may be confirmed in terms of how they manifest, whether concurrent with or subsequent to, the primary incident.

These states are associated with losses, limitations, and abnormalities of psychological function and/or physical structure or function which in turn place constraints on the individual's ability to perform the activities of daily living. They may place the individual at disadvantage relative to others in any or all of the following aspects of living—cultural, social, economic, and environmental.

Already reference has been made to the fact that the changes in health status, which result from breakdown or its consequences, need to be considered in terms of their actual or potential interference with the activities of daily living. The degree of interference is largely a reflection of the strength of the adaptive/maladaptive processes of people in their particular circumstances and environment, relative to the nature and strength of breakdown factors or consequences. When an individual's responses do not restore a state of equilibrium in respect of their activities of daily living, intervention becomes necessary.

The nature of and extent to which there is interference with the individual's ability to perform the activities of daily living will, in the main, govern the intervention process in general and the adoption of relevant modes of care in particular. Already the different modes of care have been identified when core ideas about intervention were presented. This model provides new insight to the concept of modes of care by showing their relationship to outcomes of the breakdown process or its consequences; to goal setting; and to the relationships which will result between the initiator and the recipient of care or the self-care manager.

The outcomes of breakdown processes and/or intervention may be expressed in terms of a continuum, from adequate to inadequate or to the ultimate, death. In terms of the nature of recovery the result has been portrayed as taking one of three possible paths. Firstly the least desirable, but sometimes inevitable, response has been labelled 'no integrated recovery' which invariably places the person at risk of further breakdown and/or ongoing effects of the consequences of breakdown, as identified earlier. In terms of intervention, greater emphasis may well be placed on habilitative, preventive, and then therapeutic modes of care. Rehabilitation would be a least likely mode for people who respond in this way.

The second type of response may be described in terms of 'partial recovery' because the overall response is, at best, inadequate or at worst, maladaptive. There may, however, be evidence of ability to perform single or several individual activities of daily living. The path of recovery in this case may not involve further breakdown processes (though this is a possible outcome) but instead result in a significant impact on the individual in terms of the 'consequences' alone. The mode of intervention is again influenced by the nature of response and may focus more on rehabilitative, some therapeutic and preventive activities, the relative emphasis being determined by individual needs and responses.

The third category of response has been labelled 'optimum recovery', due mainly to adequate adaptive responses, whether intrinsic or as a result of intervention or of both processes. The modes of intervention invariably are mainly therapeutic, some rehabilitative and preventive activities, with relevant goals for each mode contributing to the outcome. To make the most of optimum recovery and ensure a sustained level of the desired state of being for the individual, health promotion activities are also frequently required.

Irrespective of the nature of response and recovery path, the role-relationships between the patient/client, family and significant others and the nurse will be influenced by the choice of the relevant mode/s and goals of care.

The provision of a more detailed explanation of the elements of this model, and of how they relate to each other, has also allowed a confirmation of the internal consistency between propositions supporting this model and the conceptual elements within the framework of intervention highlighted in the exploration of the nursing activity.

The nature of interaction

Frequent reference has been made in the foregoing discussion to the issue of 'role relationships' which was considered to be of sufficient importance to be explored at the time of the initial research. The exploration at the time was limited, but highlighted the effect of the very significant concepts of dependence, independence, and control on the way the nurse viewed practice (often in terms of 'doing things to and for patients'). It was to result in taking the first step in an attempt to achieve a balance between the roles of care-giver and care facilitator (Andersen 1976, 1978). At that time it was recorded that 'nursing justified its existence in an interaction context'. An understanding of the relationships called into being as a result of intervention was essential if the activity of nursing was not to be perceived, erroneously, as an end in itself.

The ideas, which resulted from addressing this question in a limited way, are intended to stimulate detailed development of the issues raised and maybe lead to an exploration of other dimensions of relationships among nurse/patient or client and/or family and significant others.

A physical care activity, associated with respiratory problems, has been chosen to illustrate the dependence—independence concepts. A similar analysis could be carried out for care activities other than those with a physical focus (Fig. 5.7 on page 116).

A significant goal of nursing is its concern with the maintenance or restoration of independence or relative independence to the greatest extent possible. However, varying degrees of dependency can be identified along a continuum. The range of such dependency may vary from relative independence through possible needs for partial assistance, artificial support, function, or activity—substitution to 'total' dependency. The degree or range of dependency is a function or outcome of the difference between the strength of breakdown factors and individual resources and freedom to be independent.

Increasing patient dependency is paralleled by increasing nurse 'control', and in the example chosen also involves the performance of more technical and complex skills and decision making with potentially far-reaching consequences. This latter characteristic of high dependency care management is true also for the non-physical areas of care.

When a person becomes a patient and/or a client, the potential for change in position along the dependency continuum is ever present. Skill in recognizing, anticipating, and managing such change is an essential part of the care-giver or care-facilitator's repertoire in order that care, appropriate to the degree of dependency, is available at any time.

Again in the example used to illustrate the key concepts, generalizable behaviours of nursing performance have been listed as relevant to maintaining patient/client independence. They are applicable to a wide range of care activities but may not represent an exhaustive list. In addition to these general behaviours, certain procedures and/or care activities have been identified. It was recognized as critical to meaningful practice that procedures should not be viewed as ends in themselves but means directed to the achievement of ultimate goals—facilitating adequate adaptive responses and the restitution of independence or that degree of independence possible. More detailed attention was given to the problem of procedure-oriented performance. Exploration of this issue is recorded in the description of the care activity framework.

Whilst manifestations of pathological and/or psychopathological or antisocial processes may provide indicators of changing dependency states, management strategies also need to take into account the impact of role

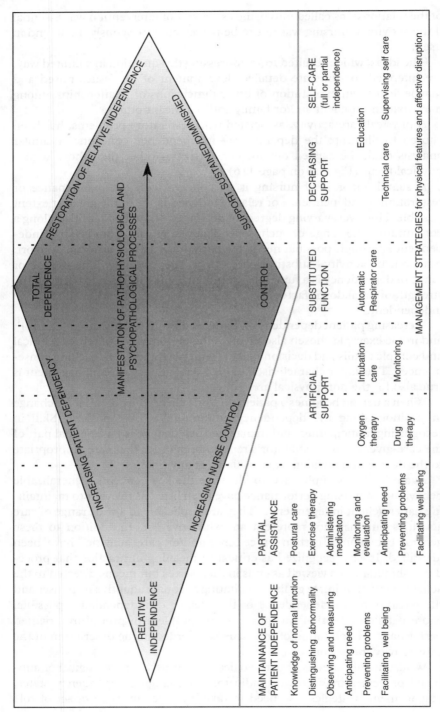

Fig. 5.7 Nurse-patient relationship. A dependency model.

changes for both the nurse and the patient. Role relationship reversals may indeed occur.

It is inevitable that total independence or even a relative level of independence will not always result from nurse–patient interaction and the application of appropriate modes and goals of care. However, whilst developing the capacity to 'let go' of once dependent patients/clients it is equally important to recognize the need for ongoing appropriate levels of support should this be needed whilst patients develop self-care skills.

Generic roles and functions

The belief that basic roles and functions could be identified and that these roles and functions would be found to be common to all fields of nursing practice was an inevitable conclusion reached at the time of conducting the initial research. The conviction grew as a result of testing the ideas out with student nurse teachers in their clinical practice arenas. As these clinical teachers practised in every specialist field of nursing, the generalizable nature of these roles seemed more than likely. A sense of urgency in formalizing the theoretical position resulted from the conditions outlined for curriculum development at the time of the transfer of nursing education into the tertiary sector in New South Wales. The abolition of separate registers and the requirements that graduates of new programmes be able to function, at a beginning level, in general, psychiatric, and developmental disability settings presupposed that it was possible to identify a generic basis to nursing.

The initial attempt to take the common roles and functions beyond the stage of simply identifying them and validating their inclusiveness, was to establish a classification system which resulted in the model, 'Intervention: Roles and Functions' (Fig. 5.8 on page 118).

Reference has already been made to the position adopted whereby the practice is held to incorporate two primary roles, 'health care giver' and 'health care facilitator'. Subsumed within these primary roles is a set of five sub-roles, clinician, manager, communicator, researcher, and educator. These sub-roles in turn give rise to seven function categories. Irrespective of the care context, nurses are concerned with the functions of making assessments; structuring a safe and conducive environment; taking clinical initiatives associated with physical, emotional, social and/or spiritual activities; communicating and interacting, managing; researching; and educating/facilitating. Major nursing functions have been classified as examples within each function category. Extensive analysis of functions supplied by registered nurses, from as many types of practice and contexts as exist, made validation of the framework possible.

Practitioners in some fields of practice will play one role and perform certain functions more frequently than others and may be required to

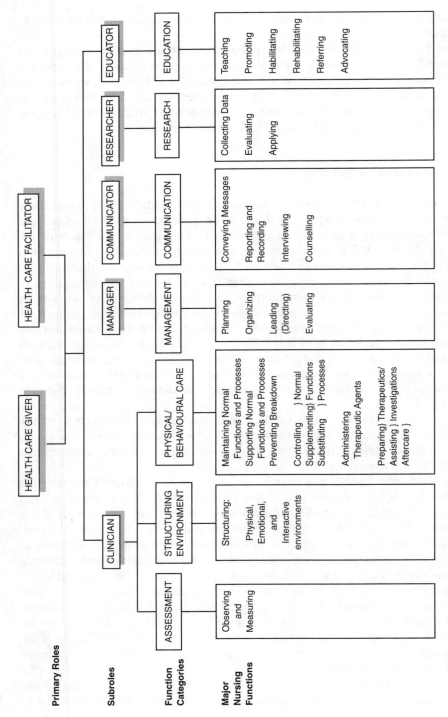

Fig. 5.8 Intervention: nursing roles and functions model.

develop more complex skills in carrying out one function or another. However general principles, in respect of each function category, can be identified and are applicable to each major function within the same category and transferable to any context or specialty practice. These principles contribute to the emerging knowledge basis of the structure of the discipline. The degree of commonality and transferability reinforce the belief in a generic basis to nursing.

Application of roles and functions to a specific care activity

The need to confirm the reliability of the framework led to its application in practice. A care activity was selected and analyzed, and the relationships among the various roles and functions inherent in that particular intervention were identified. The analysis process was taken a step further by the identification of the skills, principles, and behaviours underlying the performance of the functions, and the knowledge and concepts essential to informed practice in terms of that particular activity (Fig. 5.9 on page 120). The principles will be the same for all procedures within the same major function category, though behaviours will vary somewhat.

These two frameworks, 'Roles and Functions' and 'The Care Activity', have not only incorporated concepts previously identified in relation to intervention and nurse/patient relationships but have extended the conceptual analysis. They have done this by undertaking an exploration in some depth and detail of significant concepts, opening up understanding of their meaning in nursing and thereby adding to the process of explicating the structure of the body of knowledge basic to nursing, deemed by Donaldson & Crowley (1978) to have been neglected by nurse theorists.

No reporting of the activities which resulted in the system of interactive models just discussed would be complete without reference to the role of judgment in intervention. Not only does a judgment made in practice influence the initiation of an action or actions, that is, resolve what is to be done, by whom and how, but it also influences the quality of the activities as they are carried out. The need to modify or cut short a procedure or to seek help are examples of the application of judgment in intervention procedures.

The quality of judgment is in turn influenced by the nature of the enquiry process which culminates in judgment, the skills which are inherent in this process and the availability of knowledge and concepts relevant to the situation about which judgments are to be made. A very detailed study about the nature of clinical judgment and the skills and behaviours involved was undertaken along with the development of the theoretical basis of nursing (Andersen 1976, 1978). This study led to the decision to adopt the particular approach to nursing education known as problem-based learning. A more detailed account of the nature of judgment and the application of the theoretical models to a particular curriculum development task will be the basis of a further publication.

CARE ACTIVITY — Maintaining normal respiratory function
ACTIVITY STIMULUS — Actual or potential respiratory impairment
PRIMARY ROLE — HEALTH CARE FACILITATOR/GIVER — SUB ROLE — Clinician
FUNCTION CATEGORY — Physical/Behavioural care

PROCEDURE	MAJOR NURSING FUNCTION	ASSOCIATED NURSING FUNCTIONS	PRINCIPLES	BEHAVIOURS	CONCEPTS
Deep breathing and coughing exercises	Preventing Health Breakdown	Assessing Communicating Educating Evaluating	1 The establishment of a need 2 The establishment of a state of readiness for nurse, patient, and equipment 3 The maintenance of patient safety and comfort 4 The prevention of untoward outcomes 5 The assessment of patient's participation 6 The evaluation of the activity in terms of effectiveness and appropriateness 7 The accuracy of reporting and recording	1 C Assess patient's current respiratory status 2 C Explain procedure to patient 2 C Confirm patient's readiness 3 P Wash hands 3 P Assist patient to appropriate position 3 P Demonstrate technique 4 P Assist patient as necessary 5 C Assess/encourage patient participation 6 C Assess respiratory excursion and sputum production, as appropriate 6 C Negotiate with patient to repeat exercise 3 P Wash hands 7 P Report and record activity	Stability Ventilation Safety Comfort Dependence Independence

SKILLS: C Cognitive A Affective P Psychomotor

The details have been completed by faculty working in a team developing practice principles and skills within the present education program.

Fig. 5.9 Nursing care activity framework.

The final question in the initial series asked about the nature of the context in which nursing occurred. At the time the question was asked, there was a tendency to regard nursing as an isolated service rather than within the context of society and its various institutions. An attempt was made then to identify the various interacting sub-systems involved, and the features within those systems which influenced the provision of care in general, and in particular the ability of an individual or group of individuals to maintain a quality of life and/or respond when health-breakdown occurs. In subsequent revisions ideas about the context were taken up and dealt with in considering the amplified health model rather than as a separate entity.

CONCLUSION

A series of interrelated models and supporting propositions has been presented as the products of an extensive enquiry process. This process began as an attempt to make sense of the phenomenon of nursing; to make the essence of nursing more explicit by asking a single question. It began also in the belief that practice should drive theory which in turn should inform practice. The enquiry proceeded initially based on one 'invented' and one 'borrowed' conceptualization. However it resulted in a network of conceptualizations or structures, to use Schwab's (1964) terms, which brought together empirical practical elements and theoretical constructs or concepts. Such structures define the parameters of the syntactical structure (the terrain) and in so doing have the capacity to generate telling questions to guide enquiry, theory generation and the incorporation of knowledge into the discipline. Attention has been drawn to the systematic organization of the network of models and the interrelated nature of the concepts from model to model, satisfying the criterion of internal consistency among the various relationships.

Analysis of the processes utilized, namely: reflection on experience; questioning; abstracting and organizing answers; interpreting and establishing relationships; expressing relationships schematically and as propositions; testing theories; reviewing and revising, has resulted in a new paradigm for theory development. These processes have something to say about the syntactical structure of the discipline. They are best expressed in the form of a spiral which suggests a continuing process in that each turn of the coil, whilst allowing the structure or problem to be revisited, suggests that new insights create new understandings (Fig. 5.10 on page 122) and/or new ways of practising.

More questions need to be asked and more reflection both in and about practice needs to take place before our understanding is more explicit. However a beginning has been made in clarifying the structure of nursing—a structure which has integrity and validity. These claims can be made because the essence of the conceptualizations has stood the test of time, having been applied in the action context to review and filter practice habits

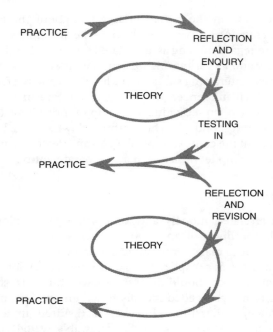

Fig. 5.10 Theory from practice: a paradigm.

and to extend nursing behaviours. Similarly these conceptualizations, though undergoing some review as a result of insights gained from the application process, have stimulated and served the needs of researchers, theorists, curriculum developers; the needs of the course revision processes; and indeed the needs of students as they have sought to make sense, not only of the subject matter, but of the phenomenon of nursing itself.

Thus the original purpose of the study (a research basis for tertiary nursing education), which caused the first questions to be asked, was achieved. However, because the processes adopted were systematic and consistent with structural analysis principles, an additional and invaluable outcome was the emergence of an embryonic discipline structure. The network of conceptualizations associated with the proposed structure should contribute, not only to an identifiable knowledge base for nursing, but to debate about that knowledge base and the processes adopted in its presentation.

REFERENCES

Andersen B M 1976 Basic nurse education curriculum. A research report submitted to the Commission on Advanced Education. Cumberland College of Health Sciences, Sydney
Andersen B M 1978 A basic nurse education curriculum evaluation project incorporating an investigation into the cognitive aspects of clinical judgment. New South Wales College of Nursing, Sydney

Andersen B M 1984 In: The Curriculum Submission to the Higher Education Board of New South Wales for the accreditation of the Diploma of Applied Science (Nursing), Macarthur Institute of Higher Education, Sydney

Armiger Sr B 1974 Scholarship in nursing. Nursing Outlook (March) 22:160-164

Benne K D 1985 Educational field experience as the negotiation of different cognitive worlds. In: Bennie W G, Benne K, Chin R (eds) The planning of change, 4th edn. Holt Reinhart Winston, New York

Dewey J 1933 How we think. D C Health, Boston

Donaldson S, Crowley D 1978 The discipline of nursing. Nursing Outlook 26:113-120

Kant I 1781 Critique of pure reason. Translation of 2nd edn by Meiklejohn 1934. J M Dent, London

Kim H S 1983 The nature of theoretical thinking in nursing. Prentice Hall International, London

Patel V, Evans D, Groen G 1989 Reconciling basic science and clinical reasoning. Teaching and Learning in Medicine 1(3):116-121

Peel E A 1971 The nature of adolescent judgment. Crosby Lockwood Staples, London

Schwab J 1964 The structure of knowledge and the curriculum. In: Ford G, Pugno L (eds) The structure of knowledge and the curriculum. Rand McNally, Chicago

FURTHER READING

Fawcett J 1978 The 'what' of theory development. In: Theory development: what, why, how? National League of Nursing, New York, pp 17-23

Toulmin S 1972 Human understanding, Vol 1, Princeton University Press, Princeton

Toulmin S 1977 Postscript: the structure of scientific theories. In: Suppe F (ed) The structure of scientific theories. University of Chicago Press, Urbana, p 600-614

6. Facilitation and self-care: developing frameworks for learning and practice

Judith Townsend

A model or framework is a deliberately simplified representation of reality. It is a way to make sense of a complex situation, a means for teasing out the central elements of an issue.

This chapter presents an account of a pilot study which explored the processes and outcomes of the development of two frameworks conceptualizing facilitation and self-care, and their operationalization. The pilot study was implemented in 1988 using participatory research (Hall 1981, Tandon 1981, Wright 1970, Rogers 1967). The population comprised registered nurse students undertaking a course unit titled 'The Nurse as Facilitator' in an accelerated Diploma of Applied Science (Nursing) which uses a problem based learning (PBL) model.

The probability statement explored through the pilot study was that 'a facilitative approach leads to self-direction/self-care'. This statement contains three components. First, a facilitative approach by a tutor causes students to be self-directed and autonomous in their approach to learning. Second, a facilitative approach by students as registered nurse practitioners leads to self-caring clients in the clinical nursing setting. Third, the same set of facilitative behaviours are appropriate and effective in both settings.

It was anticipated that an exploration of the literature would show that the wide range of behaviours/functions listed by various authors and labelled as facilitative are derived largely from a common conceptual stance. This proved to be a false assumption. Facilitation and self-care are not universally conceptualized in a way that allows for rational and informed operationalization in both educational and clinical settings.

This fragmentation generated the fourth and major element of the study which consisted of the elucidation of a fundamental statement and series of propositions which conceptualized both facilitation and self-care. In each case the statements were elaborated at three levels: a megaconcept level expressed as a single phrase which epitomized the relevant term; a superordinate concept level classified through a series of core propositions; and for each superordinate concept a subordinate concept level which was categorized through a series of behavioural descriptors.

Phase one was the initial classroom elaboration of the frameworks and the exploration of 'letting go' as a prerequisite for facilitation and self-direction.

Students rehearsed appropriate behaviours in a safe environment. Phase two was the transfer and implementation of the concepts in the clinical nursing setting.

The study is significant for three reasons. First, PBL is growing in popularity and significance as an educational method, with the acknowledgement that facilitation is the most appropriate teaching/learning strategy when self-directedness or autonomy is the desired process and outcome of learning (Little & Ryan 1988, Boud 1986, Little 1986, Boud 1985, Kaufman 1985, Barrows & Tamblyn 1980). PBL methods suggest that while it is necessary for learners to acquire and transfer knowledge from the learning to the practice setting, it is the acquisition, transfer, and application of enquiry and processing skills which is crucial for flexible and individualized decision making and intervention.

Second, there is increasing if sometimes indirect evidence that the same facilitative approach is appropriately and successfully applied in the clinical nursing setting when a self-care response in clients is preferred (Slaytor 1987, Kappeli 1986, Neufeld & Hobbs 1985, Englert 1984). Thirdly, there is a need to collect data which makes the links between the two contexts. The aim of a professional vocational education is surely to produce graduates capable of intervening in their chosen field of practice in a competent, thoughtful, rational and caring manner.

In the study the tutor adopted a co-learner position and modelled facilitative behaviours (Iwasiw 1987, Taylor 1986, Percy & Ramsden 1980). This is consistent with the major approaches to adult learning (Boud 1985, Boud et al 1985, Mezirow 1981, Knowles 1975) which suggest students should be autonomous, independent, self-directed, and self-motivated. Teaching/learning strategies take account of the learners' experiences, their readiness to learn, and the relevance of information to their needs.

Skills such as questioning, challenging, probing, guiding, assisting, mediating, and negotiating are utilised in many teaching/learning approaches and by many practitioners in a range of clinical nursing settings. Indeed the very universality, flexibility, and adaptability of these skills and behaviours, when derived from the global conceptualization of facilitation, suit a wide variety of individual learning needs and practice situations, and makes their development both vital and attractive.

THE PILOT STUDY

The PBL tutorial process

Within the classroom context a means was sought to conceptualize and operationalize the dual concepts of facilitation and self-care and then to determine their applicability to practice. The testing through participative research involved:

1. The tutor modelling facilitative behaviours with the goal of allowing students to experience 'letting go' as a prerequisite to the adoption of a co-learner position in which the locus of control largely shifts from the tutor to the learner, causing the student to shift from being tutor-directed to being self-directed.
2. Students rehearsing 'letting go' as the first level of facilitative behaviour through simulated client interactions with the goal of enabling self-care.
3. Developing and justifying conceptual frameworks for facilitation and self-care.
4. Students initiating a range of facilitative and self-directed/self-care behaviours in actual clinical nursing situations, and then analyzing both process and structure of intervention by using the facilitation and self-care frameworks through role playing and evaluating critical incidents.

Application in teaching

Having gleaned some useful information from the literature (Brookfield 1986, Schon 1983, Knowles 1975) mainly related to specific behaviours, the tutor adopted an open co-learner position. Relevant information was shared with students in session one. The roles and responsibilities of the tutor were emphasized followed by the implications this had for student responsibility and behaviour. The major input from the tutor was in generating self-directed/self-care responses each week as the concepts themselves and their application in learning and practice were explored.

The tutor shared with students some of the key concept words on which she based her behaviours. These included responsibility, control, power, autonomy, independence, ambiguity, uncertainty, contracting, negotiating, resources, safe environment, goals, participation, accountability, reflection. It was suggested that students would assume a major share of the responsibility for their own learning; that the locus of control or wisdom would transfer from the tutor to all co-learners; and that this would involve students in making their own decisions and in accepting the consequences and outcomes.

The tutor worked alongside students to provide support and demystify the process where possible, being creative, flexible, motivated, and involved in mutual goal setting and identifying appropriate resources, and above all provided a safe and secure environment within which everyone could experiment, take risks, accept uncertainty without coming to harm, and develop mutual trust and acceptance. Using this approach traditional content input became a thing of the past. As co-learners, individual and group behaviours were the subject of examination.

From the tutor's perspective acting as a role model was not an easy task in the early sessions. This involved 'letting go' of students' behaviour;

relinquishing control of the classroom environment; and negotiating goals for each week. It meant taking the chance that the probability statement was correct and that all this activity would lead in an appropriate and acceptable direction, and produce a satisfactory result by the end of semester. Such is the nature of facilitation. The tutor's behaviour needed to be consistent and she experienced difficulties remaining in the facilitator role. The difficulty in maintaining this role arose not because 'letting go' was such a problem per se, but largely as a result of constant student pressure for the tutor to conform to the traditional didactic role. Teamwork and trust between tutor and students was ultimately one of the major keys to success. As students moved through explorations and problems they were able to provide support for each other, to use their respective strengths, and to balance their performance.

Time was spent each week examining and recording individual behaviours and the group processes and interactions; identifying shortcomings and gains; and adding to the store of knowledge which supported or refuted the probability statement. Gradually the frameworks were being built. Words, ideas, phrases were incorporated, modified, discarded, reclaimed and reworked. All the time the cutting edge of everyone's knowledge about these concepts of facilitation and self-direction/self-care was advancing and being constantly tested in the classroom and subsequently in the clinical nursing setting. While there was undoubted support and enthusiasm for the approach by the tutor the same could not be said of the students in the initial weeks, although their effort to come to terms with the concepts and the approach was real and concerted.

Application in learning

Students expressed marked reluctance to engage in self-directed learning. The idea that they should take responsibility for their own learning generated apprehension and some hostility. Athough they tried, students were not particularly interested in acquiring process skills or creating behaviour change. They wanted content.

This initial student response to the PBL method and facilitation seemed the very place to start exploring the issues and to start building the frameworks. Students were encouraged and challenged to examine and reflect upon their responses and feelings. The issues explored included control, motivation, roles, dependence, and accountability. Why did they want to be controlled by the tutor? What was so appealing about dependence? Why were they at university if there was no motivation for change? The picture which emerged incorporated issues about safety and comfort, familiarity, and the known. Their ability to cope with uncertainty was very low and their previous socialization processes in traditional education and work practices had emphasized submissive attitudes and the importance of measurable achievement. They would say: 'Tell us what you want—what we should be doing or learning' , 'We feel all at sea', 'We're going round in circles'.

When no specific answers were forthcoming over time, although they were angry, they made some very tentative efforts at debating, challenging, asking questions, and disagreeing, at least in their small group work where they felt reasonably safe to open up a little. They began to back each other up, offer encouragement, and allow all group members to air their views. When this small group behaviour proved successful, they began to offer their opinions and findings firmly and with conviction in open feedback sessions. Throughout, the tutor was requiring students to examine the process, to reflect on what was happening within the classroom, and build up the theoretical construct of the frameworks.

Students saw that far from being penalized for these apparently radical feelings, behaviours, attitudes, and beliefs they were being praised; their early efforts at challenging and confronting were being rewarded. Their self concept was being enhanced and they began to take initiative, be assertive, question authority, demand involvement and control. Students began to be self-directed self-carers. They were feeling more secure as their ability to provide a mutually supportive environment grew along with their negotiating skills for determining future direction in their learning.

By this stage many of the superordinate concepts had been confirmed as appropriate and significant, and the frameworks were taking shape. As students resolved their ideas and feelings about each core proposition and its associated subordinate concepts, they internalized and rehearsed the related operationalized behaviours. The letting go behaviours became more frequent. Throughout the early process skill acquisition period the only content addressed was the concepts of facilitation and self-care. The analysis and evaluation was of individual and group behaviours and the changes occuring. It cannot be too heavily emphasised that constant reflection on the process by the students was essential to letting go and changing behaviours.

Regular informal reflection was only one means by which the behaviour change and acceptance of facilitation/self-care by students was monitored and evaluated. The formal assessment items within the unit were designed to demonstrate student understanding and internalization of the process and its application by them in learning and practice; and to enable them to conceptualize reality and to construct their frameworks. Firstly, students prepared their own flowcharts through the development of a series of statements which represented their understanding of the concepts of facilitation and self-care. These were then refined and amended as necessary over time. Finally students developed a rationale which demonstrated the comprehensiveness and universality of their statements, showed their internal consistency and highlighted the relationships between the flowcharts, which then enabled them to justify and defend the stand they had taken.

During this time the tutor followed the same process and developed her own frameworks for facilitation and self-care. These were designed to test the probability statement and derived largely from those key words devised at the beginning, since it was found that these had stood the test of classroom application. Also when the students' work was examined many commonalities were discovered although often the terminology differed markedly. So some minor accommodations were made and the frameworks were presented for the students' scrutiny. In comparing their own flowcharts with the tutor's frameworks, students were able to see that they had independently discovered and incorporated most of the elements which had been covered in the frameworks and presented a coherent theoretical concept for intervention.

The result of this was an enhanced feeling of product ownership and greater commitment to the tutorial process by which they had acquired that feeling. The critical link that students made was that the product (i.e. the frameworks) actually incorporated the process (i.e. the concepts) and allowed them to identify the behaviours necessary for implementation (i.e. operationalization). It was agreed that the frameworks had become the embodiment of a way of thinking, feeling, and acting in the classroom. Students now had the necessary knowledge and skills to incorporate the conceptual processes into their own practice.

Application in practice

Students came from diverse nursing practice backgrounds. If the initial premises were correct and the subsequent core propositions universal and generalizable, the frameworks should be applicable to any practice areas. Some of the students remained sceptical. Although ready to agree that the facilitative/self-care approach had some merit in a teaching/learning situation, they were reluctant to risk take in their own workplace. Many of the old fears and reservations emerged again, such as relinquishing control to the client; how to get all their work done if they had to negotiate care; what would be their colleagues' response to this facilitative approach; and how would management react? Making the transfer was not straightforward for many students. It required some class time to rework the process; to challenge and support; and to enable the tutor to re-establish self trust and esteem, and ensure access for consultation and support.

Following negotiation, the second piece of work undertaken by students was an applied project the outcome of which was two-fold, a role play in class and a written piece of work. The assignment required students to identify and briefly describe a critical incident from their recent practice where they could have initiated facilitation and self-care. From this incident they were to develop a situation improvement summary documenting stimuli, goals, strategies, and evaluation of care which demonstrated how they would deal with the situation using facilitation and self-care. This enabled students to recognize the stimuli to their care activity; to produce negotiated client-oriented goals; and to analyze their intervention strategies to ensure they met the criteria specified by the frameworks. Finally they were to document this analysis, justifying and defending their approach and behaviours according to the frameworks.

In order to obtain feedback from their peers and to clarify their thinking prior to writing up their work, students role played the situations in class. They negotiated with fellow students to form groups, devise their scripts, present the piece, and be ready to respond to other students' questions and comments. These role play sessions came toward the end of the semester when most students were quite comfortable with the process in the safety of the classroom.

During the role plays they displayed the full gamut of behaviours associated with facilitation and self-care, and they spent the last few minutes of each session reflecting on the process which had occured during the session. Debating and reflecting at the end of this process of role playing, the same commitment had emerged for the use of the facilitative/self-care approach in practice as was previously made to it in the educational setting. Most students were able to value facilitation and self-care as appropriate and useful, injecting innovation, flexibility and creativity into their care and enhancing the role, motivation, adaptability and self-directedness of the client.

PILOT STUDY RESULTS

The conceptual frameworks

The development and application of the dual frameworks of facilitation and self-care in both the classroom and the clinical nursing setting fulfilled the original probability statement of the study. The frameworks were found to be complementary and mutually inclusive. Each framework was regarded as informing and enlarging the other. The time sequence involved the exploration of facilitation, followed by self-care. It incorporated the development and elaboration of each framework, and examined their comprehensiveness and internal consistency, justifying relationships and testing their universality.

Facilitation—brainstorming

The initial weeks of the study were spent in brainstorming ideas relating to facilitation. Students examined the concept through the literature and through critical reflection on their own behaviour and their group dynamics. They also analyzed the application of each component to the learning or caring context. Initially students used words such as leadership, encouragement, helping, education, mediator, providing information, by example, modelling, giving support, assistance, educating, counselling, clarifying. Facilitator roles included evaluator, assessor, planner, decision maker, demonstrator, teacher. Each of these behaviours students related specifically to the roles of the nurse or tutor, and began to see similarities between the two.

Following some clarification of what these terms meant to students, further word lists appeared with phrases such as stepping back, release of inhibition, giving away preconceived ideas, two way initiation, decreasing power, increasing independence, contractual bargaining. A number of themes were beginning to emerge and students were able to cluster some of the phrases along common lines. More coherent statements were being formulated which described more abstractly how students felt about facilitation. A degree of agreement was being reached when some amalgamation and reordering of statements was done. For example:

- Set goals in accordance with patient needs
- Everyone comes to the same goal conclusion
- Goals that are self-oriented
- Supportive and agreeable environment
- Family participation
- Comfort, safety and structure in environment
- Providing comfortable surroundings
- Encouraging independence
- Educating for awareness
- Encouraging a feeling of achievement
- Encouraging personal responsibility
- Improving and identifying individual rights
- Decision making with both parties in control
- Sharing responsibility
- Promoting individuality
- Encouraging self-awareness
- Listening to problems
- Providing motivation
- Being open-minded
- Patience
- Communication skills
- Joint decisions
- Requires a compromise
- Participation of two or more parties
- Power evenly distributed
- Both parties in control
- Power of choice
- No aggression or authoritative behaviour
- Respect among all parties

From these phrases a number of key concept words became apparent and the tutor compiled a list which could be used to cluster a number of ideas. After much discussion mixing and matching phrases and key concept words, it was decided that the most appropriate were liberation and structure, control, autonomy, ambiguity, resources, contracting, environment, goals. With the tutor, students were now in a position to determine and refine the superordinate concepts; to express them through core propositions, and to examine these to elucidate the megaconcept which could encapsulate in a single phrase the distilled essence of facilitation.

Self-care—brainstorming

This concept is better known to registered nurse practitioners, so students did not have as much trouble exploring this area. The earlier process was repeated with students devising word lists, clustering like ideas, identifying emerging themes and finally extracting the key words from which the core propositions could be developed.

Early key concept word lists commonly included communication, cooperation, motivation, independence, responsibility, perception, confidence, acceptance, understanding, goal orientation. Clustered phrases included:

- Learning new knowledge and skills
- Using new equipment confidently
- Willingness to learn
- Gathering and assimilating information
- Acceptance of limitations or disability
- Better acceptance of health breakdown
- Goal orientated behaviour
- Identifies ways to deal with problem
- Motivated to achieve goals
- Confident about recovery
- Gaining independence
- Self initiated action
- Self organizing
- Behaviours are self reliant
- Does things at own pace and convenience
- More flexible approach
- Two way communication
- Non-judgemental attitude
- Increases awareness
- Seeks opinions but expresses own views
- Feels more in control

The key concept words which emerged from an examination of the thematically clustered word lists included responsibility, role change, motivation, self-concept, consultation, goal achievement, self-interest. These were discussed in detail in order to clarify meaning so that a common perspective and interpretation, and a determined sequence and logical progression, was shared.

From these key concept words came the megaconcept followed by the elaboration of the superordinate concepts each with their subordinate concepts.

The frameworks described

The facilitation and self-care frameworks described below are those which embody the interactions between nurse and client. It was indicated earlier

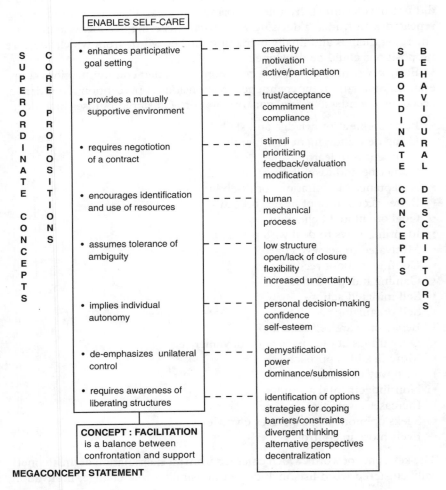

Fig. 6.1 Facilitation framework.

that the main purpose of the study was to move from the teaching/learning situation to determine the applicability of the frameworks in the clinical nursing setting. Thus the classroom interactions were the model through which the subsequent clinical elaboration occurred.

Each framework is designed with three levels: the megaconcept or single statement; superordinate concepts or core propositions; subordinate concepts or behavioural descriptors.

Facilitation framework

Figure 6.1 shows the final product for the facilitation framework.

The megaconcept. From the exploration of key words and phrases the megaconcept statement became, 'Facilitation is a balance between confrontation and support'. The notion of a balance is critical to the initial understanding of both frameworks. Facilitation is not an all or nothing concept. In every care activity the approach can be facilitative. It may be that it is only a small component of some care activities; or it may be that it is a significant and prime component of each intervention. Whatever the level or spread, the facilitator's prime goal is to allow the client to be involved in the interaction, thus coming back to the notion of balance.

Confrontation by the facilitator is used in the sense that clients need to be self sufficient, need to be able to deal with their own problems on an ongoing basis, and need to be able to understand what is happening to them. Confrontation challenges clients, and asks them to justify what they want to do and to clarify their reasoning and approach.

Support is a fairly well understood concept. Alongside confrontation people are able to support each other; provide backup and comfort; and to care about each other. The two areas of behaviour, confrontation and support, go hand in hand and should be present in any interaction in varying degrees so that the client is enabled to move forward to self-care feeling as secure as possible. The behaviour base on which all the elements of facilitation rest is that the nurse becomes a co-carer, just as in the classroom the tutor becomes a co-learner and balance is maintained.

The superordinate concepts expressed as core propositions are explored below in a logical order and may occur in this sequence, although it is more probable that they will occur in clusters moving back and forth as the situation and interaction demands.

The first core proposition indicates that the initial step in this process is to accept that 'facilitation requires awareness of liberating structures', that will allow people to break down barriers, to move outside convention and tradition, and to remove constraints which may hinder progress. Every organization has a structure which determines people's place in the scheme of things. Mostly these structures are predetermined and behaviour is constrained by sets of rules which tell people what to do and how to act. In many organizations, such as hospitals and universities, the structure is hierarchical and determines each person's level of responsibility; to whom they report their actions; how much freedom of decision making they have and in what areas; and when they should ask permission or do as they are told. In most of these organizations there is little room to move and minimal flexibility, particularly at the grassroots level.

Being autonomous, independent people and personalizing decision making means looking for an alternative structure which will allow them to participate, to step outside the traditional passive role and become proactive in their own learning or caring. This is analagous to the self-care superordinate concept of taking responsibility for one's own health. The clients generate rules which will suit their needs. This should not be so difficult given that facilitation de-emphasizes unilateral control, provides a mutually supportive environment and enhances participative goal setting.

The second core proposition states that 'facilitation de-emphasizes unilateral control'. In most interactions someone is usually in charge; someone seems to have the power to control and to direct what is happening. In behaving in a facilitative way that level of control by any one party in the interaction is limited. The idea is to share control, to put the brakes on power plays by any one person.

To achieve this it is necessary to demystify what is happening if people are to be equal partners. Creating mystery is a very common among professional people. Maintaining a unique body of knowledge says 'I'm the expert, I've got all the information, expertise and skill'. Facilitation says that sharing of knowledge and power is OK. It doesn't detract from nurses' professional position, it doesn't belittle their status. What it does is to allow other people to be part of that interaction.

This enables participants to behave autonomously, independently. The third core proposition suggests that 'facilitation implies individual autonomy'. Interacting facilitatively people need strategies that will enable them to be autonomous. The things which are significant are people's levels of confidence and self-esteem to enable them to make personally appropriate decisions.

One of the justifications for this cooperative but autonomous behaviour is that the interaction should be user friendly, otherwise it will not be of much value to the person requiring care. If clients can't make decisions which are personally appropriate, and which are useful to them in the current situation whether that is in a hospital, at home, or at work, then they will not comply with appropriate care activities. They will forget things. They will find it hard to learn new skills because these are not organised in a way they can use or in terms they can understand, so they just ignore what is happening. Perhaps days or weeks of hard work are lost because the client can't see the relevance of the request.

A facilitative interaction is not likely to be neatly packaged. It will not be straightforward or clear cut and well organized. It could be messy; it could change direction a dozen times; it might never have an ending; it might not be able to be tied up and packaged neatly. Autonomous, self-responsible people will want to go in their own direction, generating multiple strategies and outcomes. As expressed in the fourth core proposition this situation suggests that 'facilitation assumes a tolerance for ambiguity'.

People in a facilitative interaction need to be flexible, to see more than one way of achieving resolution, to think of alternatives, and to be able to deal with uncertainty if clients' autonomy is to be enhanced and the nurse's control of the situation is to be limited. Without a tolerance for lack of closure, people will be fearful and want to regain control. Then the interaction becomes rigid and people pull against each other rather than working cooperatively.

Throughout this process one of the prime external requirements for facilitating self-care is the increased provision of diverse resources. Therefore the fifth core proposition states that 'facilitation encourages identification and use of resources' either mechanical or human. When the widest range of resources is available to the client, facilitation demystifies the system. It is of no use that the nurse knows all the health care resources that are available if clients remain ignorant or if the resources are not accessible to them and clients feel they are of little value to them. Resources may be costly in time, effort or money and these and other parameters need to be accounted for when making decisions with the client.

People require adequate knowledge and skill to deal with their situation or condition. In assisting clients to a position of knowledge and power, the sixth core proposition states that 'facilitation requires negotiation of a contract'. That can be as simple as asking a client a question rather than making a statement or demand, or it can be quite formal. It can be verbal or written where the roles and functions of each person are discussed and understood; and where the direction of the interaction is determined to the satisfaction of each person.

Where a client is involved in long term rehabilitation, or where people have a chronic illness, or some sort of permanent health breakdown or disability, negotiation can be very significant. If nurses want compliance and involvement then client input will be part of the process of identifying the stimuli for intervention and determining the strategies for care. Negotiation enhances identification of those legitimately involved in the interaction; involves setting priorities for care which are mutually acceptable; and provides regular feedback, evaluation, and modification of care.

For people to move this far and beyond in a facilitative interaction they need to feel safe. If people feel afraid they will withdraw. The seventh core proposition states that 'facilitation provides a mutually supportive environment'. Trust is very important. Acceptance of where people want to be and where they want to go enhances commitment to the process and increases their cooperation with others involved in the interaction. An environment which is mutually supportive again reinforces the role of all people in an interaction, and stresses that the client, friends, family as well as the health carers should provide support and care for all others. It further emphasizes the importance of balance in an interaction.

People need to be well informed about their care, and to complete the facilitative interaction the eighth core proposition states that 'facilitation enhances participative goal setting'. Every intervention or interaction ought to be as a result of some goal that has been set. At whatever level and with whatever formality, people have some notion of the outcome when they enter any sort of interaction, particularly if they are intending to use negotiation as part of care. Outcome goals may not be the same for everybody. Ideas which can be examined are those relating to creativity, lateral thinking, motivation, and involvement so that goals are compatible and achievable for all parties.

So from starting out with the ideas of balance between confrontation and support, all of the core propositions and their associated behaviours and attitudes add together to complete the linking megaconcept statement that 'facilitation enables self-care' for everyone and the interactive cycle begins again.

Self-care framework

Figure 6.2 shows the final product for the self-care framework.

The megaconcept. Self-care is the counterpart to facilitation and returns to the idea of balance and the megaconcept statement is that 'self-care is a balance between demands and capabilities'. The behaviours, thoughts and feelings that are being balanced in self-care begin with the demands which self-care places on the individual or group. It is important for independence that people possess the ability to implement activities of daily living and meet the demands of care situations on a daily basis. People need to be able to feed and clothe themselves, to work and play, to handle money, drive a car, to communicate with others, and so on—that is, to be self-caring.

When the demands and their capabilities are in equilibrium people behave as autonomous, independent beings requiring very little reference to others in order to make decisions and run their lives. But when the demands of self-care and the maintenance of equilibrium or homeostasis increase, people's capabilities may or may not cope with the task of returning them to their former state of well being.

In many instances when a minor health breakdown occurs, people's self-care capabilities are equal to the situation and so they take some aspirin for a headache or take a day off work and go to bed to recover from the flu. In these instances people can move through the elements and stages of self-care to resolution of the situation as their own facilitator of self-care.

In other situations when a significant health breakdown occurs, there is a deficit between the demands of that situation for a return to equilibrium and

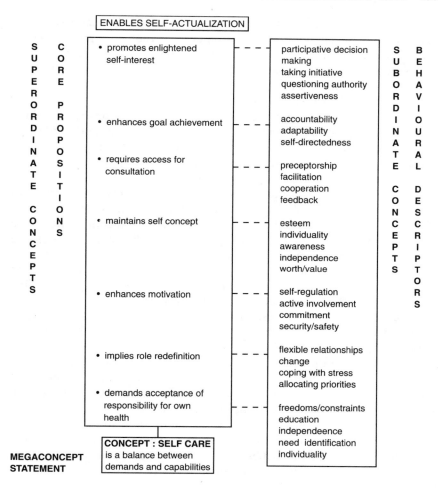

Fig. 6.2 Self-care framework.

people's self-care abilities, and they seek assistance to resolve the situation. They can still remain self-carers and be involved at whatever level and in whatever areas of daily living it is feasible for them to do so. In this instance the first self-caring act is the decision to seek help, to find the appropriate people to assist, and then to move with others through the elements expressed in the framework to situation improvement and restoration of well being.

Superordinate concepts. The first core proposition suggests that the initial element people need to accept is that 'self-care demands acceptance of responsibility for one's own health'. The word 'demands' is chosen carefully. Self-care cannot occur adequately, appropriately, or easily if people do not accept responsibility for their own health, be that psychological, emotional, social, physical, or any other dimension or domain of health that may be involved. This particularly applies to the nurse as carer because there seems to be some misconceived notion among nurses that if they spend a significant amount of time caring for themselves it constitutes neglect of their primary responsibility to the client.

People need to be cognisant of the freedoms and constraints which surround them; of areas where education may be needed; and of ideas of independence and dependence in acceptance of responsibility, which relate to safety and security. People will accept responsibility for their own well being at the level and to the degree possible for them at the time.

The second core proposition moves from health to the person and states that 'self-care implies role redefinition'. In this case the shift is from the traditional passive patient behaviours and the active controlling nurse behaviours to a more equitable shared position. Initially this may place some stress on all parties as they move into unfamiliar and possibly uncomfortable relationships. People who are to be self-carers and behave facilitatively need to be prepared to and capable of change. They should enter into flexible relationships with a range of health care workers, friends, family, and colleagues. When a self-care response is generated and the client is taking on an extended and involved role they are behaving facilitatively by tolerating ambiguity and exercising individual autonomy.

One of the most difficult of role realignments for the nurse to cope with is when the client becomes the teacher and is the one who knows more about their own condition and its treatment or care than the nurse. This is the case with many people who have chronic health breakdown problems or permanent disabilities. The nurse needs to be willing to listen and learn from the client so that normal routine is interrupted as little as possible and the continuation of self-care activities is maximized. This of course requires the negotiation of a contract and the identification and use of appropriate resources.

When the client does retain responsibility, is able to find room in which to negotiate, and defines a suitable role for themselves, then two more elements are added. The third core proposition suggests that 'self-care enhances motivation' and the fourth core proposition that 'self-care maintains self-concept'. When the client is empowered and care is tailored to suit their needs the real potential exists for active commitment to care.

One of the fundamentals for client involvement is security/safety. If the client does not feel safe—physically, intellectually, and/or emotionally—they will be reluctant to participate. They will not be prepared to take risks and to experiment with alternative approaches to care. They will retreat back to a previous safe position. A mutually supportive environment is crucial if the client is to feel safe with and trusting of others who are co-carers. In a very real sense this comes right back to the original self-care megaconcept statement, which is the search for balance between demands and capabilities through self-regulation and active involvement.

When that feeling of safety is present and everyone is involved and active in care then their feeling of worth and value are enhanced. Any care strategy which increases autonomy, confidence, and compliance within care includes behaviours which increase self-esteem, individuality, awareness, and self-worth. These elements are particularly critical when the client is in an unfamiliar environment such as a hospital, or when the health breakdown problem is new and the client is in the novice learner situation.

In the majority of instances the client will be in a novel situation which is strange and potentially threatening and the fifth core proposition states that 'self-care requires access for consultation'. While the role of facilitator and/ or expert may move between people in an interaction, it is generally accepted that in the initial stages of improving a client's health breakdown situation the health carer will have the greater knowledge and skills. The behaviours which are important in this area include cooperation, communication, a willingness to learn, the selection and acceptance of new knowledge and skills, the perception of needs, the provision of regular feedback, nonjudgemental values, and an open and sharing attitude. However, if these are not shared with the client right from the beginning of an interaction the client will not be enabled to establish self-care.

If clients are continually being told, 'No, that's wrong, that's not the way to do it'; if they feel they are being hurried or made to feel a nuisance; or are constantly reminded how busy everyone is, they will retreat to the familiar passive, compliant behaviour of 'you do it for me because you're so much better at it than I am'.

What the client needs is access not dominance—access to knowledge, time, tolerance, encouragement, patience, expertise, a sympathetic ear, or perhaps just a smile. Self-care is difficult without the facilitative behaviours which go with it. Nurses need to examine their behaviours and attitudes, to change focus from care giving which requires only minimal communication and cooperation to care facilitation which maximizes perception, creativity, involvement, and sharing. Co-caring and teamwork are important for efficient resource use.

When all earlier propositions are accepted the sixth core proposition follows logically and states that 'self-care enhances goal achievement'. It is important for a self-carer to have goals and to determine the criteria by which they can be met. So often goals are set which are very broad, too far away, or at too high a level, and so the chances of achieving them are reduced. Facilitators need to be sufficiently aware of reality and the client's expressed needs so that appropriate goals can be negotiated.

Along with the goals, the criteria should be specified so that everyone moves along the same track providing maximum support. Criteria should be determined at the beginning of an interaction; be available to everyone; and provide a means by which the success of the interaction can be evaluated and subsequent interactions or behaviours modified, altered, added, or deleted. This increases the level of accountability to all co-carers. What is done is very visible to all and people are more likely to clarify and validate what they are doing and in the process refine and enhance their approach.

The final core proposition which encompasses all preceding ones is that 'self-care promotes enlightened self-interest'. Self-interest is not selfishness, particularly if the concept of enlightenment is included. This is a rather mystical term. The path to enlightenment requires the person to look inwards and reflect, in order to eliminate self centredness and selfishness; to enable the person to grow; to assist them to focus on others and to help others. Enlightenment implies openness, generosity, purity, tolerance, kindness and a spirit of community.

To be interested in self certainly involves in part looking after one's own interests. It might mean that people have to question what is happening. They might have to be assertive to get answers, and they may need to take the initiative. But self-care behaviours enable people to do these things in a way that is positive and beneficial for everyone in the interaction and brings the process right round to the initial facilitation megaconcept statement that facilitation is a balance between confrontation and support, perhaps now seen in a different context.

It has been shown that the frameworks are in principle interconnected and mutually inclusive, and when both frameworks are put together and seen as a whole the ultimate megaconcept statement that we can make is that 'self-care enables self-actualization' (Maslow 1962). Everyone is enabled to reach toward their full human potential.

Analysis of student processes and outcomes

Along with the decision to explore facilitation and self-care via the development of appropriate frameworks came the requirement to impose certain teaching/learning strategies and behaviours on both the tutor and the students. This involved the modelling of facilitative behaviours by the tutor and the use of self-directed behaviours by the students, with each party needing to come to terms with 'letting go', its meaning and consequences, rewards and constraints, in preparation for students applying facilitative/self-care behaviours in the clinical nursing setting.

Facilitation framework

In brief, the exploration of and reflection on our own behaviours in the classroom and the development of the phrase clusters promoted the elucidation of the megaconcept statement. The initial idea was expressed that facilitation is dynamic within the health continuum and falls between given care and self-care. Facilitation as a balance between confrontation and support is nonspecific to person and place until applied in the required context and so may be used to analyze and evaluate the process and outcomes in the classroom as well as clinical nursing settings.

Student processes and outcomes. Initially students found it difficult to accept the term 'confrontation' with its connotations of them against us, of exploitation and of accusation. After considerable discussion it was accepted as a term simply meaning coming face to face with, coming to terms with, being opposite and challenging, with the reservation that it should not be seen to isolate any of the parties to the interaction.

It was emphasized through the tutor's modelling that with beginners confrontation should be minimized, with support being the major tool, but that as students became more competent and confident with the process and their own abilities the level of confrontation could be lifted. This was also the case when students transferred these behaviours into the clinical nursing context. However students also agreed that it was not necessarily a case of tutor verses students, but that much of the confronting occurs between individual students or subgroups of students with the tutor acting as the support.

'Letting go' of preconceived ideas was the first challenge to student perceptions of appropriate intervention behaviours based on facilitation. 'Letting go' was a difficult idea for students to become comfortable with initially. They had considerable difficulty reconciling such deeply held beliefs as accountability, advocacy, maintaining acceptable professional standards, ethical, legal and moral duties, and expert carer with 'letting go'. They suggested that clients would see them as lacking confidence, authority, cohesion, skill, credibility, respect, and so on.

It required a deal of discussion to clarify that 'letting go' did not mean abandoning all responsibility in a situation, or becoming totally non-directive or letting anarchy rule. It did require them to discover new ways of expressing these beliefs, and of adopting alternative behaviours which enabled all parties equal opportunity to share in these responsibilities. Without this sharing the concept of self-care is largely negated. As the concepts of facilitation and self-care are mutually inclusive it was essential to persist until students were able to find an acceptable letting go position that in itself constituted a balance.

One of the strengths of the facilitative approach and its conceptualization through the framework is that individuals can maintain different though compatible letting go positions as a prelude to adopting facilitation as their principal approach to care. Professional skills, beliefs, and behaviours can actually be enhanced by a process of adapting and incorporating them into a different cognitive structure embodied in facilitation.

With the core propositions students had two components with which to come to terms; the implications and consequences contained within each propositional statement, and the imperatives of the action verb enabling operationalization of the proposition. Terms such as demands, implies, de-emphasizes, requires, assumes, provides, enhances, and encourages, obliged students to incorporate some precision in their interpretation of the proposition and their elaboration of the subordinate concepts. Three particular core propositions generated most concern.

The first was that 'facilitation requires awareness of liberating structures'. 'What is a liberating structure?', they asked. It implies that there is openess, a breaking of traditional barriers, flexibility, receptiveness, and a willingness to explore and embrace alternatives which may not be conventional.

The second was that 'facilitation de-emphasizes unilateral control'. Many of the problems expressed by the students were similiar to those suggested in 'letting go'. The idea of limiting their own level of power and dominance generated great discomfort and resistance. Ultimately, students worked their way back to the idea of a dynamic continuum. It was not the degree of control exercised by any party that was necessarily of paramount importance but the opportunity for all parties to share control in an appropriate way. The means to determine that level of appropriateness was through 'negotiation of a contract' and 'participative goal setting'.One of the educational and clinical difficulties faced in developing the frameworks was that of necessity—the propositions were largely developed and elaborated one at a time and it was not until they were all in place that the interconnectedness could be seen.

The third was that 'facilitation assumes tolerance for ambiguity'. This created real dilemmas for the students. They could not see the relevance to nursing practice. Students verbalized two deep seated issues which were causing them most concern and which were explored through modelling and role playing. The two issues were the need to abandon long held preconceived ideas and the need to release deep seated inhibitions. This naturally generated fears which related to failure, loss of professional role and dignity, potential for ridicule, and possible loss of self-esteem. Ambiguity is created because the client is setting goals and making decisions, and their desires and responses are unknown and therefore problematic.

The breakthrough to acceptance of this proposition came when students perceived and internalized the idea that involving the client, far from detracting from their role and prestige, actually enhanced it. A dimension was added to their own thinking and behaviour which made the process of client care more satisfying; created a greater number of positive outcomes for both parties; and increased the satisfaction level of each outcome. It reduced the total nursing time required for a given interaction because of the self-care component. The challenge of the unknown became quite exciting as students' confidence in their performance as facilitators grew.

In relation to the subordinate concepts, the skill which students identified as requiring most work and improvement was communication. Negotiating a contract, providing a supportive environment, being involved in participative decision-making and goal setting, demystifying the process, and so on involved a great deal more verbal communication with the client, significant others, and colleagues. This happened on several levels and internal enquiry makes it far more likely that they will identify the real needs of the client and the demands and constraints related to the context and environment. It enables students to perceive the universality of concepts and ideas which encourages them to adapt their behaviours to multiple situations.

Self-care framework

The self-care framework discussed is the partner of the facilitation framework. The concepts were first explored as they related to self-directedness in students by continued examination of our own behaviours and reactions to the classroom situation. As we progressed the concepts were related to the clinical practice area.

Student processes and outcomes. Self-care was explored in three dimensions which related to clients, colleagues, and self. Initially students related most easily with self-care applying to clients/patients. They identified many situations and health breakdown areas where through judicious interventions clients can become independent in care. When it came to colleagues they learned that each area carries its own stresses expressed in different ways and there is the need to be mutually supportive in a community of caring. The dimension in which they were least able to identify the need for self-care or to see how it could work was in relation to themselves. Students perceived a conflict between their role as a facilitator and that of a self-carer. However, self-care can be applied to self and others where others may be colleagues, clients, family, and friends.

Students used the key words to identify the megaconcept statement of self-care as a balance between demands and capabilities, incorporating the knowledge, skills, and beliefs which can be brought to bear in order to fulfill felt needs.

People can be and are self-carers to the best of their abilities and within the constraints of the demands such care places upon them. The notion of the dependence-independence continuum was explored using students' own behaviours which swung back and forth, and then transferring the ideas to the client or others. This allowed students to explore the values and beliefs they were imposing on the framework.

In the elaboration of the superordinate concepts students had difficulty with a couple of the core propositions. The area of most difficulty was with the statement that 'self-care promotes enlightened self-interest'. The immediate reaction of students to this phrase was the idea of selfishness, looking out for number one, egocentricity. Students were enabled to come to terms with this statement through a philosophical or mystical level exploration of enlightenment. This acceptance was furthered as subordinate concepts for this proposition were described in terms such as assertiveness, taking the initiative, questioning authority, being autonomous, participating. In the end students did decide that an element of self-centredness is appropriate if the individual is to be a self-carer in today's health care system.

Mutual interactiveness of concepts among the frameworks

At the beginning students were reluctant to adopt the idea that self-care almost invariably required the intervention of another party at some level and in some way. This issue was largely resolved as students elaborated the prerequisites for self-care in their word lists. In answering such questions as: from where or whom is knowledge acquired, how are coping strategies identified and operationalized, and how are the necessary skills developed, students again came to the notion of partnership and of the mutuality of facilitative/self-care interactions.

In fact in response to these questions students started using facilitative language and behaviours in their classroom group debates without realizing it. Responses were recorded and on completion of each discussion students were urged to look at their facilitation flowcharts and were startled to see the consistency between their responses and the superordinate and subordinate concepts expressed in the framework.

Students explored much of the literature to determine whether one concept could be discovered within, or be inferred from, a discussion of the other. They discovered that invariably the literature uses both terms together although only one may be explained and analyzed, and that it seemed accepted by most authors that the two concepts belong together.

Ultimately students began to see that facilitation is more than a set of behaviours, no matter how conceptually expressed the term may be. Facilitation in its most universal conceptualization is a process of knowing and a state of being. That is, any interaction may be approached facilitatively whether it is in teaching/learning, in nursing, in any other profession or occupation, or simply on a social or family occasion. Exploration revealed that the action verbs were the key to the whole concept. Students had resisted embracing the frameworks wholeheartedly because they were apprehensive that if they adopted them they would be caused to behave that way, and they perceived situations in which they would wish to behave more directively or exert greater control, for example under emergency conditions. The exploration and definition of the action verbs enabled them to see that they were not all or nothing, that they did not prescribe actions, that they only suggested.

Students were not being asked to abandon their previous behaviour or coping mechanisms either as learners or practitioners. What was suggested was that another major role and other behaviours were being added to their repertoire. The scholarly literature and the popular media and press were making it obvious that some change was required. It is believed that the concepts of facilitation and self-care answer the criticisms and requirements that are emerging within the community.

CONCLUSION

Demand for participation by the client arises from a view that traditional professional services are too expensive or unproductive. Hospitals with their high technology approach and chronic understaffing can deal only with the worst and most acute health breakdown problems. The majority of the community is often left to its own devices with either minimal or inappropriate professional health care services because health carers have been reluctant to let go and genuinely include the client.

Nursing is in a process of role redefinition, widening of its functional base, and re-evaluating its attitudes in response to consumer demand. It would seem from the preceding study that the hitherto dominant nursing role of care giver is becoming less appropriate; the attitude of care controller less palatable; the maintenance of hidden knowledge less acceptable. If nurses are to remain a central, significant and relevant group in relation to the health maintenance and restoration needs of the individual, group, or their community a major philosophical and behavioural re-orientation is required. In part, to retain relevance nurses need to acquire new ways of thinking about their roles and functions as a basis for interactive nursing intervention. The role of facilitator leading to a self-care response is the one of choice. For students, the process of coming to terms with a new method of practice was simplified and clarified by the development and use of an interactive conceptual framework with a common set of behaviours allowing for operationalization in any setting.

In determining whether the initial probability statement was supported, the original concept was reviewed. This was, that a framework as a simplified representation of reality and as the distilled essence of a complex situation enables participants to make sense of their behaviour and that of others in an interaction. In this case the interactive frameworks of facilitation and self-care enabled students to make sense of their nursing intervention in a logical, cohesive and rational way.

In elaborating the frameworks, students did make a philosophical shift. They were able to perceive the value of incorporating facilitation/self-care concepts and behaviours into their learning and practice. They did demonstrate changed behaviours in the classroom and in the clinical nursing setting using a single set of conceptual propositions. The probability statement was supported. A facilitative approach does lead to self-direction/self-care and provides a real alternative as a method for intervention in the practice of nursing.

REFERENCES

Barrows H S, Tamblyn R M 1980 Problem-based learning: an approach to medical education. Springer, New York
Boud D (ed) 1985 Problem-based learning in education for the professions. HERDSA, Sydney
Boud D 1986 Facilitating learning in continuing education: some important sources. Studies in Higher Education 11(3):237-243
Boud D, Keogh R, Walker D 1985 Reflection: turning experience into learning. Kogan Page, London
Brookfield S D 1986 Understanding and facilitating adult learning. Jossey Bass, San Francisco
Englert J 1984 Self-care in sickness. Unpublished paper
Hall B 1981 Participatory research, popular knowledge and power: a personal reflection. Convergence XIV(3):6-17
Iwasiw C L 1987 The role of the teacher in self-directed learning. Nurse Education Today 7:222-227
Kappeli S 1986 Nurses' management of patients' self-care. Nursing Times 82(11):40-49
Kaufman A 1985 Implementing problem-based medical education. Springer, New York
Knowles M 1975 Self-directed learning: a guide for learners and teachers. Follet, Chicago
Little P J 1986 Problem-based learning. A staff-development leave report on problem-based learning in nursing and medical programmes in the U.S.A. Canada and New Zealand. Macarthur Institute of Higher Education, Sydney
Little P J, Ryan G 1988 Educational change through problem-based learning: a new role for the student and the nurse educator. The Australian Journal of Advanced Nursing 5(4):31-35
Maslow A H 1962 Toward a psychology of being. D Van Nostrand, New York
Mezirow J 1981 A critical theory of adult learning and education. Adult Education 32(1):9-24
Neufeld A, Hobbs H 1985 Self-care in a high-rise for seniors. Nursing Outlook 33(6):298-301
Percy K, Ramsden P 1980 Independent study: two examples from English higher education. Society for Research into Higher Education, Guildford
Rogers C R 1967 The facilitation of significant learning. In: Siegel L (ed) Instruction: some contemporary viewpoints. Chandler, San Francisco
Schon D 1983 The reflective practitioner. Basic Books, New York
Slaytor K 1987 Negotiating diabetes management. The Australian Nurses Journal 17(5):47-49
Tandon R 1981 The interlinkages between primary health care and adult education. Convergence XV(2):9-19
Taylor M 1986 Learning for self-direction in the classroom: the pattern of a transition process. Studies in Higher Education 11(1):55-72
Wright A R 1970 Participative education and the inevitable revolution. Journal of Creative Behaviour 4(4):234-282

7. The relationship between theory and practice in the educative process

Elizabeth Davies

Modern nursing has been plagued by a perceived disjuncture or disalignment between nursing service and nursing education (Walker & Norby 1987–88). Nursing service, or the delivery of nursing care, what nurses do, has been seen as far removed from nursing education, what nurses learn. Chinn (1988) identifies this as the education/practice gap and describes the distressing sense of 'other worldness' experienced by those nurses who must function in both education and service as they 'pass back and forth from one world to another'. A major impetus behind the desire to transfer preregistration nurse education from hospitals to the tertiary sector has been the anticipated improvement in the relationship between theory and practice.

Nurses are now striving to understand why the problem has arisen and how it is perpetuated, and to determine its possible implications for nursing service and nursing education. An examination of the literature reveals a number of possible explanations for the problem and related strategies for its solution. Nurse authors have approached the problem from perspectives which can be categorized as:

1. philosophical
2. conceptual
3. systemic
4. cultural.

A philosophical approach to the problem is taken by Walker & Norby (1987–88) who see the disalignment between nursing service and nursing education as logical and inevitable given the different philosophical base for each activity. Figure 7.1 on page 150 illustrates the differences seen to exist by these authors as a consequence of philosophical divisiveness.

It is further contended that this disalignment has contributed to problems in adjustment for new graduates as they make the transition from student to service provider. Practising clinicians, when discussing the transfer of nurse education to the tertiary sector often express concern regarding the new graduate's likely ability to be able to manage time effectively, to achieve clinical objectives in less than ideal conditions, and to be cognizant of institutional policies and procedures. This would seem to indicate that many clinicians do take a utilitarian approach and, in fact, may have little choice

	SERVICE based on UTILITARIANISM	EDUCATION based on HUMANITARIANISM
PURPOSE	Providing a health care service	Generating and imparting knowledge
FOCUS	Task achievement Task specialization Greatest good for greatest number	Freedom Individual needs Fair opportunity for each
ORIENTATION	Outcome	Process
NURSING METAPHOR	Fight against disease	Patient advocate
NURSING SCIENCE	Provision of solutions to real world problems	Debate and ambiguity concerning problem definition and resolution

Fig. 7.1 Disalignment between nursing service and nursing education.

but to do so. In attempting to find a possible solution to the problem Walker & Norby (1987–88) can only suggest that each sector engage in 'open and consistent dialogue' as they strive for maximum flexibility and creative resolution of problems.

This approach to the problem represents a much broader perspective than that taken by Wong (1979). This author takes a conceptual approach and suggests that the disparity between theory and practice in nursing results because of a learning problem experienced by students who are unable to transfer classroom learning to the clinical situation. This is seen to result in inflexibility in and frustration with clinical practice for students who view classroom instruction as 'right' and hospital practice as 'wrong'. The problem is examined only from the educational perspective. Responsibility for the development of the problem is seen to belong to nurse educators who must also accept responsibility for the solution. Such a solution, it is suggested, involves the making of necessary alterations to curriculum design and the teaching process to facilitate the transfer of learning.

This theme is carried further by other authors. Lewis (1988), a clinician, contends that, '...while nurse tutors teach theory, nurse practitioners go on nursing in the same way that they have always done. There appears to be a chasm dividing theory and practice'. While acknowledging that theoretically based nursing models can provide useful frameworks for nursing care, Lewis emphasizes that any selected framework must work in practice. Much reticence to use these frameworks results from their extensive use of jargon and diagramatic conceptualization. In describing the use of the Roy Adaptation Model in an acute surgical ward he emphasized that the '...main effort needed to be the interpretation of jargon into everyday nursing language'.

Chinn (1988), a nurse theorist, also refers to this perceived conceptual difference. She refers to the 'too hard/too easy' paradox described by Bunch (1987) which results in the assumption by many nurses '...that theory must be esoteric and far removed from daily life, if it is to be properly called theory. It must be too hard for most people to understand if it is to be taken seriously in the academic community'. The 'too easy' side of the paradox is the desire to be able to easily interpret and apply theory in a useful way. Chinn decries the disparity between knowing and doing for nurses and pleads with them to '...no longer accept the notion that we are doomed to experience fundamental gaps between what we know and what we do'. She suggests that if nurses are ever going to be able to achieve unity between their knowing and doing they must increase their conviction that this can be achieved and begin to take responsibility to heal the theory–practice split.

Systemic, or practice setting, factors can also have an influence on the way nurses perceive the relationship between theory and practice. The need for nurses to act in an appropriate manner in life threatening situations has had a major influence on nurse education, according to Bottorff & D'Cruz (1985). Even though, in most settings, these situations are rare in comparison with other nurse patient interactions, they receive major emphasis in education programs because of their grave implications. Similarly Chinn (1988) expounds that nurses would be better able to serve society if they were able to focus more on the promotion and maintenance of health. This ideal has already had an influence on the development and teaching of nursing theory. Yet, as Chinn states, nurses '...practice in an illness care system, not a health care system'. This disparity between health and illness, theory and practice, is referred to by Lewis (1988) when describing an attempt to implement a nursing model in practice. The model placed emphasis on the activities of living of the individual yet failed to include patho-physiology and the disease condition. This was seen to be incongruent with the real situation where '...the emphasis was on those situations of unstable physiology which presented threat to life'.

There is also a theme which suggests that cultural aspects of education have an effect on the relationship between theory and practice. Traditionally nurse education programs have devoted much less time to theory than to practice. At the same time there has been little or no attention given to reflecting on practice. It is suggested that this mode of teaching has a powerful socializing influence on students who come to believe that knowing why is not as important as knowing how (Bottorff & D'Cruz 1985). These authors call for an educational framework which acknowledges the context within which nursing occurs. Education, within western industrialized society, is seen by Miller (1989) to value masculine characteristics of rationality and objectivity rather than feminine characteristics of emotionality and intuition. Miller contends that this value system has had a major impact on the way nurse education programs are conducted. Emphasis is placed on scientific, linear, reductionist ways of thinking which cannot explain what happens in the practice of holistic nursing. She suggests that the recognition and inclusion of intuitive knowing in educational programs will increase their relevance and reduce the disalignment between theory and practice.

From these broad perspectives on the relationships between theory and practice in nursing, it is possible to move to a more detailed analysis of the situation. This can be undertaken from the perspectives of:

1. The balance between theory and practice
2. The nature of the theoretical component of courses
3. The correlation between theory and practice.

BALANCE BETWEEN THEORY AND PRACTICE

The amount of time allocated to theoretical instruction can be seen as an indication of the value placed on this component of nurse education. While there are variations across states, the Queensland example (Fig. 7.2) will serve to illustrate changes that have occurred over time. From 1928 to 1980, hours were mandated by legislation. The 1990 hours represent the average number of hours that have been allocated to theoretical instruction in tertiary programs. An examination of the proportion of theoretical hours to practice hours in Queensland courses may also assist in demonstrating the relationship between theory and practice (Fig. 7.3 on page 154). Average course length has been used in calcualtions, but it should be noted that there was some degree of variability in the length of courses in different hospitals up until 1970.

Course length variability could also be seen as indicative of the greater value placed on practice in comparison with theory. The length of the course to be undertaken was determined by the number of beds in the training hospital. In Queensland,from 1928 to 1965 the course length was 4 years in hospitals with more than 20 beds and 5 years in hospitals with less than 20 beds. In 1965 course lengths were set at 3 years for more than 40 beds, 4 years for between 20 and 40 beds and 5 years for between 10 and 20 beds. By 1970 all courses were of 3 years duration. This approach would seem to be based on the premise that the greater variety of cases available in larger

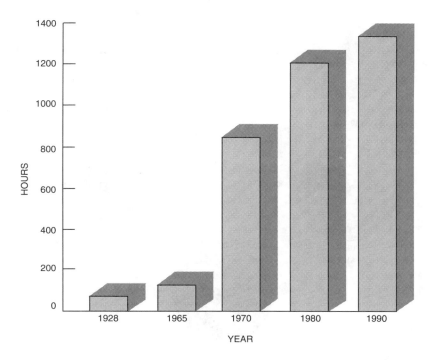

Fig. 7.2 Time allocated to theoretical instruction.

hospitals would enhance the on the job experience of the students and thereby prepare them more quickly for their role as registered nurses (Trembath & Hellier 1987). It should be noted that in the 1990 example, while course length is 3 years, the total time allocation is considerably reduced because of the change from hospital to tertiary based courses. Because of this, while the balance between theory and practice is more even, the time allocated to clinical practice diminishes markedly. Changes in the balance between theory and practice have been enormous. Theory has increased from a mere 1% in 1928 to almost 50% in 1990. This is indicative of the increasing value placed on theory and the recognition that safe, competent practice must be based on firm theoretical foundations.

THEORETICAL COMPONENT

The nature of the theory taught to students has also expanded considerably over time. This would indicate a responsiveness to changes in the nursing role by improving the relevance of theory to practice and the influence of

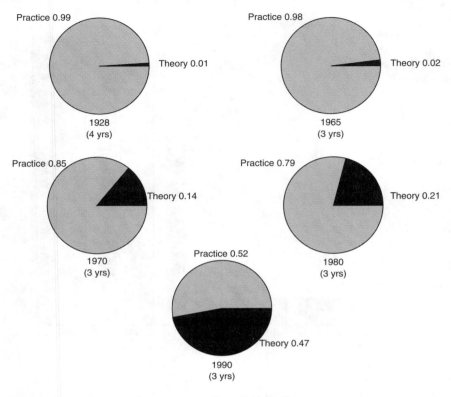

Fig. 7.3 Proportion of theoretical instruction to clinical practice.

particular philosophical underpinnings. The following Queensland examples illustrate changes in the nature and breadth of theoretical offerings.

Table 7.1 Curriculum content 1928

Topic	Hours
Medical nursing	12
Surgical nursing	12
Anatomy and physiology	12
Nutrition/hygiene	19
Practical demonstrations	6
Invalid cookery	9
TOTAL HOURS	70

Preparation based on the content outlined in Table 7.1 enabled the nurse to function in a role largely dependent on the medical officer and relied heavily upon on-the-job training. The influence of romanticism is evidenced by the emphasis on medical function and the inclusion of nutrition, cookery, and hygiene; traditional female nurturing functions.

Table 7.2 Curriculum content 1965

Topic	Hours
Principles and practice of elementary nursing	15
Anatomy and physiology	16
Medicine and medical nursing	24
Nutrition/hygiene	18
Principles and practice of advanced nursing	12
Surgery and surgical nursing	24
Elementary psychiatry	6
Matron's lectures	10
(Presented after final exams and including:	
History of nursing	
Hospital administration/finance	
Law	
Social services	
Maternal and child health	
School health)	
TOTAL HOURS	125

The approach represented in Table 7.2 showed little change in role perception. The disease orientation in such programs and the minimal focus on psychological, social, and spiritual needs reflect pragmatic philosophical underpinnings.

Some advance is apparent in the curriculum content shown in Table 7.3 on page 156. There is evidence of increasing emphasis on the psychological and social needs of patients and their developmental stage in these programs. This represents the beginning influence of humanistic philosophy. The inclusion of various medical and surgical specialties such as orthopaedics, surgery, and anaesthesia is indicative of the increasingly technical nature of nursing function as a support for the medical officer. This indicates that pragmatism was still influential and that the major nursing role, if not entirely dependent, was certainly interdependently related to that of the doctor.

By 1980 the prescriptive approach was no longer taken. Instead of listing mandatory content and hours for the revised 1200 hour nursing courses the following objectives and guidelines for content were provided (Nursing Studies Regulations 1980). The objectives of the revised general nursing course conducted by an accredited school of nursing shall be to enable the student to:

1. Attain those professional and personal attributes which are essential for the development of nursing competence
2. Gain a knowledge of the sciences upon which nursing is based in order that safe nursing may be provided within the context of total patient care
3. Determine the nursing needs of patients; formulate plans of nursing care to meet these needs; implement these nursing care plans and evaluate their effectiveness

Table 7.3 Curriculum content 1970

Topic	Hours
Nursing introduction, history of nursing, trends in nursing, ethics	12
Ward administration and law	22
Psychology	25
Social and preventive medicine	42
Pharmacology for nurses	41
Biology, anatomy and physiology	80
Nutrition and diet therapy	20
Microbiology for nurses	16
Chemistry for nurses	12
Physics for nurses	12
Paediatrics and the adolescent	25
Principles of geriatrics and geriatric nursing	10
Maternity nursing	25
Principles of psychiatry and psychiatric nursing	15
General nursing arts (including first aid and bandaging and physiotherapy for nurses)	147
Medicine, pathology and medical nursing	77
Surgery, anaesthesia, applied anatomy and surgical nursing	77
Principles of theatre technique, operative procedures and instruments	20
Orthopaedics and orthopaedic nursing	15
Gynaecology and gynaecological nursing	15
Urinary diseases and nursing	15
ENT and ENT nursing	15
Ophthalmology and nursing	10
Cardiac surgery, vascular surgery, transplantation	10
Clinical demonstrations, seminars and other educational activities	82
TOTAL HOURS	**840**

4. Assume an active role in the prevention of disease and the maintenance of health
5. Teach staff members under her control
6. Assume responsibility for further professional development.

These programs represented substantial changes in relation to philosophical, theoretical, and functional aspects of nursing. The humanistic influence is illustrated by the emphasis on meeting individual needs in a holistic manner and extending beyond the patient to the family and community. Nursing theory is not seen as a unique entity. Rather, there is emphasis on the application of theoretical concepts from related disciplines such as the biological, physical, and behavioural sciences. There is an emergence of the independent role of the nurse in assessment of needs and planning of care, in health promotion through health teaching and counselling and in self-responsibility for continuing professional development.

From 1990, with the expansion of tertiary courses in Queensland, each institution has developed and will implement their own unique courses. An analysis of these new curricula indicates that the theoretical component can be generalized into the areas of basic science and formal models for its application. These foundations are seen to be essential to prepare the graduate for practice (Fig. 7.4).

Such programs further extend the humanistic approach by the integration of content, emphasis on the individual needs of clients, and the expansion of practice settings beyond the acute care hospital. Nursing theory is recognized as separate from other related theoretical concepts. Not all programs carry nursing theory through to application in practice but each acknowledges developments in this area through nursing research. There is increasing emphasis on the independent role of the nurse through the use of the problem solving approach and the models required for health teaching, counselling, advocacy, and research.

These examples serve to illustrate that the nature of the theoretical content in nurse education programs has changed over time. The major philosophical influences have moved from romanticism and pragmatism towards humanistic existentialism. The development of theory in nursing is beginning to exert an influence and the nursing role is evolving in diversity and complexity.

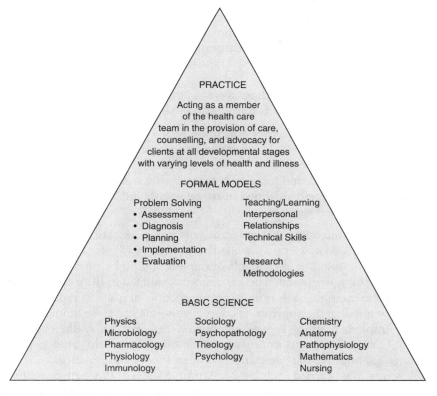

Fig. 7.4 Theoretical foundations in tertiary nurse education.

CORRELATION BETWEEN THEORY AND PRACTICE

Retrospectively, it is difficult to establish whether student nurses were given appropriate theoretical instruction before having to deal with particular situations. However, the Sax Report (1978) cites two major investigations which suggest that, in the past, correlation between theory and practice was poor. The Kelly Report of 1943 stated that, 'The nurses' practical training is not organized at present, instruction given in many cases being casual and uncorrelated, with the result that the education of the nurse is often sacrificed to the requirements of the hospital'. It appears that little change occurred in the next twenty years as it was reported by the Institute of Hospital Matrons of New South Wales in 1967 that '...emphasis has been placed during training on nursing procedures in order to prepare a nurse as quickly as possible for ward duties without providing the necessary correlated theoretical instruction'.

The general poverty and neglect of nurse education was also acknowledged by Bennett & Wallace (1978). In the pseudo apprenticeship system characteristic of hospital based programs, they proposed that academic planning was poor because it was carried out by nurses who had limited contact with the academic community. These nurses, therefore, continued to perpetuate the system from which they themselves had emerged. In addition, it was seen that efforts to improve programs were further hampered by a shortage of qualified nurse educators, high ratios of student nurses to nurse educators, and a very low standard of physical facilities such as libraries and laboratories.

These previously cited findings were supported by the final report of the Sax Committee (1978) which summarized major problems as:

1. Priority of service needs over education needs
2. Varying degrees of lack of correlation between classroom and clinical teaching
3. Inadequate preparation for service tasks during training
4. Lack of appropriately qualified nurse educators, inadequate library and other educational services.

As well as recommending that the transfer of nurse education to the tertiary sector continue, on a strictly controlled basis, Sax (1978) also recommended that existing hospital based schools of nursing should be rationalized and, where necessary, upgraded. This recommendation led to the establishment and implementation of statutory requirements for the accreditation of schools of nursing, the approval of course proposals and close monitoring of course implementation. It was anticipated that the provision of better educational facilities and improved course offerings would, among other advantages, improve the correlation between theory and practice.

A study was carried out by McArthur et al in 1983 to provide a comparative evaluation of students and graduates from college and hospital based basic nursing programs. When asked to specify aspects of their course which they felt had prepared them to work as graduate nurses, college graduates identified most frequently the patient centred course approach and the theoretical content of the course. Hospital graduates, however, most frequently identified general patient care skills. College graduates felt that theory created a greater awareness of their patients' conditions, resulted in an ability to cope with situations and enhanced understanding. Hospital graduates mentioned lack of integration as the most frequent negative aspect of their courses. They complained that lectures were often not coordinated, that the courses seemed disorganized and that, at times, they did not have the knowledge necessary to understand their practice.

A survey was conducted by Reaby (1985) to explore the attitudes of nurses in the Australian Capital Territory to nurse education. The majority of respondents ,who were either student nurses under 25 years of age or had never attended a tertiary institution believed that the apprenticeship system, characteristic of hospital based programs, adequately integrated theory and practice. However, the majority of respondents who were either nurse educators, administrators, over 25 years of age, or undertaking post graduate studies did not believe that the apprenticeship system could integrate nursing theory with nursing practice.

Figure 7.5 represents a conceptualization of the relationship between theory and practice in such training systems. The theoretical input is minimal in comparison with the practice component and only intermittent and somewhat tenuous links can be seen to exist between the two.

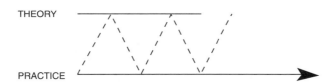

Fig. 7.5 Relationship between theory and practice in apprenticeship models of nurse education.

The major reasons for such a situation are summarized by Lublin (1985) as follows:

1. In hospital based training it is often impossible to coordinate theory and practice as students must be available to provide service within the institution
2. Less supervision is available for students
3. Hospital based students work within bureaucratic institutions which expect unquestioning acceptance of authority
4. Analytical decision making skills are not developed as there is always someone more senior available to make decisions

5. Hospital-based training is more likely to emphasize the disease process and procedural nursing rather than the psychosocial and health promotional aspects of care.

Over emphasis has been placed on the practical component of courses, the content of courses has been slow to respond to the changing focus of the nursing role and there has been an intractable problem in the planning and sequencing of clinical experience to ensure that students are theoretically prepared for the particular practice demands of the placement. In addition, institutional factors such as poor physical learning resources, inadequately prepared nurse educators, lack of clinical teaching and the intellectually stifling bureaucratic milieu have militated against an integrated relationship between theory and practice. Because of these inherent problems the strong professional move to completely alter the system for preparing nurses for practice emerged. Lublin (1985) articulated the belief of nursing's professional leaders when she concluded that tertiary education which '...is said to be based on respect for intellectual enquiry and to encourage independence and the cultivation of critical and analytical skills' would be much more effective in preparing nurses to deal with the increasing diversity and complexity of their roles.

This contention is now widely held within the nursing profession in Australia. The three national nursing organizations, the Australian Nursing Federation, the Royal College of Nursing, Australia, and the Florence Nightingale Committee, Australia, formulated policy statements that, as early as 1976, supported the transfer of basic nurse education to the tertiary sector. They have all actively lobbied to influence government decision making in this area and each supported the Commonwealth decision in August 1984 to effect the transfer over the ensuing decade. This move towards a transition in nurse education, has been based on the desire to underpin nursing practice with a firm theoretical foundation, to ensure appropriate correlation between theory and practice, and to achieve recognition and professional status. However, in its quest for these worthwhile ideals, nursing must guard against adopting a technical rational approach to professional education.

This phenomenon is seen by Schön (1987) to be based on the idea '...that practical competence becomes professional when its instrumental problem solving is grounded in systematic, preferably scientific knowledge'. The view that such an outcome would be desirable for nursing and that it could be achieved through tertiary education was expressed by Parkes (1984) when comparing hospital and college based courses of nurse education. Parkes stated that the college graduate '...practices from a theoretical base which provides reasons for selected aspects of nursing care seen to be appropriate and adequate for specific nursing situations and problems'. She also saw the tertiary education process as one which emphasized critical analysis, problem solving, decision making, and values clarification. Parkes further contended that nursing practice must grow from a scientific basis otherwise nursing care would continue to be 'deficient in quality, based on ritual and routine'.

Similar beliefs were expressed by Engstrom (1984), Adam (1985), and Marriner (1986). These authors identified the need for nursing to have a scientifically based body of knowledge as a necessary guide to clinical practice. Kim (1987) was adamant that 'The greater the empirical validity of...a scientific theory, the more effective will be the actions which are planned and guided by them'. As well as providing the basis for clinical practice the acquisition of a scientifically based body of knowledge is also seen as a prerequisite for professional status. Schön (1987) indicates that '...the relative status of the various professions is largely correlated with the extent to which they are able to present themselves as rigorous practitioners of a service-based professional knowledge and embody in their schools a version of the normative professional curriculum'. In supporting the profesional need for scientific knowledge Marriner (1986) explains that nursing's power can be increased through the use of systematically developed theoretical models as they are more likely to be successful. Similarly Kim (1987) suggests that professional practice demands logical rigour and empirical validation.

Nurse education, like all professional education based on this model of technical rationality, operates according to a hierarchy of knowledge. Students are first presented with the relevant basic science. This is followed by applied science which equips students with formal models for application of scientific knowledge. Finally students are given a practicum in which they are expected to apply basic science through formal models to deal with everyday practice problems. Figure 7.6 represents a model of this technical rational approach to education.

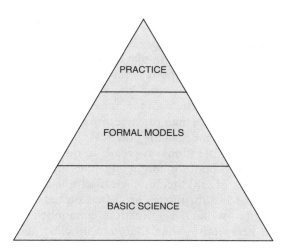

Fig. 7.6 Relationship between theory and practice in technical rational models of nurse education.

Schön (1983) proposes that there are a number of factors which must lead to a questioning of the efficiency of such an approach where theory is seen to inform practice. These are:

1. Over emphasis on the scientific rigour of knowledge at the expense of relevance
2. Failure to account for the many indeterminate areas of practice
3. Lack of recognition of the specific context and individual perceptions on the framing of problems
4. Inability to guide practice when value conflicts arises.

It is a combination of these factors which has led to a crisis of confidence in professional knowledge. It is now widely recognized that professionals must practise in divergent situations when the problems that must be dealt with are not well defined, are contextually specific and result in conflict among values.

Smyth (1988) argues that it is the often ill-defined nature or indeterminism of practice that is one of the hallmarks of professionalism. Yet professional education continued in the rigorous pursuit of knowledge which very often bears little or no relevance to the world of practice. As nurse education has moved to the tertiary sector there has been an incorporation of educational offerings from related disciplines such as physics, chemistry, psychology, and sociology. This has often resulted in the teaching of concepts that bear no relevance to nursing and that create unrealistic expectations in relation to the level of knowledge and skill to be acquired by nursing students. In addition there is often no attempt made, or an inability to apply, relevant concepts to nursing situations. Where nurses have lost or forfeited control over course content, they could be seen to have freed themselves from one form of bureaucratic and professional oppression within the hospital setting only to take on similar shackles within an educational setting.

Another issue which is of particular relevance for nursing is that of context specificity. Speedy (1989) points out that nurses need to perceive the people they deal with 'from their viewpoints within their particular contexts'. She proposes that this is based on tacit knowledge of the uniqueness and particularity of individuals. The components of caring and concern, which enable nurses to individualize their practice, are specified as not traditionally scientific yet of vital importance in the practice of nursing. It is difficult to fit such notions to a technical rational approach to nurse education. Similarly this approach fails to account for conflicting goals and values in relation to health care. In an era of rapid technological advancement and increasing self-responsibility for health, nurses are often placed in such situations. Schön (1987) points out that these situations cannot be approached from a narrow technical perspective when there are no clear and self-consistent guides to a solution.

Bevis & Clayton (1988) are also critical of the technical rational curriculum development paradigm which they see as based on the Tylerian model. They identify the major limitations as '...addiction to rule-governed behaviour, the popularity of nursing diagnosis, the attention given to competency-based education, and the dogma of prescriptive problem solving'. They question the ability of such an educational approach to provide for the development of innovative practitioners able to focus on the individual within a specific context.

The nursing profession does, however, have a responsibility to society to prepare competent practitioners. Benner (1984) acknowledges the need for strong educational preparation based on the acquisition of relevant theory and formal rules for application to ensure safe practice. However, it is also stressed that not all clinical judgements are quantifiable and objectifiable and that some skills are almost wholly irreducible to objective measurement strategies (Benner & Wrubel 1982). To enable students to move from rule governed behaviour at the appropriate time, the techniques of encouraging flexibility, focusing on the individual and the context, and feedback about the accuracy of judgements are suggested (Benner & Tanner 1987).

The use of problem solving or nursing process, as one of the formal models for applying theory to practice is also receiving professional criticism. This method to systematize practice has been widely adopted. Initial acceptance of the nursing process as a scientific approach to nursing education and practice is now being replaced by a concern that adherence to such a model may result in a mechanistic approach to care, undue emphasis on problems, and labelling of clients (Parker 1986, Bevis & Clayton 1988, McMurray 1989).

Nurses themselves are beginning to question the relevance of a model of professional education which is based on a 'view of science which attempts to eliminate the human factor' (Parker 1986). This author suggests that there is a marked shift in thinking about the scientific base of nursing. Such a viewpoint arises from a questioning of the assumptions about humans which have been incorporated into positivistic scientific methodology and which have subsequently been translated into professional practice. It is becoming increasingly common for nurse scholars (Paterson & Zderad 1970, Benner 1984, D'Cruz & Bottorff 1986, Benner & Wrubel 1989) to call for conceptualizations of the practice and education of nurses which are based on alternative approaches which value those aspects of nursing not explained by science and technology. This challenge has led to an increasing awareness and beginning acceptance of reflective practice in nursing.

It was Florence Nightingale who first expounded that nursing is both science and art (Nightingale 1980). Recently, in nurse education, much emphasis has been placed on the scientific component of nursing. This attention has focused on the application of scientific principles from related disciplines and on the development of nursing science in the form of theories for practice. There is danger that the artistic component of nursing, while highly developed in some practitioners, can be devalued in nurse education in the search for professional status and recognition. However, there is an emerging trend which pleads for the recognition of the need for humanistic and artistic elements in professional education so that theory and practice may inform each other.

The challenge for nursing is to discover strategies to achieve an appropriate balance between the artistic and scientific components of nursing. An exploration of the difference between practical and theoretical knowledge, reflection in action, and alternative ways of knowing may provide such strategies. The difference between practical knowledge and theoretical knowledge has been identified by Polyani (1962) as the difference between knowing how and knowing that. According to Polyani it is possible to develop skills or know how without being aware of the underlying theoretical principles. He has identified a number of concepts which demonstrate that it is not always possible for practical knowledge to be underpinned by theoretical knowledge. These concepts relate to maxims, connoisseurship, and tacit knowledge.

Maxims are defined as rules, the correct application of which is part of the art which they govern. These maxims are applied to improve performance but they cannot be applied until a practitioner already possesses a good practical knowledge of their art. Similarly, connoisseurship is something that can be developed only by experience and communicated only by example. Another concept developed by Polyani, that of tacit knowledge, or inarticulate intelligence, is demonstrated when experienced practitioners are able to take appropriate action in situations but are often unable to explain the theoretical basis for their action. Such an approach, as well as demonstrating that not all practice is based on theoretical knowledge, also indicates that there is theoretical knowledge to be gained from an examination and interpretation of practice.

This belief has been increasingly adopted and reflected in the work of nurse scholars (Paterson & Zderad 1970, Benner 1984, Diekelmann et al 1987). From 1960 until the publication of Humanistic Nursing in 1970, Paterson & Zderad engaged in dialogue with groups of nurses to reflect on, explore, and question their collective nursing experiences. This was based on their respect for nursing experience as a source of wisdom. As a result of this extensive dialogue they proposed that nurses reflect on and phenomenologically describe their experiences. It was seen that, in time, a synthesis of these descriptions, which they termed the 'mysteries of our commonplace', would contribute to building and making explicit a science of nursing. As a result of their work Paterson & Zderad (1970) described nursing as a transactional relationship. They proposed that it was not sufficient to educate students to be benevolent and technically competent. In addition they called for preparation of practitioners to include 'humanistic nursing practice theory' based on a resource bank which would accrue as reflective description led to an identification of common, significant themes in nursing practice. The advantages of such an approach were seen to have potential to move beyond educational preparation for the how and what of nursing practice to a stimulus for exploration and understanding.

The more recent work of Benner (1984) while based on the same belief in the 'knowledge embedded in actual nursing practice', used observational studies to identify common themes. Benner concentrated on describing the practice of expert nurses and demonstrated that it is '...impossible to learn ways of being and coping with an illness solely by concept'. She suggested that expert practice had major implications for nurse education in so far as its description and systematic recording was an essential component in the initial development of nursing theory and its further refinement and extension. While Benner acknowledged that expertise takes time to develop and cannot be taught, she suggested that sound educational preparation in the biological and behavioural sciences and in the science and art of nursing was essential to prepare the new graduate to make the best use of experience. In an earlier work (Benner & Wrubel 1982) two strategies to enhance learning for the beginner were proposed. These were the use of paradigm cases and the identification of areas that present difficulty in learning and teaching.

Paradigm cases are patient care situations that stand out because they can change nurses' previous perceptions and allow them to quickly grasp the situation and act appropriately. Paradigm cases, which are sufficiently simple and dramatic, can be used as case studies in teaching students. It has been suggested that, 'These cases often have such power that even the re-telling of them has the same learning impact as the first hand experience'. It is acknowledged that this method is already used by many clinical teachers. However, it must be recognized that it can only be effective when applied to situations where some prior understanding exists. Used appropriately this technique could be very effective in providing opportunities to increase integration between theory and practice.

The other enhancing strategy suggested by Benner & Wrubel (1982) related to the identification of areas which are difficult to learn and to teach. These are most likely to arise in situations in which context-free rules do not provide satisfactory answers. The ability to recognize and identify such situations will enable students to determine when they need to compare their judgements with those of more experienced practitioners. Such discussions can then lead to new insights and an extension of practical knowledge.

Also based on differentiation between theoretical and practical knowledge is an alternative to the technical rational model for nurse education. This is the dialogue and meaning model which has been developed by Diekelmann et al (1987). This model '... proposes an alternative way to describe what constitutes knowledge and a reconceptualization of the relationship between knowledge and skill acquisition in nursing education'.

The relationship between theory and practice in this model is described as transactional rather than applicational. Figure 7.7 represents an attempt to identify the major concepts within the model and the relationships between them. Students are permitted guided selection of clinical experience so that they can have enough experiences of a similar nature to enable them to develop some degree of expertise. The focus in clinical experience moves away from the application of previously learnt theoretical knowledge to a process of understanding the meaning and context of the nursing situation and the refinement of clinical decision-making. This model is still in its early stages of testing and as yet no evaluative studies are available.

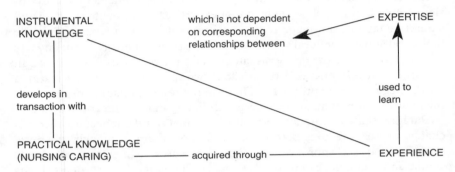

Fig. 7.7 Relationship between theory and practice in the dialogue and meaning model of nurse education.

Another approach, which could have implications for nurse education through an enhancement of the relationship between theory and practice, is the reflective practicum proposed by Schön (1987). This approach is based on a desire to develop the artistry of professional practice. The basis of the reflective practicum is '...learning by doing, coaching rather than teaching, and a dialogue of reciprocal reflection-in-action between coach and student'. The use of reflective practicums in curricula would, according to Schön '...reverse the usual figure/ground relationship between academic course work and practicum'. Rather than being tacked on at the end of a period of academic work the practicum would become a central bridge between theory and practice. Theoretical offerings may need to be re-developed to encompass broad, relevant conceptualizations open to reflection and evaluation. It would require reorganization to allocate appropriate periods of time and a rethinking of the pressures placed on students by academic work and evaluation of theoretical concepts. The status of the clinical teacher would improve and expertise in the role would be related to the level of professional artistry and the ability to empower students to '...reflect on their own processes of inquiry, examine their own shifting understandings—and compare their actual learning experiences with the formal theories'.

Not only does the reflective practicum provide opportunities for students to frame problems within the 'messy zones of indeterminancy in practice', it is also seen as a means for increasing the understanding of the organizational life of practitioners. The adoption of such an approach in nurse education, while requiring some reorganization of curricula, has the potential to increase the relevance of theoretical offerings, to deal with problems within their specific context and to enhance professional socialization.

As well as the development of the appropriate scientific knowledge and teachnical skills, the artistry of nursing is also seen to encompass the development of values, judgement, and compassion (Sward 1980). The inclusion of the study of the humanities in nursing curricula could lead to a greater measure of self-development and self-awareness in students which would enable them to apply values, insights, and creativity fostered by the humanities.

Because the two aspects of nursing practice—science and art—are unevenly balanced, so too is the educational emphasis. Wilson (1974) contends that 'The nurturing and development of the personal, human self of the nurse is the critical dimension for nursing practice'. It is therefore suggested that students be given the opportunity to explore the value systems held by themselves and others and the values which underlie nursing practice. Such understandings can create an awareness of the influence of cultural, ethical and intellectual factors on the person's interpretation of the illness experience (Sward 1980, Bottorff & D'Cruz 1985).

In urging nurses to move away from prescriptive rule driven curricula Bevis & Clayton (1988) challenge educators to find ways to '...provide the impetus for the creative, individualized, context-responsive, caring, human-services oriented, humanistic, critical-thinking, human science education that should form the basis for nursing'. They suggest that the type of learning implemented within curricula can contribute to this goal. Of six types of learning—item, directive, rational, syntax, context, and inquiry—the last three are seen to be truly educative. Syntax learning enables learners to consider the whole so that care may be responsive to the individual and the situation. Contextual learning addresses the essence of nursing and the socio-cultural context in which the discipline and its practice occurs. Inquiry learning encompasses the creative aspects of nursing which leads '...to dreaming dreams, seeing visions, and formulating ways to make them realities'.

Another area of nursing knowledge which is receiving increasing attention is that of intuition (Rew & Barrow 1987, Benner & Tanner 1987, Miller 1989). Intuition has long been alluded to in nursing practice but has been devalued as unscientific and therefore not a legitimate way of knowing. The landmark studies of expert practice by Benner (1984) firmly established the place of intuition in clinical judgement. While intuition is enhanced and refined by experience it is possible to incorporate this aspect into educational preparation. Benner & Tanner (1987) suggest that strict adherence to the use of formal models for teaching the beginner can limit the development of more flexible approaches. They refer to the skills required for intuitive judgement identified by Dreyfus: pattern recognition, similarity-recognition, commonsense understanding, skilled know-how, sense of salience and deliberative rationality. While acknowledging that there is an artistic element to these skills, an element that is unique and cannot be taught, they believe that it is possible to teach pattern recognition. This can be achieved not through formal lectures on analysis but through the use of case studies and feedback and validation by expert nurses. The very fact of learning that it is possible to make valid judgements based on intuition can potentiate the development and use of this skill.

The synthesizing process of intuition is identified as one of 'women's ways of knowing' by Miller (1989) which should be presented to students as a legitimate way of knowing. A number of suggestions are made to facilitate the use of this process in learning and teaching. These include the use of warming-up mental and physical exercises, group experience and mind-quieting activities, and mental imagery. The 'teacher as midwife' metaphor is seen as the appropriate teaching role in facilitating the students' ability to mobilize their own intuition. It is acknowledged that because this area has been neglected there is need for research into the development and effectiveness of teaching methods to foster the development of intuition.

CONCLUSION

A number of factors have emerged as significant in enhancing the relationship between theory and practice in nurse education. These can be identified as the establishment of a relevant, sound scientific base for practice; an appreciation of the context in which nursing is practised; the need for opportunities for reflection on and in practice; the difference between practical and theoretical knowledge; and the desirability of inculcating artistic and aesthetic elements in the educative process.

The emergence of the various approaches which recognize the difference between practical and theoretical knowledge and place value on reflection and the artistic, non-scientific ways of knowing has major implications for nurse education. An integration of these methods with relevant science based education has the potential to ensure that the relationship between theory and practice is one in which theory and practice truly inform each other.

REFERENCES

Adam E 1985 Towards more clarity in terminology: frameworks, theories and models. Journal of Nursing Education 24(4):151–155

Benner P 1984 From novice to expert: excellence and power in clinical nursing practice. Addison-Wesley, Menlo Park

Benner P, Tanner C 1987 Clinical judgement: how expert nurses use intuition. Americal Journal of Nursing. January, 87(1):23–31

Benner P, Wrubel J 1982 Skilled clinical knowledge. The value of perceptual awareness. Journal of Nursing Administration 12(5):11–14

Benner P, Wrubel J 1989 The primacy of caring: stress and coping in health and illness. Addison–Wesley, Menlo Park

Bennett C, Wallace R 1978 Nurse education in Australia: where to now? Australian Bulletin of Labour (March): 40–52

Bevis E, Clayton G 1988 Needed: a new curriculum development design. Nurse Education 3(4): 14–18

Bottorff J, D'Cruz J 1985 The nursing curriculum and knowledge of most worth. Australian Journal of Advanced Nursing 2(3): 9–17

Chinn P 1988 Knowing and doing (editorial). Advances in Nursing Science 10(3): vii–viii

D'Cruz J, Bottorff J 1986 The renewal of nursing education. A cultural perspective of continuities and change. La Trobe University, Melbourne

Diekelmann N, Olsen S, Jorgensen M, Crabtree A 1987 Clinical nursing knowledge research: implications for nursing education. Paper presented at Society for Research in Nursing Education, Scientific Meeting. San Francisco

Engstrom J 1984 Problems in the development, use and testing of nursing theory. Journal of Nursing Education 23(6):245–251

Institute of Hospital Matrons of NSW 1967 Report of the committee to consider all aspects of nursing. Part 1 The general nurse in the hospital environment. In: Sax S (Chairperson) Nurse education and training. Report to the Committee of Inquiry into nurse education and training to the Tertiary Education Commission. Canberra, p. 37

Kelly (Chairperson) 1943 First Report of the committee for reorganization of the nursing profession in New southWales. In: Sax S (Chairperson) 1978 nurse education and training. Report of the Committee of Inquiry into nurse education and training to the Tertiary Education Commission. Canberra

Kim M 1987 Classification of nursing diagnoses. Proceedings of the sixth National Conference. C V Mosby, St Louis

Lewis T 1988 Leaping the chasm between nursing theory and practice. Journal of Advanced Nursing 13:345–351

Lublin J 1985 Basic nurse education in CAE's—The educational evidence for transfer. Australian Journal of Advanced Nursing 2(2):18–28

McArthur J, Walsh A, Bruni N 1983 Further comparative evaluation of students and graduates from college and hospital-based basic nursing programs. Commonwealth Tertiary Education Commission, Canberra

McMurray A 1989 Time to extend the "process"? Australian Journal of Advanced Nursing 6(4):40–43

Marriner A (ed) 1986 Nursing theorists and their work. C V Mosby, St Louis

Miller V 1989 Analysis and intuition: the need for both in nursing education. Journal of Advanced Nursing 28(2):84–86

Nightingale F (1820–1912) 1980 Notes on nursing: what it is and what it is not. Churchill Livingstone, Edinburgh

Nursing Studies Regulations 1980 Department of Health, Brisbane

Parker J 1986 Introduction: changing perspectives upon nursing. In: D'Cruz J & Bottorff J (eds) The renewal of nursing education. A cultural perspective of continuities and change. La Trobe University, Melbourne

Parkes M 1984 Blueprint for change: an overview of developments in nurse education in Australia. International Journal of Nursing Studies 21(3):177–182

Paterson J, Zderad L 1970 Humanistic nursing. Wiley, New York

Polyani M 1962 Personal knowledge: towards a post-critical philosophy. University of Chicago Press, Chicago

Reaby L 1985 Basic nurse education in the A.C.T.—hospital or college based? Australian Journal of Advanced Nursing 2(3): 18–23

Rew L, Barrow E 1987 Intuition: a neglected hallmark of nursing knowledge. Advances in Nursing Science October: 49–61

Sax S (Chairperson) 1978 Nursing education and training. Report of the committee of inquiry into nurse education and training to the Tertiary Education Commission. Canberra

Schön D 1983 The reflective practitioner: how professionals think in action. Basic Books, New York

Schön D 1987 Educating the reflective practitioner. Josey-Josey, San Francisco

Smyth J 1988 The reflective practitioner in nurse education. Paper presented at the Visions Into Nursing Practice Conference, Adelaide

Speedy S 1989 Theory–practice debate: setting the scene. Australian Journal of Advanced Nursing Practice 6(3): 12–20

Sward K 1980 Precedents and prospects for the humanities in nursing. In: Spicker S, Gadow S (eds) Nursing: images and ideals. Springer, New York

Trembath R, Hellier D 1987 All care and responsibility: a history of nursing in Victoria 1850–1934. Florence Nightingale Committee, Australia, Victorian Branch, Melbourne

Walker M, Norby R 1987–88 Friendships of utility: resolving the disalignment between nursing education and nursing service. Nursing Forum 23(1): 30–35

Wilson H 1974 A case for humanities in professional nursing education. Nursing Forum 13(4)

Wong J 1979 The inability to transfer classroom learning to clinical learning: a learning problem and its remedial plan. Journal of Advanced Nursing 4:161–168

8. Nursing knowledge: processes of production

Nina Bruni

Over the past two decades in Australia several aspects of nursing have undergone change, the most public change being the introduction of tertiary-based pre-registration progams. This move has been variously interpreted by those working within nursing—its educators, administrators, and practitioners—their discussions revealing areas of agreement, disagreement, and uncertainty. One aspect which continues to spark debate is that of clinical practice, in particular the implications of theory for practice. A central concern is the issue of implementation: can theory be implemented in practice and if so, how? For many educators the answers to these questions lie in curriculum change, specifically in the inclusion of subjects relative to the students' acquisition of interpersonal and problem-solving skills and the refinement of the teaching/learning process. These arguments are informed by unquestioned, accepted understandings of what constitutes nursing (Bruni 1990).

For many practitioners however, issues of implementation are not of major concern. Rather, the appropriateness of curriculum content is questioned in terms of meeting the perceived need for students to understand the reality of the practice setting (Jenkins 1989).

However a sense of agreement appears to prevail on the conception of the rightful affiliation of the term 'profession' with nursing, for, despite some controversy over whether professional status has yet to be achieved (Speedy 1987), the term abounds in contemporary nursing literature. Such uncritical adoption of the language of professionalization is of interest and warrants analysis. This imperative derives from the many and varied beliefs associated with the concepts of the nursing profession and the professional nurse, including notions of autonomy, accountability, holistic care, and research-based practice. The concern raised by such beliefs is not one of empirical validity, specifically the question of the existence of such attributes, but rather relates to the nature of the pathway adopted for professionalization.

A reading of nursing texts (such as Maloney 1986) suggests that the pathway to professional status for nursing is predominately understood in terms of knowledge, specifically in the generation and ownership of a unique, discipline-specific body of nursing knowledge. The adoption of this discourse or interpretation of professionalization raises several questions which form the basis of this chapter. These are: first, why has the traditional knowledge base of nursing been rejected or seen as problematic?; second, what strategies or processes are proposed for the generation of an alternate or new knowledge base?; and third, what is the nature of the emergent nursing knowledge? This latter question involves exploration of the possibilities the new knowledge offers for practice and hence its degree of departure from the knowledge which has traditionally informed nursing care—knowledge made available not only through the hospital as the dominant context of care but also through nursing curricula and the educative process. Questioning the nature of contemporary nursing knowledge currently being developed in basic curricula is both timely and essential. Is it creating a nursing version of some dominant medical discourses or positing new understandings of health and care? Which understandings are dominant and why?

It is argued here that exploration of these questions is crucial if the developing discipline of nursing is to be instrumental in effecting change in health profiles at all levels of society, as suggested in tertiary curricula (Bruni 1990). For participation in change requires that power relations be recognized and addressed, specifically those involved in shaping nurses' understandings of society and the health care system—understandings which then structure their care practices. A critical analysis of the knowledge which constitutes nursing programs would provide insight into the versions of social reality accessible to nurses and may reveal areas which require refinement, inclusion, and/or deletion. This includes the area of teaching practice and the knowledge which educators produce, perhaps unwittingly, in their interaction with students. In this sense program evaluation which is focused on graduate attributes clearly misses some essential ingredients of nursing practice—the program content and the processes of its production.

Clarification of the nature of the knowledge which underpins the emergent discipline of nursing is essential if nursing is to assist in meeting the health needs of society. Such a rethink may also enable educators and practitioners to more clearly identify and articulate their differences in a language devoid of intrusive, divisive assertions of territoriality, ignorance, or elitism.

It is suggested that conceptualization of the question of nursing as a profession, the nature of professionalization ,and the role of nursing education may profitably be informed by discourse theory. In the next section a brief overview of the framework which informs the analysis is presented.

THE RELEVANCE OF DISCOURSE THEORY

The discussion of the professionalization of nursing, in particular the role and status of nursing knowledge, is informed by the theories of discourse articulated by Henriques et al (1984), Weedon (1987), and Lather (1986, 1989). Their formulations are centred on notions of discourse/language, power and subjectivity, the articulation of which appears to favour the work of Foucault.

In brief, discourse in its most general sense refers to regulated systems of statements, which as language give meaning to the world. The concept of discourse also incorporates the notion of practice, as practice is seen to be constituted by the language which informs it. As Lather (1989) writes of 'post modernisms': 'All share the focus on language as a productive, constitutive force as opposed to views of language as reflective, representative of some reality capturable through conceptual adequation'. The educator for example, who asserts that students are children, may relate to them in a manner which is authoritarian and prescriptive, informed by an understanding of children as irresponsible, undisciplined people. The identity or subjectivity of the educator is in part constituted by this discourse but also by many others including those of gender, teaching, and education. Each of these offer the educator a variety of subject positions. The problem of inconsistency of meaning or variability of attitude is hence exposed as an issue of discursive complexity—not a problem of personal irrationality or of false consciousness.

Discourses may be seen as limiting forces. But they are not closed systems. They are open to change, for they provide '...the spaces—the concepts, metaphors, models and analogies—for making new statements within any specific discourse' (Henriques et al 1984). It is argued, however, that challenges to prevailing understandings or practices must address relations of power for 'Language is a version of meaning and meaning is always political. It is located in the social networks of power and knowledge relations which give society its current form' (Speedy 1990). The dominant contemporary lifestyle health discourse (Crawford 1984) is thus seen to be constituted by, and to constitute, the power relations which sustain the dominance of medicine in the health care system (Turner 1987). In other words the dominant language of health serves the interests of social groups which have a strong power base.

Discourses of health which differ significantly from the predominant and dominant perspective, and which incorporate alternate notions of health, illness causation, and intervention, will hence remain marginal unless adopted by the controlling groups—or unless their positions of control are subverted. It is within this framework that the questions posed earlier regarding nursing knowledge are explored.

PROFESSIONALIZATION AND NURSING KNOWLEDGE

The emergence of the drive for the development of nursing knowledge is seen to be linked to the issue of the professionalization of nursing. However the links are not clear cut, their complexity deriving from the diverse interpretations of what constitutes a profession. The logic of exploring understandings of profession in order to explain the issue of change is well argued by Friedson (1983) who states: 'Without some definition of profession the concept of professionalization is virtually meaningless, as is the intention to study process rather than structure'. An outline of several discourses of a profession is therefore offered. This highlights the diversity of understandings attributed to terms commonly voiced by nurses, and argues for the need to deconstruct their meanings rather than the common plea for unity based on definitional consensus. The futility and illogicality of a consensus approach is seen to lie in its disregard of the social construction of meaning.

The term profession has been applied to nursing in Australia for many generations (Bruni 1985). Notions of the profession of nursing, professional nursing practice, professional accountability ,and professional socialization abound in contemporary texts including curricula, informing subsequent discussions or analyzes of proposed developments or requisite need. It is suggested that uncritical use of the professional label creates the commonsense understanding that nursing is indeed a profession—an understanding which is henceforth both unquestioned and unquestionable. As Weeks (1982) argues, each discourse has '...its own modes of distinguishing truth from falsity': in commonsense discourse the presumption of inherent truth is implicated in its claim to be 'natural, obvious and therefore true'. Moreover, as Weedon (1987) points out, such discourse constitutes or shapes the very reality it presumes. The practice of using the term profession, both in talking and writing about nursing, is seen as part of this constitutive process interwoven, it is suggested, with discourses of loyalty to nursing and nurses.

However, commonsense notions of nursing as a profession do not preclude an understanding of nursing as developing and professionalizing— that is moving towards a desired state. This apparent contradiction is evidence of a variety of discourses informing the dialogue.

The desired professional state is predominately understood within the trait discourse, which articulates an array of characteristics deemed to be displayed by professional occupations. Amongst those traits commonly cited are: a unique body of knowledge, altruistic service, a code of ethics regulating practice, lengthy socialization, and automomy of practice (Friedson 1983, Maloney 1986, Richman 1987). A functional explanation of the existence of the professional occupation, that is its positive contribution to the maintenance of society, underpins the identification of these traits. Within this framework the function of medicine may be cited as that of 'cure'. The rationale for the performance of this curative function by medical practitioners is their perceived expertise in the area of health care—deriving from their possession of a unique, scientifically validated body of knowledge relative to bodily cure. Decision-making is hence identified as the prerogative of doctors whilst nurses are understood to work in complementary roles as '...data-gathers for medical decision-making and as implementors of medical decisions based on a priori theorizing' (Bruni 1989). This interpretation implies that nursing contributes to societal health by assisting doctors to perform their highly valued function.

Cited professional traits of nursing are portrayed as interdependent, each necessary for the existence of the others. Texts informed by this perspective suggest that the traits represent the features of law or medicine. According to Richman (1987) nursing has appropriated the professional model of medicine in order to emulate the occupation. But as Weedon (1987) points out, dominant discourses which govern the organization and practices of social institutions, such as hospitals, are under constant challenge as people seek to resist, and so change some aspect of their reality. In adopting the trait model of the professions, nurses are thus seen to be challenging the meanings and practices of the dominant medical discourse of health care management which in part has shaped their occupation.

In seeking to professionalize, the traditional role of nursing is transformed. Informed by notions of highly valued uniqueness, expertise, and autonomy, the submissiveness of nursing becomes unwarranted and untenable. Traditional functional areas are reinterpreted and new claims are made. Thus health promotion has been identified, as well as rehabilitation, as an appropriate functional area of practice, and the caring role revalued and re-acclaimed as the essence of nursing.

However there is little to suggest that writers within nursing have acknowledged various problems identified with this approach. Its lack of attention to process, in particular the historically specific conditions in which medical dominance emerged, and the illusory image of unity amongst the traits and within the occupation which supposedly exhibits them, question its descriptive capacity and reveal its analytical inadequacy (Dingwall & Lewis 1983, Richman 1987, Willis 1989). The discourse however remains dominant in nursing, and nurses so informed endorse the relocation of nursing education from hospital-based programs to the tertiary sector, enrol in variously located educational programs to develop their knowledge-base, and use the language of professionalism. In these terms nursing is professionalizing.

Despite the transformation of some elements, the politically conservative functionalism of the medical discourse remains. The discourse of professionalization appropriated by nursing does not challenge the exisiting occupational hierarchy, but rather seeks merely to relocate nursing to a new and higher level. The relocation discourse, which focuses on the generation of nursing-specific knowledge, does not address relations of power between medicine and nursing, but posits a process of change which is internally focused—the challenge to change residing within the occupation of nursing. In this sense it constitutes a reformist discourse of change. Moreover whilst new subject positions for nurses are created—such as academic, health care facilitator, and autonomous practitioner—these are (as will be discussed later) presented as operating in environments which appear to be devoid of power relations. As such they pose no substantial threat to the health care hierarchy since nurses so informed will engage in practices which are not directed at challenging medical power or their own power base. In this sense the oppositional status of this discourse of professionalization is limited, and its political conservatism revealed.

Critical structural discourses of professionalization which explore power relations between nursing and medicine are offered by theorists external to nursing. Focusing on relations of class, gender, and sovereignty, nursing is conceptualied as an oppressed, subordinated occupation, its members unable to exercise autonomy in their practice (Game & Pringle 1983, Willis 1989). Changes in the educative, practice, and administrative arenas of nursing are seen to reflect changes in the division of labour, as for example the product of technological developments in medicine (Game & Pringle 1983), whilst notions of control based on expertise and autonomy of practice are understood as ideological constructs which serve to mystify prevailing relations of inequity (Game & Pringle 1983, Richman 1987).

Turner (1987) offers a post structural analysis of medical dominance, arguing for the constitutive power of medical knowledge. In examining the various perspectives on the professionalization of nursing, Turner looks at the use of metaphor and homology which suggests that nursing is the rightful occupation of women. He argues that naturalistic or essentialist gender discourses and the family metaphor are powerful forces which shape the subjectivity of doctors and nurses and so sustain relations of inequity between them. He also points to the conservative force of the scientific discourse for '...the knowledge of the doctor... [is] ...scientific, while the actions of the nurse are merely manual and practical'.

Turner (1987) also identifies a discourse of complaint amongst nurses, one which is evident in the Victorian report of the *Study of Professional Issues in Nursing* (Marles 1988) as complaints about a lack of autonomy in the workplace. He questions the radical intent of these complaints suggesting that 'Complaining is symbolic and consists of collective gestures against authority ..[and that]..Despite the nurse's symbolic encroachment on the space of medical authority, the objective situation of nursing is maintained and her powerlessness preserved'. However whilst complaining may be symbolic of discontent, the nurses' strike of 1986 did go beyond the level of symbolic critique. But the strike action did not constitute a threat to the hierarchical structure of the care facilities in which the nurses practised, but challenged the government to uphold its promise of an improved career structure for nurses (Gardner & McCoppin 1989), arguing that the professional status of nurse practitioners was at stake. For some, winning the battle perhaps provided proof of their belief that nurses formed a powerful, professional group.

Within Australian nursing literature there is evidence of the emergence of critical theorizing about the status of nursing. Several approaches are briefly reviewed here to indicate their diverse implications for the achievement of change in nursing. Jenkins (1989) for example, argues that control and self-regulation are essential for professional status, and asserts that medical practitioners '...have acted repeatedly to perpetuate the handmaiden role for the nurse, to oppose improved education for nurses and to restrict the role of the nurse in Australia'. She maintains that existing control mechanisms (both internal and external) over education, practice, professional status and renumeration must be 'reviewed, revised or amended' to ensure that self-regulation is achievable. To this end she believes that consensus amongst nurses on desired goals and priorities is essential. But, as mentioned earlier, this suggested resolution strategy denies the social construction of discourse and hence the inevitability of divergence. Given the complexity of nursing, its variable contexts of practice, and its composition along class, gender, age,and ethnic lines, diverse voices are inevitable, although some will be more dominant than others.

In identifying the lack of professional recognition of nursing, Dunlop (1988) focuses on the dimension of care, arguing that its devaluing prevents the achievement of such recognition. In order that caring be appropriately revalued, she claims that structural forces which constrain the carer must be identified, '...the social and political structures in which people are expected to care'. She also maintains that there is a need to degenderize the work of caring—not to see it as the prerogative of a predominately female profession such as nursing. She does not, however, identify the requisite change strategies.

Concern with the humanistic domain of nursing is also expressed by Retsas (1988). Like Dunlop he rejects the conceptualization of nursing as devalued women's work and similarly maintains that reductionist empiricism cannot capture the meaning of nursing. Drawing on the work of Habermas, he argues for the use of 'the dialectic method' as a way of critically exploring how individuals create the social reality of nursing. He maintains that a distorted view of nursing has been created in part by the use of scientific language appropriated from medicine. Use of the dialectic method will enable this distorted language to be unravelled and so create the possibility that the true humanistic dimension of nursing is revealed. His emphasis on humanistic meaning as the essence of nursing practice suggests that his work is framed by a naturalistic or essentialist discourse of nursing which is offered uncritically, as itself beyond deconstruction.

The work of Speedy (1987, 1990), however, invites exploration of the discursive context of meaning as this relates to the power of the language of nursing. She cogently argues for a feminist analysis of professionalization asserting that nurses are an oppressed group, their oppression deriving from their status as women in a patriachal society. The dominant language of professionalization is, she asserts, 'male' and as such it '...tends to encourage consideration of the male as the norm and devalues women/nurses by their exclusion' (l987). Such sexist language, she argues, informs nursing texts, resource materials, and conceptual frameworks for education programs. Given the present structure and ideological governance of nursing it cannot, she maintains, become a profession. Speedy (1987) believes that feminist insights into the constitutive power of language can assist in changing the subordinate status of nurses. She posits the need to deconstruct patriarchal discourses of nursing and create new languages which would shape different practices and relationships.

In the next section, several pathways for the generation of nursing knowledge and their implications for change are explored. It is suggested that the dominant strategy remains that of positivist research, disguised perhaps by the addition of some elements of the language of social research.

THE NEED FOR NURSING KNOWLEDGE: PROCESSES OF GENERATION

The discursive context within which the push for new nursing knowledge was generated, has been identified here as that of professionalism. The complexity of its development is increased by the numerous and varied agendas of those who perceived the need for new knowledge. These agendas are implicated in questions regarding the nature of nursing, its function and processes of practice, and the origin of knowledge; questions which are linked to notions of expertise and hence control. An exploration of such questions indicates the diverse paths along which the discipline is being taken.

The definitional debate over the nature of nursing has generated a variety of labels for the occupation. Most frequently heard are those of 'a science', 'an art', and 'an applied discipline'. The practice of applying all three to capture its variable essence appears to have been adopted in curricula (Bruni 1990). Exploration of their meaning reveals their degree of compatibility and the spaces from which new discourses are emerging. Their impact on the development of the discipline is also exposed.

The professionalization discourse outlined earlier asserts that professional expertise resides in the possession and application of scientific knowledge unique to the occupation. Appropriation of this notion has informed nurses of their need to adopt the language of science; that knowledge unique to nursing could, and should be generated in this tradition; and that this knowledge-base should then inform practice. The discourse of science subsequently incorporated in the nursing progarms was, until recently, that of the empiricist, positivist tradition (Dunlop 1988, Restas 1988, Speedy 1990). Its appropriateness was unquestioned since its application did not reject the bio-medical knowledge base which has traditionally constituted the knowledge and practice of nursing, but rather sought to increase its depth, breadth, and application. These goals however, unwittingly perhaps, devalued the knowledge and practice of nurses not affiliated with the tertiary-based scientific community. Practitioners were seen as 'unscientific practical doers'. A status discourse of inequity between the professional and non-professional nurse was generated.

The endorsement of empiricism was, as Retsas (1988) argues, also based on its perceived correctness, its conceptual self-evidence, and indeed on its commonsense appeal. The power of this type of knowledge also reflected the assumption 'that scientific knowledge was incompatible with all other forms of knowledge and understanding and that, unless all other forms of knowledge followed the scientific method, they could not be viewed as legitimate bodies of knowledge in their own right' (Retsas 1988). Its sense of legitimate truthfulness is also seen to derive from its maleness—as a dominate patriarchial discourse (Speedy 1987, Hagell 1988), its appropriation hence reaffirming and constituting gender-based relations of control within the educative and health care systems. The generation of knowledge unique to nursing was thus initially sought through the conduct of empiricist research. Notions of theoretical neutrality, objectivity, control, and measurement informed design, methodology, and data analysis—with appeals to the need for vigilance and rigour.

However, challenges to the empiricist tradition have emerged from nurses whose understanding of nursing was differently informed—who perceived it as an art, a humanistic discipline concerned with processes of caring, a holistic practice. Despite the diverse interpretations of these terms, areas of commonality and divergence can be identified which suggest links with empiricism but also indicate the spaces within which reverse critical discourses of nursing and research are emerging.

The process by which new or reverse discourses are produced is understood as one of appropriation, whereby elements—concepts, ideas, or assumptions—are delocated from one discourse and relocated within another. In this process of recontextualisation the new item may be transformed (Bernstein 1986), its meaning arising from its new, but pre-existing, discursive context. Assumptions of shared meanings attached to the same words employed in different disciplines is hence as problematic as is the assumption that meanings are constant over time (Lather 1989). Rather, relativity of meaning is explored in terms of the relations of power in which the element is located, its constitution seen not merely as a product of its cultural milieux. In this sense the new languages of nursing research are seen as political, as constituting or challenging existing patterns of control.

Understandings of nursing as the professional practice of caring have been explored by Dunlop (1988) in a discussion of the 'science of caring'. Her work reveals the incorporation of a language of caring within a foundational empiricist discourse which reduces the elements of caring to discrete variables. The assumption underlying this approach is that '...caring can be operationalized in some way as a set of behaviours which can be observed, counted, and measured' (Dunlop 1988).She decries the work of Watson & Leininger conducted in this tradition as '...attempts to describe caring in terms of sets of context-free variables'. Hagell (1988), who similarly maintains that caring is the definitive feature of nursing, argues that if nurses continue on this scientific path, '...they will lose what is critical to nursing—caring—because science cannot conceptualize caring nor can caring be measured, only experienced'. Her research, which was concerned with methods of developing nursing knowledge, explored the methodologies of Masters' theses from a Canadian Faculty of Nursing completed between 1980 and 1984.

Hegell's (1988) concern for the delimiting impact of positivism is expressed in her assertion that many of the studies began by posing questions that could generate knowledge. However, her analysis revealed that they rarely addressed the question initially posed but reconceptualized it, so that the research problem became the development of a tool to measure the phenomenon of concern. This process is seen to negate the possibility of generating knowledge new to the discipline of nursing, for potentially exciting, innovative propositions become reformulated within inappropriate and constricting frameworks. Her work indicates that attempts to move in a new direction may be circumvented, as the dominant discourse of research continues to inform the practices of discovery.

However, reverse discourses of knowledge development have been generated. The re-emergence of caring in an attempt to revalue an area found to be difficult to quantify, has generated various research discourses and notions of care which range from naturalistic discourses to radical feminist ideology critiques of care (Dalley 1988). Critical discourses nevertheless remain marginal. Descriptive exploratory and interpretive phenomenological research designs have been developed and applied, frequently in the grounded theory tradition. The value of this tradition for nursing research has been cited as its exploratory potential, for example its relevance for the study of previously unresearched areas, particularly the practice areas of nursing, and also for the study of issues on which previous research has been inconclusive (Chenitz & Swanson 1986). As such, its appeal to a new discipline could be understood as one of self-evident commonsense.

Its perceived implications for knowledge development, described in terms of the possible outcomes of its application, are '...a coherent theoretical framework which elaborates the important elements of the problem being investigated...[but]...More frequently, however grounded theory research results in the identification of concepts or variables which...require more rigorous testing in different situations and contexts' (Battersby & Hemmings 1990). Embedded in this understanding are empiricist notions of emergent truth, the decontextualization of data for analysis, and an implication that grounded theory research constitutes a precursor to the more rigorous practices of positivist empiricism. This inherent orthodoxy is further evidenced in the concerns about the approach voiced by adherents of grounded theory. These are summarized by Battersby & Hemmings (1990) as: researcher bias, the collection and analysis of large volumes of data, the criterion of theoretical saturation, and judgements about data relevance. Implicit in these problems is the issue of researcher bias—the notion that the human researcher contaminates her/his data base, which paradoxically is initially contextualized. Data trustworthiness has hence been pursued through the practice of triangulation, with collaborative data sought from multiple sources, utilizing a variety of techniques (Lather 1986). Notions of methodological rigour continue to be reiterated in an attempt to mirror the supposed neutral objectivity of statistical analysis.

Many research discourses which have accompanied different understandings of nursing hence remain variously attached to empiricism, their development exposed as a process of appropriation and transformation. This limits the development of new discourses of nursing as implicit assumptions remain dormant, rather than being exposed for critical review. As Opie (1989) explains, the process involves '...a filtering of the "new" through the old so that the new is suppressed in favour of the old, and the potentially destabilising impact of new knowledge is subverted by a process which permits the established view to retain its dominance'. In nursing research the tendency to overlay qualitative perspectives on quantitative assumptions has meant its failure to escape the shackles of positivist science (Retsas 1988).

However, approaches to nursing research are being proposed which constitute radical, oppositional discourses rather than modified versions of positivist empiricism (Dzurec 1989, Speedy 1990). These acknowledge the humanness of the researcher as an integral aspect of the research process, whose world views inform her/his understandings of research. The need to deny the researcher's framework or seek redress for personal bias through disclosure is hence untenable (Angus 1986). As Gitlin et al (1989) argue in an analysis of the politics of method in educational research, 'To say that the ethnographer is never neutral is too simple...for it suggests that the problem of realism could be solved by including a paragraph stating the researcher's orientation and methodological decision points'. Rather, knowledge is never neutral nor is the process of its creation. Research is thus not a neutral process of discovery but is implicated in the relations of power which its understandings and practices constitute, and which in turn sustain the discourse.

In arguing for a relationship between knowledge and power, critical researchers dismiss interpretive research as limited, lacking the explanatory power to adequately contextualize data. Interpretive research fails to address the constitutive or generative social processes and accepts the identified interpretive frameworks as definitive explanatory perspectives. The need for critically informed nursing research relates not only to the importance of understanding the impact of nursing knowledge and care practices, but to the perceived need to alter situations of inequity. Such research Speedy (1990) argues '...ought to be directed toward the emancipation of our patients and clients by the removal of unnecessary and unjust constraints'. The role of such research is thus emancipatory and empowering (Lather 1986). The issue of the powerfulness of the researcher also needs to be addressed.

The question of control also emerges in exploring the notion that knowledge is not the prerogative of the academic, the nurse researcher, or theorist, but also resides in the practitioner and informs her/his practice. Whilst this argument may be articulated by practitioners in their rejection of imposed frameworks to 'guide' and so improve their practice, it is also heard amongst academics, such as Benner & Wrubel (1989), who articulate discourses of nursing knowledge which challenge notions of cognitive rationality and empirical validity. Central to this new theorizing about knowledge development in nursing are the concepts of self-reflexivity and intuition, variously interpreted and inter-related.

Clinical intuition, relative to the 'content' of the practitioner's knowledge and/or the process of its development, is defined as '...a process whereby the nurse knows something about a patient that cannot be verbalized, that is verbalized with difficulty, or for which the source of knowledge cannot be determined' (Young 1987). The need to defend this conception from empiricist demands for proof have perhaps resulted in defences which entail notions of inherent 'female' ability. However the concept of reflexivity, the process of self-reflection aimed at the determination of insight and knowledge to guide practice, denies this possibility since the process is understood as a skill which can be acquired or learnt. The cognitive basis of this interpretation therefore questions its degree of difference from empiricist rationality. Moreover the appropriation of female language suggests that its endorsement poses no threat to prevailing gender-based relations of power. The nature of its contribution to the improvement of nursing care is thus questioned. Indeed whilst it may generate some discussion on process aimed at closing the theory/practice gap, it begs the question of the nature of that gap. Differences in meanings and practices are contextual and discursive; bridge-building which is not so informed will collapse or lead its workers and users on a fruitless path.

This review of the pathways for the generation of nursing knowledge posited in nursing literature, in particular contemporary Australian texts, has indicated some of the areas of difference and development. More importantly it has highlighted the marginality of discourses which could provide insight into the politics of nursing knowledge and practice. The possibility of this profile being altered is explored in the next section where the content of several basic curricula is examined. This discussion draws on a preliminary analysis undertaken in 1990 of the philosophies and rationales of four basic programs (Bruni 1990). It indicates that individualistic discourses predominate, delimiting the boundaries of mainstream nursing knowledge. This suggests that the process discourses, which inform the practices of both teaching and clinical practice, may not achieve the desired course objectives as nursing, nurses, and their clients remain decontextualized and depoliticized.

PEDAGOGIC DISCOURSES OF CONTENT AND PROCESS

Before exploring the selected areas of the four basic programs, the educational discourse which frames them is outlined. This indicates an assumption of technical neutrality which dominates the meaning of the educational process thereby effectively 'containing' the development of critical perspectives relative to the teaching process, as well as to the content of these programs.

Nurse education is introduced in curricula in terms of its perceived functional mandate: to provide the appropriate context for the students' acquisition of competencies relative to the registered nurse role as a reflective first level practitioner. This mandate is based on the notion that education must respond positively to societal change, meet its demands for new skill development, as well as effectively meet existing needs. Education thus provides the mechanism by which change can be met and requisite adaptability achieved. The educational agenda is not perceived as problematic or contentious; indeed it is offered as self-evident and taken for granted. To achieve its mandate, the program is charged with providing relevant learning experiences which will assist students to effectively integrate knowledge and make appropriate clinical applications.

The role of the educator is to promote an optimal learning environment. She/he is perceived primarily as a resource person rather than as a transmitter of knowledge, for the student is ultimately responsible for developing and consolidating her/his knowledge-base. Requisite teaching skills are those pertinent to the effective and efficient management of learning contexts, of curriculum development and of subject areas. The need to be critically informed about content areas is perhaps taken as read, as a commonsense attribute of the good teacher. In any case the curriculum, the requisite teaching tool, is available to inform the teacher of the areas to be covered.

Analysis of the curriculum provides insight into the content to which students are exposed and which subsequently structures their possibilities for future practice, perhaps through their challenging of it and by developing oppositional discourses. The curriculum is thus not understood as a neutral instrument to be effectively and efficiently processed by equally neutral educators. Both are implicated in the production of knowledge which, as argued earlier, is never context free.

In unravelling the discourses which constitute the curricula, a reading of the four concepts adopted as central to nursing is offered: those of the nurse, client, health, and environment. The concept of environment is considered first since its meanings highlight the reliance in the curricula on commonsense knowledge and the absence of critical frameworks.

Environment

Nursing is portrayed as a part of society which is modified or influenced by social structures and processes. Their pressure is deemed responsible for the need to generate new curricula and so ensure that nurses have the requisite expertise. A number of substantive areas of social change relative to health and nursing care are listed. These include an increased complexity of health and illness in society with a subsequent alteration in people's expectations about care; increased knowledge about health and illness; advances in medical technology; and a growing emphasis on holistic care and personal responsibility for health. The question of the relationship between these areas, and with nursing, is not addressed. Rather, the posited changes are presented as undisputed facts whose interdependence is seemingly self-evident. No critical insight into the dynamics of society is offered. Indeed their presentation as common-sense knowledge seemingly negates the need for critical reflection on their existence and on the need for nursing to respond to them. As Weedon (1987) explains, 'Commonsense consists of a number of social meanings and the particular ways of understanding the world which guarantee them. These meanings...become fixed and widely accepted as true irrespective of sectional interests'.

Nursing is thus presented in the curricula as being located in an environment whose needs are changing. Nursing's response is one of adaptation, to assist in meeting the existing and emergent needs through the production of graduates who are able to fulfill new requisite functions and be adaptable. Such language promotes conformity at all levels, demanding an uncritical acceptance of change—initiated elsewhere—with a corresponding demand on nurses to accommodate to it.

The nature of nursing is also informed by discourses of professionalism and caring. Such understandings are equally depoliticized with regard to the context of practice, its content, and the process of practice; that is, power, as a relationship, is not implicated. At the level of practice, contexts such as the community or the family are taken as given; conceptualized within functional consensus frameworks within which the nurse is located. Practice is principally located in an interpersonal context—in other words the occupation of nursing is reduced to an interpersonal nexus in which the nurse and client are the main actors. As Crawford (1980) notes in his ideology critique of health care occupations '...the social context is most often reduced to the immediate context of interpersonal relations and "psychological atmospheres"'. This transformation is accompanied by the reduction of the occupation of nursing to the nurse. This is evident in each text: to talk of nursing is to talk of the nurse. Other health care personnel, for example the physiotherapist or dietician, are not identified as relevant to the context, content, or process of the encounter.

Nurse

The subject position of the nurse within this individualized and personalized environment is constituted by notions of professionalism and caring. Both discourses variously contribute to understandings of the content and process dimensions of the practitioner role. As a professional the nurse is portrayed as occupying a position of autonomy and equity vis-a-vis her interactions with other health care professionals. Notions of collegiality and teamwork signify a departure from her former status of subservience and dependence. Interaction with the recipient of nursing care is also described in a language of equity, the word client denoting her/his acquisition of decision-making power, formerly denied to the patient. Indeed the use of the label recipient is questionable since the nurse is regarded as a facilitator, her role being to assist the client to make decisions rather than to promote the patient's compliance to pre-empted decisions. This role is based on an understanding of nurse/client difference which reflects the nurse's unique possession of health care knowledge and skills. Such notions are presented in the curricula as undisputed commonsense knowledge about the attributes and practices of a professional nurse.

Notions of care also constitute the subject position of nurse. Care, whilst signifying the humanistic rather than scientific processes of nursing, denotes those activities or skills of interpersonal caring. The concept of care is operationalized as a series of concrete acts or steps, the discursive practices of the caring nurse. These are termed the nursing process. The concept of process is thus reified as a prescriptive set of steps (those of assessment, planning, implementation, and evaluation) through which the professional, caring nurse progresses in order to resolve an identified health problem. The subsequent transformation of this process tool into care-plans further reveals the creation of a seemingly new language of practice, but one which is based on the orthodoxy of scientific premises. As such it does not signify a radical departure from traditional medical discourse, and potentially locks the practitioner into a prescriptive, linear mode of practice. Within this discursive context, care as a process of practice is not incorporated in a gender specific discourse. The subject position of the caring nurse is hence made available to the male since its connotation of being an unnatural male role is removed.

The implications of the nursing process discourse for teaching practices are significant, but are concealed by an acceptance of the discourse of teacher as neutral facilitator. However, the process discourse may function as a discourse of management, structuring relations between teacher and student as teaching practice becomes focused on the accurate delineation of the process stages or on the development of care plans. This interpretation is suggested by studies of problem-solving in secondary school subjects (Singh 1988, Unger 1989). This research suggests that this process approach to problem-solving denies students access to knowledge derived from their own experience whilst the empiricist analysis it entails excludes the possibility that differently informed questions would be asked and be appropriately explored. As a discourse of care, the nursing process effectively removes the immediate context of practice from concern.

Client

As indicated earlier the discourses of professionalism and caring imply that the client is an equal partner in the health care team with input in the process of care, albeit appropriately structured by the expert nurse. Nurse/client interaction is understood in terms of communication processes devoid of political intent. This negation of power is compounded by the discourse of individual rights which represents the client as a person with ultimate freedom of choice and autonomy of action, whose rights of self-determination and individual responsibility must be acknowledged and respected. The assumptions underlying these notions are unquestioned, their endorsement seemingly unquestionable. Abstraction of the client from her/his social context is also implicit in the notion of the client's uniqueness, her/his holistic essence. This stress on individual difference exhorts the nurse to conceptualize and care for clients as discrete, isolatable entities: the social construction of their subjectivity is effectively denied.

Health

Assumptions of individual responsibility and autonomy, encapsulated in the concept of self-help, underlie the notions of health which inform the curricula. Health is extended beyond the disease-illhealth/health dichotomy to encompass the notion of wellness. The state of well-being is evidenced behaviourally. A relative lack of wellness arises when the person engages in behaviour which is dysfunctional for the attainment of prescribed human needs deemed essential for optimal wellness. Such behaviours are termed risk-taking, with the probability of illness increasing if this type of behaviour is sustained. The nurse is charged with facilitating the requisite change in the client's lifestyle. The imperative to change thus lies with the client as does the ultimate right of choice. The dominance of empiricism is further suggested by an emphasis on the meaning of health as self-control, the ability to stop engaging in negative behaviours and the degree of control a person exhibits being measurable in terms of her/his discrepancy from the norm. Nursing research informed by this conception of health will follow the scientific method of causation determination and measurement. Crawford (1980) indicates that health may be interpreted to mean release, that is the opposite of control with an emphasis on the attainment of emotional well-being. This approach suggests the relevance of qualitative approaches for the assessment of a client's level of wellness, albeit marginalized by the seemingly more objective approach.

Assumptions regarding the location of health and its treatment suggest that the discourses of health in these basic curricula do not constitute a radical departure from the biomedical discourse. Health remains located at the level of the individual in terms of both its causation and resolution. Whilst the person's social/cultural context may be identified as an element in her/his environment, this social variable is transformed into an aspect of her/his lifestyle (Pearson 1986). Social dimensions of health, such as class, gender, age, or ethnicity, are negated by their reduction to issues of individual preference or choice (Crawford 1984). Health remains privatized, medicalized, and devoid of political meaning (Tesh 1988).

THE FUTURE OF THE DISCIPLINE

This exploration of the constitution of nursing knowledge suggests that the emerging discipline of nursing is shaped by the discourses of scientism and professionalism. These discourses have informed the processes of its development and the content of its knowledge base. Nursing research for example, has been conducted primarily in an empiricist tradition, based on the premise that subsequent theoretical formulations should guide practice. Tertiary-based programs hence produce graduates whose practice has been developed within these perspectives. Furthermore the analysis suggests that the traditional knowledge base of nursing practice has not been replaced, but rather has been modified and developed. The lifestyle discourse of health for example, incorporates the empiricism and rationalism of the bio-medical discourse; health remains privatized and medicalized.

Strategies for achieving change within the health care arena implied by mainstream contemporary nursing theory hence do not constitute a radical departure from previous approaches. Efforts directed at achieving change in a client's behaviour based on the assumption that an appropriately informed person will alter her/his risk-taking activity, fail to acknowledge the social constitution of the person's knowledge and practices. A client's subjectivity or identity is multidimensional, being a product of the many positions made available in the discourses she/he accesses. Behavioural change is hence not simply an issue of altered cognition, for the individual is constituted and so governed by discourse. Change must therefore be directed towards the alteration of some aspect of the discursive context in which the individual is located. As Crawford (1980) points out, whilst interventions informed by notions of cognitive rationality may overcome a client's specific deficit, it cannot be assumed that any resultant change will be sustained or that the client will have the skills pertinent to the achievement of change in other areas of her/his life which affect health. The development of such skills would be predicated on a discourse, or frame of reference, which asserts their need; such discourses are not dominant in contemporary nursing texts.

The knowledge which constitutes or informs nursing texts is revealed as neither innovative nor intrinsically different to that which previously informed practice. These assertions derive from an acknowledgement that nursing, nurses, and clients are located in networks of power relations. These relations of power shape the perspectives in which these social entities are located, and these in turn sustain the relevant power relations. Hence not only must issues of theoretical or practical interest in nursing be contextualized, the context itself must be politicized. The power relations involved in nurse/client interaction, for example, need to be identified and interaction conceptualized as in terms of their dynamics. A discourse of communication concerned principally with verbal and non-verbal skills is thus seen to sustain the dominant position of the nurse by effectively denying her dominance. The client's perception of the nurse's power, however, shapes the client's pattern of communication. A critical discourse of communication which addresses the interdependence of power, discourse, and subjectivity would generate interventions which entail these dimensions, including a restructuring of the prevailing power relations. Such a discourse informs the practices of critical researchers who reject the notion of an objective, neutral researcher.

The development of nursing knowledge has been explored in terms of the appropriation of knowledge generated in other discipines, such as medicine. In this process the new, introduced elements, are recontextualized within the existing dominant discourses. This process may transform them, altering their meaning and so perhaps destroying their critical potential. New developments such as care plans may thus contain the very elements or pocesses against which their development was aimed.

The discourses which dominate the content of contemporary nursing knowledge are those of scientism and professionalism. These have shaped the central concepts of nursing theory: the nurse, the client, health, and the environment. Nursing is understood to be practised in an interpersonal context in which the problematic issues are those of effective interaction/communication between the nurse and client. Curricula and the educative process are also informed by the dominant discourses; they are conceptualized as unbiased neutral tools and processes. Knowledge and power are not viewed as necessarily linked. An analysis which assumes a mutually constitutive relationship between knowledge and power reveals the conservative character of contemporary nursing knowledge. Its discourses offer no challenge to relations of power prevailing between occupational groups or individuals involved in the provision of health care. Their continued endorsement and/or uncritical modification will ensure that nursing will not have a dramatic, new or radical impact on health care.

The potential for challenge does, however, exist in any discourse for discourses are not coherent, unified, closed systems. They contain spaces within which challenges can be, and are made as people oppose some aspect of the context in which they are located. Hence nurse administrators, clinicians, and educators continually generate oppositional discourses as they reject and attempt to change some aspect of their work environment. However, unless they are informed by discourses which acknowledge power relations, the strategies of change they develop and employ can have minimal impact. The possibility of such action is, moreover, questionable since critical discourses of nursing are marginal and marginalized—evident in curricula as elective subjects or subjects/units of relatively minor weight. Given the social constitution of health, clients, and nurses, the generation of alternate nursing discourses is imperative, but their development must proceed with caution. The constitutive power of new discourses (their languages and concomitant practices), must be explored prior to their adoption. For they may sustain, rather than challenge, the status quo albeit framed within new concepts and terminology which has a nursing flavour.

If nursing knowledge is to produce practices which do challenge the prevailing status quo, implicit assumptions of theoretical neutrality and objectivity must be exposed and challenged. Tesh's (1988) concern for public discussion about the assumptions which should guide the formulation of health policy is indeed pertinent: 'There is no science uninfluenced by politics. This is a plea to get the politics out of hiding'. Nurses concerned with the development of the discipline of nursing should heed this plea.

REFERENCES

Angus L B 1986 Research traditions, ideology and critical ethnography. Discourse 7(1): 61-77
Battersby D, Hemmings L 1990 Grounded theory in nursing. Paper presented at Nursing Research in Action Conference, Adelaide
Benner P, Wrubel J 1989 The primacy of caring. Addison-Wesley, Menlo Park
Bernstein B 1986 On pedagogic discourse. In: Richardson J G (ed) Handbook of theory and research for the sociology of education. Greenland Press, London
Bruni N 1985 The professionalization of nursing. Unpublished M.Ed. Studies Thesis. Monash University, Melbourne
Bruni N 1989 Self-help, health promotion and change: a question of compatibility. Paper presented at the 11th National Royal College of Nursing, Australia Conference, Perth
Bruni N 1990 Holistic nursing curricula: towards a reconstruction of health and nursing. Unicorn 6(2):100-108
Chenitz W C, Swanson J M 1986 From practice to grounded theory. Addison Wesley, Menlo Park
Crawford R 1980 Healthism and the medicalization of everyday life. International Journal of Health Sciences 10(3):365-388
Crawford R 1984 A cultural account of 'health': control, release and the social body. In: McKinlay J B (ed) Issues in the political economy of Health Care. Tavistock, New York
Dalley G 1988 Ideologies of caring. Macmillan, London
Dingwall R, Lewis P 1983 (eds) The sociology of the professions. Macmillan, London
Dunlop M 1988 Science and caring—are they compatible? Shaping nursing theory and practice: the Australian context. Monograph 1. Lincoln Department of Nursing, La Trobe University, Melbourne

Dzurec L C 1989 The necessity for and evolution of multiple paradigms for nursing research: a poststructuralist perspective. Advances in Nursing Science 11(4):69-77

Friedson E 1983 The theory of professions: state of the art. In: Dingwall R, Lewis P (eds) The sociology of the professions. Macmillan, London

Game A, Pringle R 1983 Gender at work. Allen & Unwin, Sydney

Gardner H, McCoppin B 1989 Emerging militancy? The politicization of Australian allied health professions. In: Gardner H (ed) The politics of health: the Australian experience. Churchill Livingstone, Melbourne

Gitlin A, Seigel M, Boru K 1989 The politics of method: from leftist ethnography to educative research. Qualitative Studies in Education 2(3):237-253

Hagell E 1988 Nursing and science: a critical analysis. Paper presented at Pathways to Progress Conference, University of Wales College of Medicine, Cardiff

Henriques J, Holloway W, Urwin C, Venn C, Walkerdine V 1984 Changing the subject. Methuen, London

Jenkins E 1989 Nurses' control over nursing. In: Gray G, Pratt R (eds) Issues in Australian nursing 2. Churchill Livingstone, Melbourne

Lather P 1986 Issues of validity in openly ideological research: between a rock and a soft place. Interchange 17(4):63-84

Lather P 1989 Postmodernism and the politics of enlightenment. Educational Foundations (Fall):7-28

Maloney M M 1986 Professionalization of nursing: current issues and trends. Lippincott, Philadelphia

Marles F 1988 Report of the Study of Professional Issues in Nursing. Government Printer, Melbourne

Opie A 1989 Qualitative methodology, deconstructive readings, appropriation of 'other' and empowerment. Paper presented at TASA Anual Conference, La Trobe University, Melbourne

Pearson M 1986 Racist notions of ethnicity and culture in health education. In: Rodmell S, Watt A (eds) The politics of health education: raising the issues. Routledge & Kegan Paul, London

Retsas A 1988 Towards a dialectic understanding of nursing. Shaping nursing theory and practice: the Australian context. Monograph 1. Lincoln Department of Nursing, La Trobe University, Melbourne

Richman J 1987 Medicine and health. Longman, London

Singh P 1988 Computer education: recontextualizing the information processing model of learning. Paper presented at Australian Association for Research in Education, University of New England, Armidale

Speedy S 1987 Feminism and the professionalization of nursing. Australian Journal of Advanced Nursing 4(2):20-28

Speedy S 1990 Never mind the width, feel the quality. Paper presented at the Nursing Research in Action Conference, Adelaide

Tesch S N 1988 Hidden arguments: political ideology and disease prevention policy. Rutgers, New Brunswick

Turner B S 1987 Medical power and social knowledge. Sage, London

Unger Z 1989 Ideological bias in school texts: discourse theory to the rescue. Paper presented at the TASA Annual Conference, La Trobe University, Melbourne

Weedon C 1987 Feminist practice and post-structuralist theory. Blackwell, Oxford

Weeks J 1982 Foucault for historians. History Workshop 14(3) 106-119

Willis E 1989 Medical dominance. Allen & Unwin, Sydney

Young C E 1987 Intuition and nursing process. Holistic Nursing Practice 1(3):52-62

9. The contribution of feminist research

Sandra Speedy

INTRODUCTION

Nursing has a history of shunning the principles of feminism. Or has it? Explicit feminism appears to have been rejected by all but a few nurses. Nevertheless, an examination of the concepts which are currently guiding the development of nursing and nursing knowledge suggest that feminist principles, whilst not necessary recognized as such, are becoming more and more influential. This augurs well for the development of the discipline of nursing because feminist principles are congruent with those principles espoused by nurses today, including the ethic of care, nurturing, the centrality of the patient or client, the dialectical relationship between carers and cared for, and a healthy questioning of the appropriateness of traditional 'scientific'modes of thinking and research. The discipline of nursing is thus developing along, if not a parallel track, then one which is incorporating principles within its knowledge base which are surprisingly feminist.

This chapter will consider the value of the contribution of feminist research to nursing research and practice, recognizing the centrality of caring as integral to nursing. It is necessary first to examine understandings of feminist research. Feminist research is research guided by an understanding of feminism and feminist principles. Before addressing the issue of feminist research and its contribution to nursing research and practice it is necessary to comment briefly on feminism and the principles on which feminist research rests.

FEMINISM AND FEMINIST PRINCIPLES

Feminism involves an active desire to change women's position in society and is a social movement which works towards these changes. 'It is the way of thinking created by, for, and on behalf of women, as "gender-specific". Women are its subjects, its enunciators, the creators of its theory, of its practice and of its language' (Mitchell & Oakley 1986). The major tenets of feminist theory include (Stanley & Wise, 1983) a number of beliefs, as follows.

Women are oppressed

The experience of female oppression is the *raison d'être* of feminist theory and feminist research approaches. However, there is no unanimity in the women's movement or in feminist theory as to the causes of the oppression of women. Consequently, there is no one view or approach which we can call feminist research. When the historical development and transformation of feminist theory over the past 50 years is considered, four major orientations are apparent:

- *Radical feminism* holds that gender exploitation is the original and most profound form of exploitation and is the archetype of all oppression;
- *Socialist feminism* views gender, racial and class oppression as varying but related manifestations of capitalist economic exploitation;
- *Liberal feminism* maintains that barriers to women's liberation can be eliminated without changing the economic structure and those changes can occur within 'the system' through reform and education;
- *Cultural feminism* is a separatist position that maintains that women cannot achieve liberation in a patriarchal culture; liberation can only occur within a matrifocal culture (Eisenstein 1984).

Each of these orientations differs in its explanations about the causes of female oppression. As a result they all espouse alternative approaches to women-centred analysis, to the social construction of inequality, and to the means by which social justice (through social change) can be achieved.

No matter what 'type' of feminism one adheres to, there is a common acceptance that women are oppressed. The oppression of women is a fact, is undeniable, but is able to be changed. This oppression has negative consequences for everyone in society, including children and men, because while in the 'sexual political system...men are in some sense women's oppressors...they are themselves oppressed by their own status as oppressors' (Stanley & Wise 1983).

The personal is political

A second tenet of feminist theory is captured in the phrase 'the personal is political'. This phrase refers to the fact that 'every aspect of our personal circumstances as women, and as nurses, grows out of, and creates, larger political realities in the world' (Chinn 1989). The concept embraces a number of issues. It relates to the experience of oppression, which is a shared experience among women. For feminists, personal experiences cannot be invalidated because they are 'personal'; if they can be felt, they are real. This necessitates rejection of 'objective reality' interpreted from a masculinist perspective because it '...denies validity to women's understandings of women's experiences, because they are "merely" subjective, rooted in the particular' (Stanley & Wise 1983).

In essence, 'the personal is political' refers to the fact that power and its use can be examined from the standpoint of women's personal lives, whether these are affected by the economy, family relationships, or social systems in general.

Consciousness-raising

The third tenet of feminist theory involves the concept of consciousness-raising. Through the process of consciousness-raising, women learn to perceive the world in a different way; they move from a masculinist perspective to one that is feminist. This means that...'women's understandings...are transformed so that we see, understand and feel them in a new and quite different way, at the same time as we see them in the "old" way' (Stanley & Wise 1983).

This 'double vision' of reality, and women's experience of it, is central to the consciousness-raising process as it exposes the contradictions present in life. It also sensitizes and heightens women's awareness to the social construction of meaning. Consciousness-raising is therefore 'based on knowledge rather than some form of personal insight or psychological "high"' (McCormack 1981).

These theoretical 'givens' are the premises on which feminist research methodological principles are based. Provided this research methodology takes account of the tenets cited above, it can be categorized as feminist. It should be noted here that other authors, in particular Cook & Fonow (1986) include two additional central characteristics of feminist methodology. These are: concern with ethical issues and an emphasis on empowerment and transformation. A key element with respect to ethical issues is the use of language which perpetuates women's oppression and subordination. Another is professional gate-keeping practices, 'particularly those which prevent publication and dissemination of feminist research' (Cook & Fonow 1986), but also those practices which influence topic selection, research funding, hiring of personnel, promotion, and tenure. Other ethical dilemmas include intervention in respondents' lives and the question of withholding needed information from women subjects (Webb 1984, Oakley 1981). Empowerment and transformation will be addressed in a later section, but it is noted here that the object of generating information and knowledge is to create alternatives to oppression.

THE CONCEPT OF FEMINIST RESEARCH

There are diverse views of what constitutes feminist research. Kelly (1978) states that research is feminist if it is undertaken for feminist reasons. This means that, regardless of the approach (whether empiricist, interpretive, or critical), the research is feminist providing it is driven by feminist principles.

Although acknowledging the importance and appropriateness of a feminist research approach, Kelly warns of the dangers of rejecting human attributes if what are sometimes viewed as 'masculine' attributes are considered unacceptable guides to research. She states that '[r]ationality and objectivity, the ability to reflect on our actions, are important human attributes, which can be seen as the fullest development of our intellectual capabilities, and we should not lightly disown them'.

Lather (1987) suggests that '...to do feminist research is to put the social construction of gender at the center of one's inquiry'. This requires gender to become the organizing principle of research, whose ideological goal is to 'correct the invisibility and the distortion of female experience'. The ultimate aim is to alter the unequal social position of women in society. This is a view similar to that of Klein (1983), who defines feminist research as that which takes '...women's needs, interests and experience into account and aims at being instrumental in improving women's lives in one way or another'.

Spender (1976) argues that feminist research must question the whole basis of knowledge in our culture and rejects the accepted male definitions of 'good', 'poor', 'relevant', or 'irrelevant' knowledge. Stanley & Wise (1983) agree, and maintain that feminist research explores the bases of the everyday lives of women using feminist principles. They insist that 'feminist social science must begin with the recognition that the personal lived-experience underlies all behaviours and actions'. This requires that women must 're-claim, name and re-name [their] experience and thus [their] knowledge' of the social world which they inhabit (Stanley & Wise 1983). The present world is conceptualized from a perspective that is male derived and hence distorted for women in society.

Feminist research can also be conceived of as multiparadigmatic. As Lather (1987) suggests, feminist empirical efforts are by no means the only approach to feminist research. While some efforts operate out of a traditional positivist paradigm, others are guided by an interpretive or a critical social science approach. For example, a statistical survey on the frequency of endometrial cancer in women over the age of thirty represents an 'empiricist' piece of feminist research. An 'interpretive' study could examine the meanings that women attach to menopause. Feminist research that explores women's construction of the birthing experience with the aim of creating changes preferred by these women can be classified as following a 'critical' research approach.

There is not 'one' feminist research methodology. What is held in common however, is that feminist scholarship, and hence research, seeks to address women's lives and experiences in their own terms, which requires that theory be grounded in the actual experiences and language of women (du Bois 1983). This requires the adoption of a woman-centred approach, in order to discover and uncover the actual facts of women's lives and experiences. These facts have, in the past, been inaccessible, distorted, misunderstood, and ignored. It is only in recent times that feminist researchers have begun to observe, name, and describe the experiences and realities of women.

The feminist literature debates the issue of research *on* women and research *for* women (for example, Duffy 1985). Research *for* women tries to take account of women's needs and interests, and endeavours to improve women's lives in some way. It 'struggles with the political realities in research and society' (Duffy 1985). Stanley & Wise (1983) are adamant that feminist research specifically *on* women, that aims to increase the volume of knowledge about women, should not be confined to this; it must be concerned with all aspects of social reality, and all participants in it. However, they emphasize that research *by* women is 'absolutely fundamental to feminist research'. This leads them to the position that men cannot be feminists because they cannot possess a 'feminist consciousness'. This consciousness is '....rooted in the concrete, practical and everyday experiences of being, and being treated as, *a woman*' (Stanley & Wise 1983). The implication here is that feminist research can never be conducted by men, because they are bereft of a feminist consciousness. This prevents them from viewing reality in the way women do. This type of logic implies that women cannot understand men either, since men view reality differently. If we accept the basic paradigm inherent in critical theory (derived as it is from male thinking) and analyze it using a feminist perspective, we ought to be able to increase our levels of shared understanding of both women and men. This entails constructing a view of what it might be like to experience the existence and reality of the opposite sex. Whilst this does not necesssarily result in a feminist consciousness, it may lead to the development of shared meanings across female-male boundaries.

Returning to the question of who can conduct feminist research, as alluded to above, Kelly (1978) proposes that as long as research is undertaken for feminist reasons, it can be done by anyone adhering to feminist principles. Bernard (1973) suggests that only those persons who can move out of the androcentric definition of society—those who have had their consciousness raised in relation to feminism—can conduct feminist research. This would not appear to exclude either gender.

Calloway (1981) argues for feminist research to shift the centre from which knowledge is generated, by looking at *human* experience from the *point of view* of women. This, she asserts, would deepen understanding of the whole of human experience—both female and male, and embue the whole of cultural history with greater depth. This view is problematic for some feminists who adhere strongly to the principle of centralizing women and their experiences within the research. In fact, if women and their experiences are not central, then the research is not, by definition, feminist. However, she does assert that '...before women could develop new directions evolving from female experience, we have had to take a critical stance against the dominant models of scholarship which place male at the centre and female as peripheral and which confer on males the powers to define and interpret not only themselves, but females as well'.

These are some of the issues that occupy feminist researchers. Closely linked to these issues is the question of traditional research methodologies, and the limitations these impose on alternative forms of research.

LIMITATIONS OF TRADITIONAL SOCIAL SCIENCE RESEARCH METHODOLOGY

Many feminists reject the idea that traditional research methods are appropriate for research on and for women. Because it builds on a 'consensual (patriarchal) construction of reality', positivist-empiricist research is unacceptable to feminists (du Bois 1983). She continues, asserting that 'feminist science-making withdraws consent from given constructions of what is to be known and how. We reject dichotomies between science and the maker of science, between observation and experience; we reject the idea that the task of science is to examine a given, fixed reality of which we are observers, not participants'.

Critical social theory is concerned with enlightenment and emancipation, and with transformation from oppressive conditions. The relationship of feminism to critical theory is readily apparent. As Lather (1987) points out, in feminist inquiry '...empowering methods, including dialogue and reflexivity, contribute to consciousness-raising and transformative social action'. Clearly, what the Frankfurt School sought to achieve was to transform the society of 'man', without changing the paradigm of 'man-is-the-norm' (Klein 1983). Androcentricity being the norm, feminists now need to do the work for women the Frankfurt School has, and is doing, for men. Klein continues, indicating that a 'feminist approach to knowledge, however, defines as an indispensable prerequisite women's right to a place among those who create and transmit knowledge on our terms and meeting our needs'.

This cannot be done unless there are marked changes to the approach taken in research. Some of these changes will now be indicated. It should be noted that there are many male researchers who also hold the view that positivist research, in particular, is limiting and inappropriate for many kinds of research. This view is therefore not confined to feminist researchers.

Traditional ways of doing research are masculine ways, which treat the male as the norm, as the recognized frame of reference for all human beings. It is often assumed that results obtained from male-only samples can be generalized to women. Furthermore, examination of the mainstream social science research literature indicates that women have been either ignored or are invisible. They have been effectively excluded from male culture. Often their experiences have been distorted and misinterpreted. In fact, the '...androcentric perspective of social science has rendered women not only unknown, but virtually unknowable' (du Bois 1983).

It is just these deficits that feminists wish to alter. Klein (1983) argues that feminist research will enable feminists to name their paradigm. This is empowering, as it works towards legitimizing the process and the outcomes. Traditional research methodologies which do not focus on women or treat their experiences as valid cannot achieve this.

Traditional research claims to be assumption and value-free. It claims to be rational, objective, replicable, and generalizable. Most feminist research-ers (and others) do not believe it is possible, or appropriate, to do research in this way. They point out that science and research involve naming and framing the questions, selecting the methodology, and interpreting the results. These are all expressive of a dominant culture, conveyed via a language which is frequently masculinist. Experimental research is typically isolated in a clinical laboratory in order to 'objectify' and 'neutralize' outcomes. Feminist researchers assert that this denies social and contextual factors, 'stripping them of the very complexity that characterises the real world' (Parlee 1979). This 'context-stripping' is ahistorical and acultural. It denies the grounding of an individual's experience in reality, and relation-ships between individuals. Researchers are forced to deny the basic human-ness of their subjects so that 'objectivity' is attained. Feminist researchers believe that there is no simple separation possible between the 'researcher' and 'subject'—or the 'knower' and 'known' (du Bois 1983).

Traditional or empiricist researchers counterclaim that feminist research-ers are biased, subjective, and heavily ideological. Feminists agree that their work rests on feminist principles and that they reject the subject/object dichotomy. But they claim to apply rigor and honesty to their work. As Webb (1984) points out, feminist research is scientific in terms different from 'objective science'. It is reflexive, honest, and rigorous in that it takes gender into account, and insists on examining the experience and existence of women. She adds that the 'only way of knowing a socially constructed world is by knowing it from within, and all research methods use the researcher's consciousness as an instrument of data collection and analysis, usually without acknowledging and facing up to this'.

This counterclaim (of bias and subjectivity) raises an important issue which has been hotly debated by feminists. Some feminists who reject traditional research methods simply because they are masculine argue for the development of new research techniques. They reject objectivity and rationality because these characterize the traditional approach. They em-brace subjectivity and personal experience because they are characteristics of feminism. Both Kelly (1978) (noted above) and Keller (1980) view this as a dangerous and inappropriate way to proceed. By rejecting all masculine defined research, Keller argues that we subvert the aim of a feminist critique of science. She points out that we affirm the definitions of masculine and feminine imposed on us by the patriarchal culture (that is, masculine as objective and scientific; feminine as anti-scientific and subjective). Two outcomes are then likely. First, 'we run the risk of romanticizing the feminization of women's culture' (Keller 1980), and second, it changes nothing, leaving 'masculine science' to men. In fact, it '...invites scientists to cease worrying about the possible ambiguity of their definitions, criteria, etc. and permits the return of a monolithic definition of science—as objectivist, as instrumentalist, and as masculine'.

Keller concludes her argument with the observation that the characterization of feminine as opposite to rationality and objectivity is dangerous and confusing. She warns feminists that this approach will promote 'the return of a monolithic definition of science' (Keller 1980). McCormack (1981) promotes the view that empiricism is the major problem faced by feminists. She states that 'it is not the malevolence of man but the malevolence of method that constitutes the true obstacle [and] that if the majority of social scientists were women the situation would not be significantly different'.

Lather (1986a), while committed to the examination and development of new research paradigms, argues for greater systematization in establishing the trustworthiness of data. She asserts that failure to develop accountability in methodology and data analysis will jeopardize attempts at new theory building and 'will not improve the chances for the increased legitimacy of the knowledge they produce'. Lather's discussion focuses on the development of minimal standards for 'ideological research', issues that cannot be ignored by feminist researchers.

FEMINIST RESEARCH METHODOLOGY

Lather (1987) asserts that feminist research is multiparadigmatic because it can operate out of a variety of research paradigms, providing it is based on feminist principles. She adds that some feminist research uses 'a conventional, positivist paradigm, [while] an increasing amount operates out of a critical, praxis-oriented paradigm concerned with both producing emancipatory knowledge and empowering the researched'.

Few feminists argue for a distinctive feminist methodology, although one noted feminist researcher, Reinharz (1983) argues for the adoption of a particular mode, known as 'experiential analysis'. This methodology seeks 'an alternative set of assumptions from the objectivist mainstream morality-methodology, and stemming from perceived contradictions of inadequacies in certain research methods...'. Reinharz proceeds to articulate the method involved in experiential analysis which she views as a collection of interacting components. These components are: examination of assumptions, personal preparation, problem formulation, data gathering and stopping, data digestion and presentation, and policy questions. Most feminist researchers however, argue for flexibility, for 'methodological borrowing' (Cook 1982), and the development and refinement of new and varying methods of collecting data.

Cook & Fonow (1986) discuss a range of creative and innovative feminist research methodologies that may be adopted, depending on the situation being studied. Feminist methodology does, however, incorporate three interrelated aspects. These are: a dialectical relationship between subject and object of research, a concept known as intersubjectivity; the centrality of women and their experiences; and the perception of contradictions and subsequent transformative action. These will be briefly elaborated upon.

Intersubjectivity

This refers to the dialectical relationship between subject and object of research, discussed by Westkott (1979). Intersubjectivity refers to the dialectical relationship between subject and object. Klein (1983) supports this view, elaborating that intersubjectivity allows the researcher to '...compare her work with her own experiences as a woman and a scientist and to share it with the researched'. It requires that the researcher and the subject be regarded as having the same status as participants or collaborators in the research. This necessitates 'subjects' being involved in considering the moral and political implications of the research, which in turn creates an obligation to maintain honesty between researcher and researched. For the feminist researcher and subject there is active participation in the actions, movements and struggles for women's emancipation. This is neatly summarized by Lather (1986a) when she comments that the 'methodological task is to proceed in a reciprocal, dialogic manner, empowering subjects by turning them into co-researchers'.

In summary, feminist research recognizes the subjectivity of the researcher and the researched and denies the possibility and value of 'anonymity, impersonality, detachment, impartiality and objectivity' (Webb 1984), which characterizes a traditional, empirical approach.

Centrality of women and their experiences

This refers to the fact that women's experiences are examined and regarded as valid for study. The process by which this occurs has three major components. First, it involves reflexive and self-reflective thinking by both researcher and researched. Second, there is analysis of events and experiences through immersion in the data. Third, interpretation of realities must occur. This process clearly demonstrates the importance of the slogan, 'the personal is political'. Adherence to a critical theory paradigm also requires subsequent transformative action to be taken.

Perception of contradictions and action

This refers to the fact that the feminist research process must result in the perception of contradictions. Inherent in the realization of contradictions is the potential for empowerment. This is followed by subsequent action against the perceived oppressive elements of reality. For Cook & Fonow (1986) this means that 'research must be designed to provide a vision for the future as well as a structural picture of the present'.

One method by which this can be achieved is by the study of women's individual and social history. Mies (1983), for example, suggests some methodological postulates for feminist research. These include a recognition of conscious partiality, achieved through partial identification with the researched; adopting a systematic 'view from below' to avoid domination of the researched; active participation in actions, movements and struggles; the 'conscientization' of both researchers and researched; subsequent problem-formulating methodology accompanied by the study of women; and the collectivization of women's experiences.

These postulates led Mies to an applied methodology which was then tested on an action group known as 'Women Help Women' in Cologne in 1976-1977. This grew out of an initiative responding to violence against women in the family as a campaign was begun to help women find shelter from brutality in their families. The procedure was as follows:

1. An initial meeting of women was held and a position paper drafted which asked social welfare for a 'safe house'.
2. Social welfare replied that a 'safe house' was unnecessary; the group was told to do a survey and develop a case for what was needed. The group could not afford an expensive survey.
3. The group organized a street action with posters, photos of battered women, newspaper clippings, and signatures collected from passers-by about the need for a women's house for battered women. At the same time, people who came to their stand were interviewed about their experiences and their views of wife-beating; this provided initial data for the study.
4. The street action was published in the press which the municipal authorities found hard to ignore; women responded to the publicity and began to ask the group for help. Social welfare were forced to conduct their own study and uncovered a large and increasing need. A suitable house was found and the government provided a subsidy.

Mies (1983) points out that the problem had to be 'created'; there had to be a challenge to the status quo and persuasion that in fact there was a problem. The study also indicated that there had to be partial and egalitarian involvement of all participants. In addition, there was discussion and 'socialization' which formed the basis of raising women's consciousness as a starting point for emancipatory action. This methodology was effective in that it produced a sought-after outcome. It demonstrates the importance of 'grounding inquiry in concrete experience rather than in abstract categories [and reflects] women's historical identification with the concrete, everyday life of people and their survival needs' (Weskott 1979).

Feminist research: a summary

Having surveyed in some detail the characteristics and principles of feminist research and the varying positions adopted by feminist researchers, the following summary is offered.

There are three major principles inherent in feminist belief systems which inform feminist research. These include: recognition of the fact that women are oppressed, which necessitates an examination of the reasons for oppression, in order that changes be made; the personal is political, which acknowledges and accepts the value of women's experiences; and consciousness-raising, which results in alternative views of the world from a women's perspective. These three principles inform feminist research.

Feminist research is characterized by a variety of methodological stances, conceptual approaches and strategies, but must be based on the feminist principles indicated above. The methodology may embrace all types of research requiring reason and it has three characteristics. The first characteristic described was intersubjectivity, and it was noted that subject and researcher were in a dialectical relationship during the research process. This involves rejection of the notion of 'total objectivity' and distancing of researcher and researched. The second characteristic of feminist research methodology was the centrality of women and their experiences. As Lather (1987) notes: 'to do feminist research is to put the social construction of gender at the center of one's inquiry'. This means that gender is the basic organizing principle.

The third characteristic of feminist research methodology was the perception of contradiction and action as a research outcome. Once contradictions are noted, empowerment is achieved, and action can then be taken. This corrects the invisibility and the distortion of female experience in ways relevant to ending women's unequal social position. Feminist research derives from an ideology, which creates difficulties for 'traditional' researchers. However, it is an ideological underpinning that is rigorous and valid, as well as imperative for women's research and nursing research.

A FEMINIST PERSPECTIVE ON NURSING RESEARCH, THE ROLE OF CARING IN NURSING PRACTICE AND THE DEVELOPMENT OF NURSING THEORY

But what of the connections between feminist research, nursing research, the concept of caring in nursing practice, and the development of nursing theory?

Nursing research

It is a commonly held belief about feminist research that it is concerned with and confined to researching women's issues, and in the context of nursing, women's health. Obviously, a major and vital role is fulfilled by adopting a feminist research perspective when researching women's issues and health. But feminist principles can also offer an alternative paradigm to the dominant patriarchal view when addressing nursing theory and practice issues, as they allow for the examination of human experience from the perspective of and for women. This is of immense value in itself, but also equips nurses with the knowledge, and hence the potential, to develop deeper understandings of female/male experience and our combined socio-cultural history.

A literature search reveals that very little nursing research is informed by feminist theory. Further, very little nursing research addresses the health concerns of women. Dunbar et al (1981) reviewed the major nursing research journals for the period 1970 to 1979 and found that only 19% of 371 nursing research reports related to women. More than half of these studies addressed the maternal role of women, rather than other health related issues. The authors express concern that nursing has 'followed a disease-oriented focus in selecting problems of critical inquiry' (Dunbar et al 1981), and stress the importance of nursing in examining its role as a contributor of knowledge about women. They conclude by recommending that 'nursing [as a profession composed largely of women] should take the lead in the critical investigation of women's health for establishing a sound theoretical basis for practice'.

In a later study, Bernhard (1984) reviewed 90 reports published in '*Nursing Research*' during the years 1962-1967 and 1977-1982 to establish whether any of these were feminist in nature. Using eight criteria, no study could be so categorized. The author reporting this study (Duffy 1985) expresses major concerns at this finding. She notes that when 'feminist research is not conducted or published, potential knowledge is lost. What remains is the knowledge developed in the traditions of male science [which] biases the data that influence decisions in practice and research'.

There is a variety of reasons why nursing research should be informed by a feminist perspective. Current knowledge about women and women's health contains distortion of facts arising from gender stereotyping. All nurses are familiar with the saying that 'women patients are much more difficult to nurse because they are so dependent' the obverse being true of men. Or that 'men do not need as much reassurance as women because they are more emotionally resilient'. Such distortions operate against the best interests of both female and male clients and patients. It limits nurses and doctors to views which are of questionable accuracy, and which have implications for medical and nursing diagnoses, treatment, and care. In such cases, both female and male clients may be disadvantaged. Furthermore, a feminist perspective critically questions medical dominance over patients and health care providers, and creates the consciousness-raising essential for change. Feminist nursing research will also provide an important counter-balance for existing bio-medical research on, for example, menopause (MacPherson 1983) and other conditions such as endometriosis and hyster-ectomy. Nurses can also conduct research on the value of caring on patient outcomes and disseminate these findings widely.

Nursing practice and the concept of caring

Hagell (1989) suggests that nursing knowledge must keep sacrosanct the humanness of the nurse-patient relationship, which requires contextualization and centredness of nursing knowledge. This requires an acknowledgement of values and a focus on personal experience. The importance of caring must be highlighted here. Diekelmann (1990) questions the practices within our nursing culture which make caring impossible. She relates this to the lack of caring shown to students by nurse academics and suggests a range of strategies to avoid practices that she argues are competitive and power driven, both in academia and in nursing practice. In recent times, nursing has turned its energies toward embracing the caring concept as a unique expression of nursing practice (Benner & Wrubel 1989, Watson 1985, Leininger 1984, 1988, Dunlop 1988).

Diekelmann (1990) calls for this to be extended to nursing education, and a feminist approach to nursing research will extend this aspect into research practice. This view is supported by Tanner. She stresses that nurses must nurture and cultivate their caring practices, that these practices must be protected from assault. Tanner (1990) is convinced that some caring practices are obscured by dehumanizing and abstract language, while those recognized are either not valued, cannot be described in language, or are not made completely explicit. Webster (1988) further articulates the challenge: that of integrating the values of both caring and self-care in ways which are clear enough to nurses and others that they cannot be distorted and used as weapons against us.

Tronto (1987) interjects a note of caution, reinforcing Webster's (1988) concern that adopting the caring concept in nursing could be used against nurses. She argues that while an ethic of care is of vital concern to feminists, this debate should not be raised in gender terms. It is clear that some attachment to the notion of caring in nursing has been located in the fact of gender, that is, that most nurses are women, that nursing is uniquely about caring. She notes that the simple assertion of gender difference in a social context that identifies the male as normal contains an implication of the inferiority of the distinctly female. Nursing must examine carefully its adherence to the care concept as central to its identity, for as has been shown previously, such notions are regarded as secondary and 'unscientific'.

Notwithstanding such concerns, Miller (1988) observes that nursing has become 'increasingly interested in preserving nursing's feminine values and heritage as a women's profession'. This has occurred as a consequence of nursing valuing human caring encompassed in a humanistic, nurturing role and for the less conservative, a celebration of the 'uniquely feminine'. Miller views nursing as moving toward 'a stronger sense of community and colleagueship whereby nurses are learning how to network and consult each other, and to use each other's special knowledge'. This movement is also apparent in approaches to research within nursing; the acceptance of a wider range of viewpoints and methodology for nursing research is traceable in the nursing literature. In particular, the increased use of qualitative methodology for nursing research is apparent. It is no accident that feminist research is more likely to be qualitative than quantitative in nature, since the qualitative approach 'captures the more salient features of women's social world as the self-reports of women's own experiences of health/illness, family life, work in and outside the home, sexuality, friendship, and aging reveal important data' (MacPherson 1983).

This view is supported by Meleis (1986) as she traces the trend away from cure, illness, prescribed tasks, and the duality in relationships between the person delivering the care and the person receiving the care. She defines the focus as moving to a consideration of the concepts of care, environment, and the perception and meaning of the situation of individuals, encouragement of active participation in care, and collaboration of all those involved in care. Meleis asserts that all these appear to be conditions that have grown out of the feminist movement and out of feminist methodologies, which in turn have been influenced by existential philosophies and phenomenology. If this is so, it suggests that nursing may be adopting espoused feminist principles without being aware of them.

Chinn (1989) has a consistent history of promoting feminist principles in nursing. She believes that nursing's patterns of knowing and feminist thinking can be coalesced to form a whole, which will effect a revolutionary change in the health care system, and which will enact the 'fullness of our passion, intellect, and moral activity'. She notes the similarities between feminist principles and nursing theory and practice. Feminists agree that personal experience leads to the refinement of theory, which itself feeds back into experience ad infinitum. Theory is not abstract and unrelated to the facts of experience.

To illustrate, Chinn elaborates the notion of 'praxis', suggesting that feminist ideas are integral to feminist praxis, just as nursing ideas are integral to nursing praxis. She continues: 'whether we call it practice-oriented theory, bridging the gaps between education and practice, or putting an idea into practice, we are describing praxis'. Nursing praxis has dialectical tension, is interactive, and involves reciprocal shaping of theory and practice. Its aim is to produce emancipatory knowledge and empowerment of those in our care.

While Chinn suggests that incorporation of the best of feminist insights will empower all women and all nurses, this is more difficult than appears on the surface. One of the major problems with feminism and nursing is that the latter has failed to embrace feminism for a variety of reasons. These include fear, ignorance, all feminists being identified with the "vocal lunatic fringe", and the belief that accepting feminism implies loss of favour with dominant groups. In the case of nursing, it is clear that many nurses derive power from their subordinate relationship with doctors, a superordinate group. To espouse feminist views and values is seen to place that relationship in jeopardy. Another major difficulty is the social context in which nurses are required to work.

As Moccia (1988) points out, nursing has the task of caring in a society that devalues such activities. She quotes a number of authors who provide analyses that highlight the difficulties of caring within bureaucracies and systems, including the health care system. Moccia also notes that caring activities are difficult and rare because of the 'dominant ideology and the power relations designed to maintain the status quo'. She concludes that it is not difficult to understand that individuals (in this context, nurses and patients) must limit their caring for each other, and thus fail to realize the full potential of their relationships. Her recommendation from this analysis is that nurses must reform the current health care system, or create a new one. This will best be achieved by operating from a feminist informed perspective; hence the value of being conversant and accepting of a feminist ideology.

MacPherson (1988) provides a perceptive feminist analysis of the caring concept. She notes that liberal feminists stress the individual motivations for caring, whereas radical and socialist feminists have a wider, social perspective. Liberal feminism ignores conditions and power relations in the contexts where nurses do their work, although it argues for equality and rights within the health care arena. It suggests that the basis for caring stresses individual discretion and values, acknowledging that the nurse's right to care should be given equal consideration with the physician's right to cure. This individualistic orientation is exemplified in the work of Noddings (1984) and Gilligan (1982). Noddings asserts that '...women should retain their natural orientation and find ways to make it work for them, and perhaps for others as well...[this requires]...that a woman remain in touch with her deep feminine psychological structure and bring its great strength into the public world of work'.

But returning to MacPherson's (1988) analysis, she maintains that the radical feminist view indicates that nursing's ability to operationalize the caring ethic is seriously undermined by the social context in which nursing is practised. This is one reason why nurses find themselves unable to care, or leave nursing altogether. Radical feminism aims to uncover the hidden sources of coercion and domination that are embedded in the nurses' lived-experience. In terms of caring, it addresses the concepts of patriarchy, misogyny, women's health problems, nurses' involvement in iatrogenic medical activities and nurses' relationships with each other, focusing particularly on horizontal violence. Caring can develop to its highest order when feminist insights are gained from such analyses.

The bringing of a feminist perspective to the development of nursing knowledge, and theory development in particular, is also fruitful.

Nursing theory development

The development of nursing theories is a major component of nursing knowledge development. Nursing theories have been proposed for varying situations and clientele, and have been in existence for some time. They are beginning to be questioned in a highly critical fashion. Lundh et al (1988) query their usefulness, and suggest that nursing theories are 'rules for action [that] appear trivial and largely a matter of common sense'. They further suggest that theories require the nurse to function in a way that requires manipulation and problem-solving. They view nurses as having to 'emerge as an omnipotent "big mother"'. This does not allow for the active participation and involvement of patients and clients in their care. Such an approach is not congruent with a feminist perspective. Furthermore, with such omnipotence also comes a distancing that prevents understanding of patients' situations. This militates against caring and nurturing, and cannot lead to adequate nursing treatment and care. In fact, it also prevents relevant research questions being asked, thus jeopardizing the future development of nursing as a discipline.

Moccia (1988) proposes that the low level of success of nursing knowledge development can be attributed to the fact that nursing's identity has been derived from the values and mores of the dominant ideology. It should be noted that, until recently, nursing's knowledge was (and to a large extent still is) based on the development of nursing theories. Moccia believes that it is possible that nursing theories would be relevant and more usable if they derived from the lived-experience of nurses who are predominantly women. Caring and sharing may bring to the surface the form of 'tacit knowledge' that is communicated through the practical work of everday nursing which has long traditions within nursing care. Such possibilities may also help nurses ask the 'right' research questions, which, as previously indicated, current nursing theories tend not to do. The similarity with feminist principles and the potential for a positive contribution from a feminist perspective is readily apparent. Again, the ideas espoused by Chinn (1989) with respect to the dialectic between nursing theory and practice, and feminist praxis have relevance here. Nursing theories cannot be imposed from on high by nurse academics who have little or no relationship with nursing practice.

It is clear from the foregoing that research does not exist in a vacuum. Heron (1981) points out that, among other things, it is a way of exercising power over persons. Its focus therefore must be 'a critique of domination, a recognition of those existing structures that exploit, alienate, and repress people' (Hedin 1986). It is a political enterprise 'embedded in the patriar-chal social structure and values that it helps to reinforce' (MacPherson 1983). The development of nursing is dependent on rigorous and relevant research, deriving from the theory and practice of nursing. Nursing research that does not take account of feminist principles and theory will fail to ask the appropriate questions and deliver valued knowledge.

CONCLUSION

This chapter has examined the contribution that feminist research could make to nursing research, theory, and practice. An examination of feminism and feminist beliefs was necessary as a foundation for discussing and defining feminist research. These beliefs include: that women are oppressed; that the personal is political; that consciousness-raising is necessary for a change in belief structure. Feminist research was represented as frankly ideological, having some unique characteristics which differentiate it from other forms of research. These include, for example, the interconnection between the researcher and the researched; the centrality of women and their experiences; the perception of contradictions and action. The question was addressed: Why has feminist research become a vital and important alternative to current forms of research? The reasons addressed lie in the belief system which informs feminism, the 'emergence of feminist, new paradigm and qualitative methods and philosophies as linked aspects of a strengthening of female values within society' (Wilkinson 1986), and by the sheer inadequacy and inappropriateness of traditional forms of research, which have been recognized for some considerable time. What feminist research can offer nursing is research that is more connected than traditional forms, while still embracing excellence.

This chapter also offers a feminist perspective on nursing research, the development of nursing theory, and the role of the caring concept in nursing practice. The phenomenon of caring was explored, and some cautionary comments made about the potential for the concept of care being used against nurses and women. Whilst caring is vital for nursing practice, research and theory development, it is prudent to consider it from a variety of perspectives, including feminism. Feminists are concerned that a focus on caring as uniquely nursing and 'naturally' feminine will result in further devaluing of women and nurses unless this focus is coupled with an awareness of power relations in the health care system and in the wider society.

It is in nursing's best interests to understand and incorporate the contri-bution which feminist principles and feminist research can offer nursing research, theory, and practice. Feminism offers a different and appropriate perspective from which to develop the discipline of nursing. It provides a frame of reference which is an alternative to the current world view. Feminist principles have the potential to create a paradigm shift for nursing and in the process, a more life-affirming world (Chinn 1989). It can offer timely and new historical and sociocultural perspectives which allow nurses to question and, if necessary, change our approaches to patient care and teaching. Another valuable outcome will be the creation of greater understanding of the female experience. Given that most nurses are women and the majority of patients are of the same gender, this is imperative. A feminist perspective will facilitate the recognition and ownership of women's wisdom, and avoid its use in ways that are distorted.

In summary, 'doing feminism' in nursing

...is a process of thinking and acting in a manner that challenges institutionalized power relations and relations of domination in the social reality of nursing. Its implications are important for the social institution and discipline of nursing, as well as for social definitions and practices of health. The promise of feminism is the possibility of transforming the social world, toward affirmation of women's lived experiences and active participation in the construction of reality ...the promise becomes the possibility of transforming personal and social lived experiences and meanings of health and health care (Smith 1988).

There are few other contributions to nursing that have such potential for developing the discipline of nursing. Nurses are now ready for that challenge.

The author acknowledges that some components of this chapter appeared in the *Issues and Methods in Research Study Guide*, published by the South Australian College of Advanced Education, Adelaide, South Australia, 1990.

REFERENCES

Benner P, Wrubel J 1989 The primacy of caring. Stress and coping in health and illness. Addison-Wesley, Menlo Park
Bernard B 1973 My four revolutions: an autobiographic history of the ASA. In: Huber J (ed) Changing women in a changing society. University of Chicago Press, Chicago
Bernhard L A 1984 quoted in Duffy M E 1985 A critique of research: a feminist perspective. Health Care for Women International 6:341-352
Calloway H 1981 Women's perspectives: research as revision. In: Reason P, Rowen J (eds) Human inquiry. John Wiley, London
Chinn P L 1989 Nursing patterns of knowing and feminist thought. Nursing and Health Care 10 (2):71-75
Cook J A 1982 The development of feminist methodology: issues and practice in three academic disciplines. Paper presented at American Sociological Association Annual Meeting, San Francisco.
Cook J A , Fonow M M 1986 Knowledge and women's interests: issues of epistemology and methodology in feminist sociological research. Sociological Inquiry 56 (1):2-29
Diekelmann N 1990 Nursing education: caring, dialogue and practice. Journal of Nursing Education 29 (7):300-305
du Bois B 1983 Passionate scholarship: notes on values, knowing and method in feminist social science. In: Bowles G, Klein R D (eds) Theories of women's studies. Routledge & Kegan Paul, London
Duffy M E 1985 A critique of research: a feminist perspective. Health Care for Women International 6:341-352
Dunbar S B, Patterson E, Burton C, Stuckert G 1981 Women's health and nursing research. Advances in Nursing Science 3:1-16

Dunlop M 1988 Science and caring: are they compatible? Conference Proceedings. Shaping nursing theory and practice: the Australian context. Lincoln School of Health Sciences, La Trobe University, Melbourne, p 16-22

Eisenstein H 1984 Contemporary feminist thought. George, Allen & Unwin, London

Gilligan C 1982 In a different voice: psychological theory and women's development. Harvard University Press, Cambridge

Hagell E I 1989 Nursing knowledge: women's knowledge. A sociological perspective. Journal of Advanced Nursing 14:226-232

Hedin B A 1986 Nursing, education, and emancipation: applying the critical theoretical approach to nursing research. In: Chinn P L (ed) Nursing research methodology: issues and implementation. Aspen, Rockville

Heron J 1981 Philosophical basis for a new paradigm. In: Reason P, Rowan J (eds) Human inquiry. John Wiley, London

Kelly A 1978 Feminism and research. Women's Studies International Quarterly 1:225-232

Klein R D 1983 How to do what we want to do: thoughts about feminist methodology. In:Bowles G, Klein R D (eds) Theories of women's studies. Routledge & Kegan Paul, London

Keller E F 1980 Feminist critique of science: a forward or backward move. Fundamenta Scientiae 1:341-349

Lather P 1986a Issues of validity in openly ideological research: between a rock and a soft place. Interchange 17 (4):63-84

Lather P 1987 Feminist perspectives on empowering research methodologies American Educational Research Association, Washington

Leininger M M (ed) 1984 Care: the essence of nursing and health. Wayne State University Press, Detroit

Leininger M M (ed) 1988 Care: discovery and uses in clinical and community settings. Wayne State University Press, Detroit

Lundh U, Soder M, Waerness K 1988 Nursing theories: a critical view. Image: Journal of Nursing Scholarship 20:36-40

McCormack T 1981 Good theory or just theory? Toward a feminist philosophy of science. Women's Studies International Quarterly 4 (1):1-12

MacPherson K I 1983 Feminist methods: a new paradigm for nursing research. Advances in Nursing Science 5 :17-25

MacPherson K I 1988 Looking at nursing and caring through a feminist lens. Conference Proceedings. Caring and nursing: explorations in the feminist perspectives. Denver, p 25-55

Meleis A I 1986 Theory development and domain concepts. In: Moccia P (ed) New approaches to theory development. National League for Nursing, New York

Miller K L 1988 A study of nursing's feminist methodology. Conference Proceedings. Caring and nursing: explorations in the feminist perspectives. Denver, p 56-77

Mies M 1983 Towards a methodology for feminist research. In: Bowles G, Klein R D (eds) Theories of women's studies. Routledge & Kegan Paul, London

Mitchell J, Oakley A (eds) 1976 What is feminism? Blackwell, London

Moccia P 1988 At the faultline: social activism and caring. Nursing Outlook 36 (1):30-33

Noddings N 1984 Caring, a feminine approach to ethics and moral education. University of California Press, Berkeley

Oakley A 1981 Interviewing women: a contradiction in terms. In: Roberts H (ed) Doing feminist research. Routledge & Kegan Paul, Boston

Parlee M B 1979 Psychology and women. Signs: Journal of Women in Culture and Society 5 (1):121-133

Reinharz S 1983 Experiential analysis: a contribution to feminist research. In: Bowles G, Klein R D (eds) Theories of women's studies. Routledge & Kegan Paul, London

Smith S 1988 A feminist analysis of constructs of health. Conference Proceedings. Caring and nursing: explorations in the feminist perspectives. Denver, p 340-362

Spender, D. 1976 quoted in Kelly A 1978 Feminism and research. Women's Studies International Quarterly 1:225-232

Stanley L, Wise S 1983 Breaking out: feminist consciousness and feminist research. Routledge & Kegan Paul, London

Tanner C A 1990 Caring as a value in nursing education. Nursing Outlook 38 (2):70-72

Tronto J C 1987 Beyond gender difference to a theory of care. Signs: Journal of Women in Culture and Society 12 (4):644-663

Watson J 1985 Nursing: human science and human care. A theory of nursing. Appelton-Century-Crofts, Norwalk

Webb C 1984 Feminist methodology in nursing research. Journal of Advanced Nursing 9:249-256

Webster D 1988 Mental health: the politics of self-care. Conference Proceedings, Caring and nursing: explorations in the feminist perspectives. Denver p 181-211

Westkott M 1979 Feminist criticism of the social sciences. Harvard Educational Review 49 (4):422-430

Wilkinson S (ed) 1986 Feminist social psychology: developing theory and practice. Open University Press, Milton Keynes

10. In search of an Australian identity

Jocalyn Lawler

In this chapter I want to explore some of the notions associated with alleged universal and protoscientific aspects of nursing which have been imported, promoted, proselytized and imposed on clinicians in Australia. And I will also argue that clinically grounded research, whether it is conducted with patients/clients or nurses, is more likely to help us articulate our particular Australian style and contributions to the discipline than the adoption of imported ideas and styles of practice. The importation of ideas in the last two decades has been motivated, in part, by nurses' wishes to overcome medical dominance on the one hand, and on the other hand, articulate what distinguishes nursing from all the other occupations in which some form of caring is central. We have been asking ourselves a number of crucial questions and among them are these: What is universal (or unique) to nursing and what is specific about it at the workface? How can we organize autonomous practice? How can we define it and defend it against erosion? How can we market it? How can we explain it to others? How can we overcome the ignorance which surrounds it? How can we document it so that we can show others what we do? How (or can, or will) we turn it into a science so that it will look familiar to others who have grown up in a scientized society? How and where will we find the language to express what we know to be 'real' about nursing? and How will we overcome our discomfort about the inadequacy of positivist scientific paradigms for nursing?

THE INTELLECTUAL DOMINANCE OF AUSTRALIAN NURSING BY IMPORTED IDEAS

In international affairs, the United States of America has had a dominant role, particularly since the Second World War. North Americans have exported their culture, products, dreams, and ideas. Nursing has not been immune from this influence, indeed, if anything we have been very heavily influenced to the extent where some people believe that if something has happened in North American nursing or health care, then it will almost certainly happen here. North American ideas tend to be seen as internationally relevant and like the English and Spanish in other historical periods, the

211

North Americans have spread their influence around the globe. I want to explore this influence on nursing in Australia, that is, to tease out some of the details of nursing as a universal but culture-bound activity.

If nursing is a universal phenomenon, then we need to ask what its central and distinguishing features are, and if nursing is also culturally influenced, we also must ask how that is expressed in practice and what the relationships are between the universal and culturally determined qualities of nursing. That is, how do we integrate the universal with the particular contexts of care? I have argued elsewhere (Lawler 1991) that

> nursing is fundamentally and centrally concerned with the care of other people's bodies, but it is care provided in a particular context. Physical body care and comfort are provided for those who are completely dependent on other people—the unconscious, the senile, the paralysed. But varying degrees of body care are required for most patients, according to their particular state of dependence. Nurses also help people with the experience of living with and through what is happening to their bodies during illness experience, recovery and dying—times when the body can dominate existence. Nurses are, therefore, centrally concerned with the *object body* (an objective and material thing) and the *lived body* (the body as it is experienced by living people). They are more concerned with integrating the object body with the lived body. This is what I have termed *somology*, that is, understanding the body as an integration of the object body (the thing) into experience so that it is simultaneously an object, a means of experience, a means of expression, a manner of presence among other people, and a part of one's personal identity.

What I have described as somology, which is stylistically typical of experienced and expert practitioners, allows an integration of the physical with the socio-cultural and personal aspects of being but it is only possible if the nurse is concerned for the experience of 'the other'—a situation which is typically called caring and which is universal and fundamental in nursing. It is also an interpersonal business in which the two parties have a reciprocity of outlook and perspective.

> When nurses practise somologically they not only take account of the physical body (a thing) and the body as it is experienced, lived, and felt by the patient but they also integrate these two aspects of human embodiment. For example, if we take a scenario where a patient has a gangrenous foot and is therefore also systemically ill from the toxicity of the gangrene, in simple terms the nurse can do one of three things: (1) practise objectively and reductively by focusing attention on the obvious signs and symptoms, document them and compare them with previous observations in order to arrive at a judgement about progress—all of which can be done sympathetically and kindly, but the primary attention is directed at pathology; (2) concentrate on the patient's lived experience and attend to the feelings associated with the problem and provide medication to relieve headache and nausea, leaving to others (medical practitioners) the problem of pathology; or (3) practise in a way which integrates the pathological problem of a gangrenous foot into lived experience so that the patient's situation is seen compositely (Lawler 1991).

In what we could call (for convenience) Type I nursing outlined above, the emphasis is on what can be objectively (meaning 'scientifically') determined, irrespective of whether that is physiological, psychological, social or what-ever—a stylistic approach to care which is necessary in some form. In Type II nursing, the emphasis is on the patient's feelings, experience and human-ness, typical of a humanistic approach to care—which is also stylistically desirable. In my view, neither Type I nor Type II is characteristic of nursing at its best, nor characteristic of experienced and expert practitioners. Those who promote the scientific approach, however, tend to emphasize and promote Type I nursing—an approach in which the viewpoint of the nurse is dominant; those who promote Type II nursing tend to over-emphasise the perspective and experience of the patient. These are people about whom the joke is made (sick though it may be)—that such nurses may not be able to stop the haemorrhage, but they are able have deep and meaningful discus-sion about what it feels like to bleed to death.

In Type III, or somological, nursing care, there is shared meaning about what is happening and neither party imposes 'reality' on the other except in circumstances where the patient's recovery is compromised.[1] If the nurse knows what the patient thinks (believes) is happening, or if the nurse in some way(s) incorporates the patient's perspective, then it is possible to practise somologically. In this sense successful care becomes, in part, a partnership. When we transpose this situation to the profession more generally, we do not necessarily see a shared perspective with those who write about nursing and those who practise it. As Australians we do not necessarily share the same world view as nurses from the USA who do most of the promotional work about a science of nursing—we are culturally two different groups and that means we do not necessarily share the same world views, nor do we live and practise in the same socio-cultural contexts. Additionally, the sort of part-nerships between nurse and patient which occur in somological care are not typical of the ways in which the scientist and the 'subject' interact. If nursing embraces a scientific model, then of necessity, the nurse will presume to know *for* the patient—an approach which is more in keeping with medical and patriarchal models. I do not think this is what nurses, particularly feminist nurses, or patients want.

In recent years, the North American style of scientific 'reality' has been imposed upon nursing discourse in this country, that is, there has been the presumption to know *for* us. There has been little reciprocity of perspective between those who have promoted 'scientific' nursing and those who have been supposed to make it work in practice. In emphasizing what can be objectively determined we have adopted, more or less, an approach which leans on the pathological and the physical, predominantly because that is what one is able to see as objective reality—the more experiential elements have consequently been relatively displaced or dislocated from a central

---

[1] See Lawler (1991) for a discussion of how nurses will sometimes attempt to shift patients' definition of reality when recovery is delayed by an inability to face some form of objective physical reality, for example, the denial sometimes associated with acknowledging the effect(s) of paraplegia.

position, at least on paper. Alternatively, the more humanistic concerns have been expressed in objective language which tends to make them sound a bit ridiculous or awkward—at least in the Australian context. For example, the nursing diagnosis, 'distress of the human spirit', is laughable in our (white) culture. In practice, though, experientially based concerns have not been displaced, but any tool which concentrates on what is 'seeable' for a systematic documentation of the objectively real will make what is 'feelable' problematic. And we know from practice that nursing care is also about what is felt—by the patient and/or the nurse.

The academic discourse on the discipline, which is dominated by nurses from the USA, has reflected a growing emphasis on the perceived 'need' to develop and scientize nursing knowledge. We have been encouraged—extolled even—by most of the North Americans and their Australian followers to embrace positivist scientific models, and with them reduction, objectification, quantification, and taxonomic and linear thinking. We have been encouraged to see scientific knowledge and scientific nursing practices as universal and highly desirable features of the discipline—indeed some have gone so far as to argue that it is only through traditionally scientific methods that we can develop the knowledge base and standing (that is, the status) of the discipline. While much of nursing practice can be studied by quantification, measurement, and positivist enquiry, individual patient perspectives and perceptions are also important, especially if we are committed to patient-centred care. But within positivist approaches patients' experiences of illness can become peripheral or unresearchable. Although nursing has, of necessity, accommodated more technologically and scientifically oriented health care, it has also retained a concern for the care and comfort of patients but, in the academic literature, this commitment has taken on some ideological, rhetorical, and philosophical qualities as notions of 'scientific' nursing have tended to override non-quantifiable elements in nursing.

During the last decade Australia has been intellectually colonized by ideas from the United States through:

1. The large volume of print material generated by writers from the USA and sold in Australia—a form of traffic in information which is not reciprocated
2. The Australian myth that imported things are necessarily superior to the 'home-grown' variety
3. The steady stream of visiting (often invited) North American 'experts'.

There are a number of consequences and responses to this process of epistemological imperialism, not all of it to our disadvantage. However, what is of relevance to this discussion is that, although there is a trend, both locally and internationally (including the USA), away from scientism as a methodological standard, we have seen the relatively generalized and unquestioned adoption of some of these notions of 'scientific' nursing. I want to explore three imported ideas in more detail—the nursing process; patients' needs and the ubiquitous hierarchy of needs according to Maslow; and nursing diagnoses.

Imported notions of 'scientific' nursing

The nursing process

The nursing process was marketed as a sure way to practise nursing scientifically (for example, Mauksch & David 1972, Humphris 1979, Marriner 1983) and humanistically (La Monica 1979). As an instrument which promised the potential for concrete, objective, and verifiable effects of nursing care, it was indeed a breakthrough. Nurses would at last have hard evidence for the value and outcomes of nursing care—they would have evidence that some change(s) occur, as a result of nursing acts. There was to be some level of predictive and reproducible action that could be demonstrated objectively and which could be shared by written means. Such benefits were and are seen as having great potential, especially if the nursing process could also be marketed and used as a tool to make practice humanistic.

There are, though, some interesting paradoxes in the nursing process and what it is supposed to facilitate. It mimics medicine and the stylistic qualities of medical decision-making at a time when we are supposedly trying to break away from the dominance that the medical model has had over nursing. Its positivist-reductive style is typical of 'scientific' disciplines but nursing is simultaneously constructed around notions of holism—the two approaches are philosophically and methodologically opposed to each other. It is possible that the patient can become or be reduced (at least on paper) to a set of problems, needs, or diagnoses (both medical and nursing), yet the nursing process is said to be humanistic by accommodating feelings, emotions, and ways of being in the world. The taking of a nursing history also exposes the patient to the potential for what could be called a 'nursing gaze'—to adapt a term from Foucault (1976). That is, in documenting patients' needs there is potential for the patient to be the subject of unnecessary surveillance about matters which are arguably no business of the nurse—an act which is anything but humanistic.

More seriously for the long term interests of the development of the discipline of nursing, the nursing process does not allow for lived body experience (Parker 1988, Gadow 1980, 1982, Benner & Wrubel 1988, Lawler 1991). In my view (Lawler 1991) the essential and fundamentally distinguishing feature of nursing which separates it from other health occupations, including medicine, is that nursing is concerned with helping people live in a body which is damaged, disfigured, or dysfunctional. It is an existentially oriented style of practice without which nursing cannot be qualitatively differentiated from medicine which focuses on the body as a mechanical entity to be tinkered with and fixed—like any other machine. While nursing embraces methods, such as the nursing process, which can be seen as 'watered down' medicine, it can only be quantitatively differentiated from other health oriented occupations. And we have suffered long enough under that misconception. In practice, however, we can see that nursing is qualitatively different from medicine. It is in the practice setting that we ought to look for notions on which to build the discipline, and there were many indicators of this when the nursing process first arrived in this country but we did not necessarily recognize the signals for what they really were.

At the workface, the nursing process met with opposition, reluctance, and at times extreme resistance on the part of some clinicians who said, among other things, that: it was a waste of time; it was just paperwork; it was OK for beginners; it made no difference to the way nurses did their work; it did not evolve from 'real life' practice. In effect the nursing process was a style of practice which promised to 'elevate' nursing to the status of science, it was an imposition, and it was jargonistic. Many clinicians, especially the more experienced, responded with scepticism—a fairly stereotypical Australian characteristic, but also one which was well grounded because, although clinicians were not heard at the time, each of the things they criticized was later supported by research and critiques from established academics. If something does not 'ring true' to the practice environment then, in my view, something is wrong—perhaps seriously wrong. In the case of the nursing process something is seriously wrong.

Henderson's (1982) criticism that the nursing process denigrated the knowledge which clinicians derive from experience sounded familiar to clinicians. Once Benner's (1982) work on the nature of expert clinical knowledge became known we were able to have real evidence that there was something seriously mismatched between expert clinical decision-making and the sort of decision-making which the nursing process required. That our best clinicians had been saying this seemed not to have made much difference. However, we are now able to say, because of the (proper) evidence, that the nursing process has not lived up to its promise and that it is unlikely to do so.

The resistance of registered nurses to the nursing process was initially thought to be little more than reluctance to change, but over time and with experience people rejected simple explanations and, we have become aware of some of the reasons why experienced practitioners find difficulty with the nursing process. By far the most serious criticisms are coming from those who have subjected it to positivist investigation. An increasing number of studies are indicating that the nursing process is not having the effects it is designed to produce; there is little, if any, evidence to support the view that it is an adequate means of documenting practice; and it also seems that it has no demonstrable effect on nursing practice (Richards 1987, Ferguson et al 1987).

When it has been tested with positivist methodologies, on which the concept is based, the nursing process is a relative failure. Its failure, however, has not meant that it is being disregarded. Having introduced the instrument and grown accustomed to its presence (however dormant or ineffectual), there is a reluctance to give it up because there does not seem to be anything to put in its place—a situation which raises administrative and legal questions about documenting care, particularly if one considers the practicalities of submitting nursing services to accreditation processes. What has happened in practice, in Australian hospitals, is that the nursing care plan has become a part of the patient record system, but its daily use and its representation of the nursing care is often more cosmetic than anything else; or it undergoes rapid re-working in the lead-up to hospital accreditation, following which attention to it dies down again.

The ineffectiveness of the nursing process in practice has, however, served not only to heighten our understanding about the complexities of nursing but also to demonstrate and reinforce that practice is the most robust test of all. In my view, the nursing process failed because it was not derived from practice; it was imposed and as such it has a foreign and alien presence. If the promised benefits of the nursing process had been forthcoming we would have made great scientific progress. But if nursing practice does not fit a traditional scientific (positivist and reductive) model and we forcefully transform it, we fundamentally and centrally change the nature of the discipline. I am unconvinced that this is what nurses (or their patients/clients) want because we have retained notions associated with being humane, holistic, humanistic, and patient-centred. What nurses seem to have wanted with the nursing process was not science itself necessarily, but rather what science could make possible—that is, greater visibility, higher status, more access to research funds, and a more valued place is society. These are the real issues and the push for scientific knowledge can be seen more as a means to an end than as an end in itself. Turning nursing into a science sounds fine and the benefits which could flow, as they do to other sciences, would be to the advantage of the discipline.   However, this transformation may come with costly concessions such that the discipline ceases to retain its core regard for human experience, support, care, and comfort—both physically and in other respects.

We can, however, learn a great deal from the push for scientific care if we sift through the fallout from, and underlying intentions of, the nursing process, one of which is the notion of patients' needs.

Patients' needs and Maslow's hierarchy

One of the central, powerful, and pervasive concepts underpinning the nursing process is the notion that the patient has needs which the nurse can: (a) assess, usually by using Maslow's hierarchy of needs (1943); and (b) frame into nursing diagnoses. That the nurse is also expected to meet (all of) these needs opens a Pandora's box beyond the scope of the discussion here. The business of assessment has also revealed itself to be very problematic, for example, in the case of pain assessment the nurse's own experience of pain will influence decisions about the extent of patients' distress (Holm et al 1989). Given the breadth of things with which nursing is concerned, any form of assessment of a potentially infinite number of needs will be a complicated business. Nevertheless, it has been the most highly developed aspect of attempts to establish scientific nursing.

So-called 'need' theory, which underlies what is to be assessed, has been integral in texts, curricula, and ideology in a relatively unquestioned and uncritical way in Australia since the late 1960s and 1970s. Little, if any, evidence can be found, though, to ground this notion either in practice or in what patients want from health care. Rather, these needs have generally been defined by nurses with some guidance form the Maslow hierarchy and, like other elements in 'scientific' nursing, they have been imposed on our construction of the way the discipline should be conceptualized, taught, and practised.

The concept of 'needs' is a problematic one on which there is a developing literature, particularly with respect to the extent to which an adequate definition is compounded by the problem of perspective, which is itself complicated by such complex issues as class, culture, gender, age, language, values, education and economic reality, among other things. However, the Maslow model continues to have currency, perhaps because it is a systematic model which addresses physical and existential entities, and also because it feels comfortable to those who use and promote it (Lawler 1983). As a tool to aid the understanding and assessment of needs, it has limited applicability and it suffers from a middle class North American bias, among other things.

Maslow's notion of basic needs was built on functionalism, holism, and Gestalt and psychodynamic theory within psychology (Maslow 1943). Maslow believed, as a Freudian, that unconscious motives are more important in determining human behaviour than conscious motives and, because he accepted the Freudian notion of the unconscious, he also accepted that basic needs are relatively universal among cultures. He claimed that his

... classification of basic needs makes some attempt to take account of the relative unity behind the superficial differences in specific desires from one culture to another. Certainly in any particular culture an individual's conscious motivational content will usually be extremely different from the conscious motivational content of an individual in another society. However, it is the common experience among anthropologists that people, even in different societies, are much more alike than we would think from our first contact with them, and that as we know them better we seem to find more and more of this commonness. We then recognize the most startling differences to be superficial rather than basic, e.g., differences in style of hairdress, clothes, tastes in food, etc. Our classification of basic needs is in part an attempt to account for this unity behind the apparent diversity from culture to culture. No claim is made that it is ultimate or universal for all cultures. The claim is made only that it is relatively *more* ultimate, more universal, more basic, than the superficial conscious desires from culture to culture, and makes a somewhat closer approach to common-human characteristics. Basic needs are *more* common-human than superficial desires or behaviours (Maslow 1943).

Maslow prefaced his 1943 remarks with a comment that his theory was to be seen as a 'suggested program or framework for future research and must stand or fall, not so much on facts available or evidence presented, as upon researches yet to be done'. Nearly fifty years later there is little research which is supportive of the theory. In a review of the place of Maslow's need hierarchy in nursing theory in 1983 (Lawler 1983), I could find little evidence to support its validity, particularly as a generalizable cross-cultural concept. It does not fit Aboriginal Australians and it does not fit non-materialistic people, but it probably does reflect the same value system and world view of academic North American nurses who publish so much material in which Maslow's model is integral (Lawler 1983).

Little research has been done to overtly validate the Maslow model for nursing practice, even in those cultures where it may have some relevance. It continues to be accepted unquestioningly and incorporated even more deeply into 'scientific' nursing now that nursing diagnoses are becoming more topical. For example, in their study to clinically validate nursing diagnoses for the chronically ill, Hoskins et al (1986) tell us that they used Maslow's model because it 'presents a logical organization of needs' and as such it was acceptable to them as part of a validity study. This sort of claim about the Maslow model is by no means an isolated example in North American writings about need theory.

One rare study (Davis-Sharts 1986) which examined cross-cultural patterns in the relationship of physical needs (sleep) and safety supposedly subjected the Maslow model to scrutiny. The author claimed not only that the Maslow model is 'generally accepted by the scientific community' and that 'it...is highly generalizable and is not based on cultural boundaries in its attempt to explain basic needs of all human beings', but also that her results 'demonstrated...initial worldwide empirical evidence to support Maslow's need hierarchy'. Despite her claims, Davis-Sharts's study does not establish support for the model, rather only that humans use behavioural methods to thermoregulate and that the majority of cultures she studied engaged in some form of pre-sleep protective behaviours. These actions are interpreted, by her, as support for the Maslow model. She uses the argument that 'regardless of climate, prior to sleep onset thermoregulatory behaviours *reflecting the prepotence of physiological needs* occur more frequently than behaviours to provide protection' [italics added]. All that seems to have been demonstrated is that behaviours which relate to physiological need for sleep are more likely to be thermoregulatory than security oriented. This does not necessarily provide evidence for a hierarchical model. Nor does it demonstrate that the two (physiological and security needs—ranked first and second on the Maslow hierarchy) are related. The argument appears to be one where two co-existent behaviours have been interpreted as causally related behaviours.

The Davis-Sharts study and the Maslow model illustrate two important things. First, we can see how a major theoretical cornerstone, such as the Maslow model, can operate as a blindfold. So well are the notions of need and need hierarchy inculcated into nursing literature that, as fundamental assumptions, they are not questioned, even in studies which purport to test them. In many cases, researchers start from the belief that the model is sound and then go in search of supportive evidence, which is what Davis-Sharts has done. This is not a problem only for nursing, it is much more a function of dominant ideologies. I consider that the dominant ideologies, epistemologies, and methodologies which we have been attempting to integrate into a more sophisticated discourse and approach to practice in Australia have, in the main, originated in the USA and that they are not necessarily transportable across cultural boundaries. This is an issue which we need to address in addition to the more generalized problem of the paradoxes, illogicality, and misconceptions of the imported notions themselves.

Second, the Maslow model is typical of many other 'good ideas' which we have imported in that we have gone about the business of authenticating nursing practice arsy-versy. We have tried to transplant new concepts of practice into the clinical environment and we have not, as a typical approach, systematically studied clinicians or clinical practice as a source of rich and valuable material, nor have we studied the 'natural' environment as a potential host to see if some of these transplanted notions will take. We have not, therefore, valued our own clinical knowledge base but have tried to transform it by imposed styles of 'scientific' nursing. For example, many clinicians will tell you that the Maslow model works better (but not well) if you turn it upside down. Perhaps this is because the model was, like many other things which are applied to nursing, developed from studies on people who were not physically ill. Indeed, much of what has been adapted to nursing from the social sciences generally has not taken account of the problematics of extrapolating from the healthy to the ill.

More recently, we have seen attempts in Australia to adapt need theory to fit more comfortably with what is possible and/or desirable in the context of nursing, especially in nursing curricula. In the USA there is an emerging literature on consumer satisfaction which links patients' expectations (i.e. patient defined needs) to satisfaction with health care and with nursing care in particular (Ventura et al 1982, Linder-Pelz 1982, Doering 1983, Friedman 1986, Abramowitz et al 1987, Eriksen 1987, Carmel 1988) and there is also important work on what patients perceive as caring on the part of the nurse (for example, Oberst 1983, Larson 1984, *Topics in Clinical Nursing* 1986, 8 (2)). What these research findings imply is that patients' judgements are influenced by what they perceive to be the manner and personal approach of the nurse, and patients are not necessarily as interested in things which the nurse is extolled to assess and diagnose. It seems that patients' perceptions of care are linked to the immediacy of their situation and the capacity of the nurse to be humanely and caringly responsive to their situation. We should be cautious, though, of transposing this work too readily into the Australian context because there are cultural differences in the propensity to register dissatisfaction or satisfaction with health care (Carmel 1988) and there are important differences in health care systems.

However, there is some poignant and relevant anecdotal material which seems to indicate that there are universal qualities about the experience of illness and its relationship to what is perceived as good nursing care. This is valuable material because it indicates the extent to which individual differences will override the generalized social constructions of patients' needs which flow from the application of need theory. That is, there seems to be a tendency to see all patients as having the same needs. Clearly they do not. The following account by a North American nurse educator who had had bilateral mastectomies for carcinoma illustrates the tension between individual experience (which need theory is supposed to acknowledge and accommodate) and need assessment as it has been imposed on nursing.

Chemotherapy was, for me, intravenous hell. I'd receive my chemotherapy in the doctor's office, get an injection for nausea, then go directly to the hospital, where I'd go through the admission process. In my hospital room, I'd take off my silicone prostheses and my wig, put on a gown, get my Hickman hooked up to an intravenous...line, and start throwing up...I learned that it was important for my nurses to meet me at *my* point of need...[and] it became increasingly important to me that they respected my embarrassment over my distorted body and bare head. I felt naked, stripped, and humiliated...I didn't want to socialize. Of course I needed nursing care, but in the early days of my illness I also needed their respect for quiet times with my family and for time alone.

Even though the nursing care plan called for psychological assessment (and a nursing instructor or supervisor may have been outside my room insisting that the nurse get it), *my* need was for privacy. My support system was strong. To assess me for more than that was an invasion of my privacy. "How does it feel to have cancer?" for example, was an inappropriate question. It may have met the nurse's need; it didn't meet mine (Turkett 1987).

Some of the other difficulties in focusing on needs are: a tendency to construct the patient as necessarily dependent on the nurse; need assessment functioning as a reductive and objectifying procedure; a tendency to overdetermine 'problems'; and the issue of context—what is a problem for one person may not be the same problem for another. Nevertheless, the notion of needs has become firmly established as a central organizing theme in much nursing literature, in textbooks, and in curricula. It has also been translated into the more elaborate taxonomic construct of nursing diagnoses.

Nursing diagnoses

Nursing diagnoses represent a very 'scientific' approach to nursing in that they seek to identify and label a potentially endless taxonomy of possible problems which the patient may have and which are believed to be reasonably the business of the nurse. Nursing diagnoses are a distinctly North American invention exported to the rest of the world and they are a worry for several reasons.

There are serious questions about why nursing requires a classification system of diagnoses, what purpose(s) they will serve and who will validate them (Thomas (1987); and there are other issues which should make us cautious about the taxonomy of nursing diagnoses. First, they epitomize science in a way which is not necessarily suited to or adequate for nursing as a practice discipline which also espouses holism. Second, what does one actually do with the diagnosis—that is, how does it influence nursing actions if at all? This question is particularly pertinent if one considers the literature on the ineffectual nature of the nursing process, from which the system of nursing diagnoses evolved and in which it is still grounded. Third, there are questions about the validity of nursing diagnoses (Rasch 1987). Fourth, there is still the age-old problem—that measurement alone does not necessarily influence the outcome of anything. Fifth, nursing diagnoses seem to require the nursing process, if only as a background context and there are problems enough with the nursing process.

For the purposes of the discussion here, however, there is a sixth, and far more serious consideration which concerns the whole politico-economic infrastructure of health care funding in the United States and the relationship of nursing diagnoses to Diagnostic Related Groups and cost allocation (or, more accurately, cost containment). Vincent (1985) argues that the development of nursing diagnoses has become urgent in the USA as a direct result of the need to adequately cost and account for nursing care, that is, quantify it, at a time when the cost of health care generally is a serious social and economic problem. Like other western countries, Australia has a problem in relation to containing the cost of health care, but we should be cautious of taking on methods designed to authenticate practice for economic reasons and yet simultaneously argue that we are doing it for the good of the discipline as a branch of specialized and researchable knowledge. If all we are doing by transforming nursing into a quantifiable science is responding to a set of externally imposed politico-economic pressures, the problem we face is a rather slippery one.

We can reasonably ask if the push for positivist methods in nursing is little more than yet another response from a traditionally female, relatively invisible (Lawler 1990), and poorly valued occupation against a male dominated, male defined, scientifically, and curatively (not preventively) oriented health care system. It is science *per se*—a predominantly male enterprise—and its adaptation to medicine and health care which has created the cost problem. One can reasonably ask if we are looking in the wrong place if we expect science to save us from a problem created by science in the first instance, particularly during times when science itself is coming under serious scrutiny from pressure groups, especially those concerned about ecosystems and the global environment.

In reducing nursing to a set of diagnoses we could well follow the same pathway as psychology with the development of diagnostic categories for behaviour. We run the risk of making nursing just another positivist discipline because we will allow the methodology to impose reality on our knowledge and ultimately on what we teach and how we practice. What we take to be nursing knowledge will be determined by the methods we employ to articulate it. As an undergraduate psychology student I was always searching for the people-oriented aspects of what I learnt. I learnt, though, that certain questions were located outside the discipline, not because they were not of interest or relevance to a discipline concerned with the human condition, but because they could not be adequately tested. This meant they could not be quantified or measured scientifically. One of the harshest criticisms I often heard of Freud, for example, was that he was 'unscientific'. Be that as it may, few can dispute his influence on the social sciences, particularly psychology. Where nursing is concerned, the very essence of the discipline concerns things which cannot be adequately tested in the positivist sense—pain, grief, nausea, relief at waking up from anaesthesia, gratitude, and feelings of comfort and safety in the presence of a good practitioner.

IMPOSED EXTERNAL 'REALITY' AND THE AUSTRALIAN CONTEXT

Australians are believed, stereotypically, to have an independence of thought and action and irreverence for authority which makes them appear naturally sceptical and easily amused—perhaps as a legacy of our strong Irish heritage. We are also thought to be unimpressed by ideas which do not reflect real life situations and we are not much interested in jargon which attempts to dress up phenomena. Nor are we thought to be concerned with things which are pretentious and ostentatious, except for the purposes of ridicule and amusement. We have a rich and wonderful range of words and phrases that are explicit, overt, often humorous, and inclined to be direct. And our linguistic style is matched by stereotypically relaxed and direct, if not brash, behaviour. Our style of nursing practice is, necessarily, a reflection of our culture. We must take this into account when we articulate and practise nursing and when we apply imported ideas.

In my view, our Australian cultural lens ought to be applied to imported ideas so that we can analyze their potential for adaptation in the Australian context—and we are increasingly coming to understand the importance of context in nursing. However, context is not simply an issue in relation to the situation of individual patients/clients but also in the more generalized sense of community and culture. To this extent, therefore, we can engage in dialogue internationally about the problems we share and the solutions we apply, but there is a limit to which we can transplant nursing ideas and the discourse in which they are embedded. Socially grounded ideas relate to the lived-experience of people and the social environments in which those experiences are given meaning.

The discourse of North America is not the same as that of Australians, though we share many commonalities, including the fact that we are English speaking. However, as any traveller to a foreign country, even an English speaking one knows, some translations or interpretations of particular meanings are necessary in ordinary everyday interactions. Therefore, we ought to anticipate similar problems in respect of practice-related concepts because our linguistic and cultural differences will both unite and divide us, particularly in a discipline which is so heavily influenced by the contextual aspects of situations in which nursing care is delivered and received.

In the long term, we will do well if we value more seriously and research our own practice and practitioners in their natural environments. My own research with clinicians has been a humbling and enriching experience in this regard but in this country, as in many others, nurses are largely invisible and their work is often overlooked, misunderstood and poorly valued. I wonder whether as nurses and colleagues we are also guilty of not valuing and respecting our worth and work individually and collectively. This could in part explain why we look to the USA for wisdom and guidance about how to extend the discipline. However, if we do not develop our own knowledge base within the context of the Australian community—a community which differs in important ways from North America—we will increasingly absorb North American ideas, language, and culture. Like Australian children who watch *Sesame Street* on television, we will start to speak American and we will adopt methods designed to suit their situation(s) and not our own.

CONCLUSION

How as Australians we view the world and how we want to be cared for as patients/clients will reflect the way we live and die. We cannot, in my view, continue a relatively unquestioned adoption of imported ideas and not systematically explore, understand, and value our own practice and its interface with the international nursing community. In taking our place internationally and accepting responsibility for the future direction(s) of our discipline, we must contribute original research and ideas. This means being more critical of imported ideas and turning our attention to our Australian colleagues, their practice, and research.

We cannot answer the questions which plague nursing as a discipline unless we know how our best practitioners acquire knowledge and use it. We cannot hope to take our place as full participants in international debates, nor reserve for ourselves the right to consume their work, critically or uncritically, unless we also make original contributions. Research which examines what it is that nurses do when they care for others has the potential to tell us what differentiates nursing from other disciplines which are also involved with forms of care. Without such work to export, nurses will face the sort of situation which economists call a balance of payments problem— that is, imports exceed exports—and the consequences of that leave us at the mercy of world events.

The relatively large number of phenomenological[2] works currently under way or recently completed here promises to tell us a great deal about the characteristics of Australian nursing practice. By its nature, phenomenological work seeks out how people see the world and make their experience(s) meaningful; it is, therefore, ideally suited for the task of unpacking what our practitioners do when they nurse people. In the case of my most recent research (Lawler 1991), I was able to render visible knowledge that nurses had in their heads, so to speak, but which had not been formally articulated. What I discovered, and what I came to call *somology* is not the sort of knowledge one reads in North American texts (nor texts from other countries for that matter), nor is it necessarily the sort of knowledge which has been formally taught. That is not to say that it cannot now be taught and discussed.

What I documented about the ways in which nurses help a patient/client live in a body which will not work properly, does not resemble nursing diagnoses, nor can it be expressed in words which are 'at home' on a nursing care plan. However, it is the sort of knowledge which feels familiar to clinicians, even relatively inexperienced ones. There are many Australian nursing scholars' works which are attempting to 'colour in the invisible' (as one of my colleagues Cathy Carmont so beautifully put it). I interpret this to mean that the elements and essence of our discipline are already in existence and well established. That we have been successfully practising nursing for centuries is proof enough. What we require now is work which will draw out those features, name them (even if we have to make up new words), refine them, and invest them back in practice. I do not think, however, that this can be achieved by continuing the heavy emphasis on scientism. On the contrary, I believe the more productive work will come from the phenomenologists and Australia seems to be abundantly supplied with them. I think that is to our advantage.

---

[2]   I am using this term in the very general and collective sense to embrace works which take an interpretive, qualitative approach and I include in this definition specific theoretical stances such as ethnomethodology, grounded theory and such like.

REFERENCES

Abramowitz S, Cote A A, Berry E 1987 Analyzing patient satisfaction: a multianalytic approach. Quality Review Bulletin 13 (4): 122-130
Benner P 1982 From novice to expert. American Journal of Nursing (March): 402-407.
Benner P, Wrubel J 1988 The primacy of caring. Addison-Wesley, Menlo Park
Carmel S 1988 Hospital patients' responses to dissatisfaction. Sociology of Health and Illness 10 (3): 262-281
Carmont C 1991 Personal communication.
Davis-Sharts J 1986 An empirical test of Maslow's theory of need hierarchy using hologeistic comparison by statistical sampling. Advances in Nursing Science 9 (1): 58-73
Doering E R 1983 Factors influencing inpatient satisfaction with care. Quality Review Bulletin (9 Oct): 291-299
Eriksen L R 1987 Patient satisfaction: an indicator of nursing care. Nursing Management 18 (7): 31-35
Ferguson G H, Hildman T, Nichols B 1987 The effect of nursing care planning systems on patient outcomes. Journal of Nursing Administration 17 (9): 30-37
Foucault M 1976 The birth of the clinic. Tavistock, London
Friedman E 1986 What do consumers really want? Healthcare Forum 29 (May/June): 19-24
Gadow S 1980 Existential advocacy: philosophical foundation on nursing. In: Spicker S F, Gadow S (eds) Nursing: images and ideals. Springer, New York
Gadow S 1982 Body and self: a dialectic. In: Kestenbaum V (ed) The humanity of the ill: phenomenological perspectives. University of Tennessee Press, Knoxville
Henderson V 1982 The nursing process—is the title right? Journal of Advanced Nursing 7: 103-109
Holm K, Cohen F, Dudas S, Medema P G, Allen B L 1989 Effect of personal pain experience on pain assessment. Image: Journal of Nursing Scholarship 21 (2): 72-75
Hoskins L M, McFarlane E A, Rubenfeld M G, Walsh M B, Schreier A M 1986 Nursing diagnosis in the chronically ill: methodology for clinical validation. Advances in Nursing Science 8 (3): 80-89
Humphris M R 1979 The nursing process: an application of scientific method. Australian Nurses Journal 9 (4): 30-31
La Monica E 1979 The nursing process: a humanistic approach. Addison-Wesley, Menlo Park
Larson P J 1984 Important nurse caring behaviours perceived by patients with cancer. Oncology Nursing Forum 11 (6): 46-50
Lawler J 1983 Ousting Maslow from nursing. The Australian Nurses Journal 13 (1): 36-38
Lawler J 1990 The body, dirty work and nursing: toward understanding the invisibility of nursing care. Proceedings of the XII National Conference of the Royal College of Nursing, Australia, Sydney
Lawler J 1991 Behind the screens: nursing, somology and the problem of the body. Churchill Livingstone, Melbourne
Linder-Pelz S 1982 Toward a theory of patient satisfaction. Social Science and Medicine 16: 577-582
Marriner A 1983 The Nursing Process. A Scientific Approach to Nursing Care. 3rd edn. Mosby, St.Louis
Maslow A H 1943 A theory of human motivation. Psychological Review 50: 370-396
Mauksch I G, David 1972 Prescription for survival. American Journal of Nursing 72 (12): 2189-2193
Oberst M T 1983 Patients' perceptions of care. Cancer 53 (May 15 supplement): 2366-2373
Parker J M 1988 Theoretical perspectives in nursing: from microphysics to hermeneutics. Third Nursing Research Forum, Lincoln School of Health Sciences, La Trobe University, Melbourne, (March)
Rasch R F R 1987 The nature of taxonomy. Image: Journal of Nursing Scholarship 19 (3): 147-149
Richards D A 1987 The nursing process: the effects on patients' satisfaction with nursing care. Journal of Advanced Nursing 12: 559-562

Thomas S 1987 Nursing diagnosis: what is it? Australian Journal of Advanced Nursing 4 (3): 41-48
Topics in Clinical Nursing 1986 8 (2)
Turkett S 1987 From the other side of the side rails. Nursing Life (May/June): 9
Ventura M R, Fox R N, Corley M C, Mercurio S M 1982 A patient satisfaction measure as a criterion to evaluate primary nursing. Nursing Research 31 (4): 226-230
Vincent K G 1985 The validation of a nursing diagnosis: a nurse consensus survey. The Nursing Clinics of North America 20 (4): 631-640

11. Phenomenology: a window to the nursing world

Lesley Wilkes

Phenomenology is an approach to viewing and researching lived-experiences within a world. In order to determine the importance of phenomenology to nursing an understanding of the nursing world and other research paradigms used to explore this world need to be examined.

NURSING IN ITS WORLD

As nursing moves into the 1990s nurses are seeking to remove the blooming, buzzing confusion of making sense of their world (Pearson 1989). They are trying to intertwine the dichotomy of theory and practice.

Practice is a 'lived-experience' and as such involves not only the nurse but other health professionals and at the centre the client (the nursed). It involves human beings experiencing and interacting. Theory has many meanings. Scientific literature refers to theory as a specific set of related doctrines (hypotheses, axioms, or principles) that can be used in making specific predictions and detailed explanations of natural phenomena (Laudan 1977). Laudan goes on to define more general testable sets of doctrine as conceptual models. Both of these appproaches are ways of seeking a common denominator, meanings of the world one lives in, ways of conceptualizing reality (Adams 1985).

The inseparability of these two domains of theory and practice in a practice oriented profession such as nursing is discussed by Speedy (1989). She states that the rewards of keeping them intertwined will allow nurses to develop multiple understandings of their world, and she goes on to suggest that in order to formulate knowledge about nursing practice by research, the theory-practice relationship is critical.

Nursing needs to identify what it is, how it is lived, what health is, what care is from both the point of view of the nurse and the nursed. Caring is a word often used in nursing but as yet there is no consensus as to one definition. Leininger (1985a) states that the cognitive components of caring tend to be examined rather than the internal (intersubjective) structures of caring which are essential to the nurse and the nursed. Certain humanistic attributes of caring, e.g. sympathy, compassion, trust, empathy, support, protection, have been labelled as caring; but what meaning do they have for the nursed? What is the reality of the nursed? Only through an analysis and synthesis of the experiences of the nurse and the nursed will an understanding of nursing and caring evolve.

Nursing, as a human science of human beings and human interaction, implies holistic care. The nursed is seen as a social, psychological, spiritual and biophysical being. In its most abstract form holism (wholism) is seen as the totality of human experiences. Specifically related to health, holism goes beyond the notion of cure—it is more than cure, it is well being. Well being exists when a person is integrated and in equilibrium with her/his environment (Bruni 1989). In holistic nursing the nurse is the facilitator of care.

Carper (1978) sees three types of knowledge vital to holistic nursing practice: ethical knowledge, personal knowledge, and aesthetic knowledge. Ethical knowledge relates to the matters of duty, rights, obligations, and morals necessary for clarifying values and in advocating for the nursed and practice. It is communicable by language but it is not public, verifiable, or common as there are legitimate disagreements existing.

Personal knowledge is an awareness of self and others in relationships. It involves encountering and actualizing self—self awareness, i.e. honesty. It advocates freedom and choice (Kramer 1990). Aesthetic knowledge is knowing by subjective acquaintance, abstracting the particular rather than the general. Carper (1978) states that this is immediate knowing based on the gathering of the specific and unique into a balanced and unified whole, integrating these particulars and acting in relation to projected outcomes. It embodies the use of past experience and knowing. It is an expression of what expert nurses do—old knowledge and experience evolves into new knowledge in a unique situation.

Holism implies that if the parts are separated the whole no longer exists. If nursing is holistic it should be explored and analyzed by research methods that look at the lived experience and describe it. In holism there is no completeness of structured knowledge; it is practically unachievable. Holism supports the idea that there are multiple descriptions of the same phenomenon. It recognizes that there is a limitation of language in establishing meaning of lived-experience.

The uniqueness of the world of nursing stands on its appreciation of caring and holism. This appreciation needs to be studied to expand the knowledge of this world. Both of these concepts imply that there are multiple descriptions of the same phenomenon depending on the individual, the situation and the language. In the nursing world different research paradigms have been used to seek understanding. The next section explores these paradigms and how they allow researchers to seek multiple meanings for holism and caring whilst maintaining the intertwining of theory and practice.

RESEARCH PARADIGMS

There are three major paradigms utilized in nursing research. These are the positivist, the interpretative, and the critical theory approaches (Allen et al 1986, Pearson 1989). The positivist philosophical approach argues that only sensorially apprehended experiences can form the basis of valid knowledge and that accordingly knowledge can be advanced only by means of observation and experiment (Cohen & Manion 1985). In research this philosophy is concerned with quantitative appproaches, i.e. theory is developed and tested. Theory and practice are separate. This research selects particulate variables, controls, experiments, and prescribes meanings and chacteristics. Nursing is no longer holistic, care is controlled. Leininger (1985a) states that quantitative research focuses upon the empirical and objective analysis of discrete and preselected variables that have been derived a priori as theoretical statements in order to determine causal relationships among variables studied. Empirical research using control would have difficulty in assisting an understanding of holism or care, or intertwining theory and practice in nursing. It can be used to study some processes in nursing, e.g. physiological changes in illness, but other aspects of human beings, human experience—culture, values, and beliefs—may need to be explored in other ways.

The second research philosophy, the interpretative paradigm, has developed because of dissatisfaction with the positivist approach in the study of humanism. This approach is directed towards providing 'interpretative' accounts of phenomena rather than law-like generalizations. There are varied approaches in this philosophy, but all agree that the social world can only be understood from the standpoint of the individual actors rather than the actors identifying cause, predicting outcomes, and allowing control. Carr & Kemmis (1983) express it thus: human actions cannot be observed in the same way as natural objects. They can only be interpreted by reference to the actors, motives, intentions, and purposes in performing actions. To identify these motives and intentions correctly is to grasp the subjective meaning the action has for the actors. This philosophy gives rise to qualitative research.

Leininger (1985a) states that these approaches refer to methods and techniques of observing, documenting, analyzing and interpreting attributes, patterns, characteristics, and meaning of specific, contextual, and gestaltic features of phenomena under study. In this approach theory and practice are inseparable; nursing can be seen as holistic. As Allen et al (1986) state, theory in context is used to understand rather than to form principles or conclusions, and is drawn from practical activity and knowledge. Research approaches using this paradigm will explore different types of knowledge that the positivist approaches do not allow and will thus add to nursing knowledge as a whole. Examples of methods in this paradigm are: symbolic interactionism, grounded theory, ethnography, and phenomenology.

The third paradigm is the critical theory approach. This goes beyond the interpretative and positivist approaches by totally integrating theory and practice. It seeks to identify and criticise disjunctions, incongruities, and contradictions in people's life experiences. It focuses on critical self-reflection coupled with action and change. It is overtly political and is directed towards personal and social transformation rather then scientific description (Candy 1989). Before this approach can be achieved an understanding of the reality of the world under investigation is needed.

If nursing is considered holistic, caring, involving human beings experiencing and interacting, the interpretative approach to research will help nurses to grasp the totality of events, situations, and experiences and fit them together for themselves and others, especially the nursed. This approach will help to document unknown features of the construct of nursing practice. Phenomenology is one of these interpretative approaches.

PHENOMENOLOGY

A definition

Phenomenological research is the study of lived-experience. Its purpose is to seek a fuller understanding through description, reflection, and direct awareness of the many facets and integral meanings of a phenomenon. It is the ministering of thoughtfulness (van Manen 1984a). Phenomenology begins with human experience.

Historical perspective

Phenomenology is not only a research method, it is a philosophy. It arose in Germany in the late 19th century from a perceived need to understand human science (mental, social, historical) which was different from natural science (physical, chemical, behavioural, and animal). It therefore required interpretation and understanding (hermeneutics) rather than external observation and explanation as used in natural science. Human science involves the disciplines of humanities, social science, and nursing, where the interpretation and meaningful expression of the inner cognitive and spiritual aspects of human beings (holism) in social, historical, and political contexts is sought (Ray 1990). The phenomenological method crystallized in reaction to the denigration of philosophical knowledge and objectivication that was taking place in relation to human science (Omery 1983).

Historically the 'Phenomenological Movement', as described by Spiegelberg (1965), has three phases: the preparatory phase; the German phase; and the French phase. Cohen (1987) describes the preparatory phase as the method of inquiry instigated by Franz Brentano (1838-1917) in the second half of the 19th century. Brentano provided two ideas essential to later phenomenology. The first is inner perception—the ability to be aware of one's own psychic phenomena. The second is discussed intentionality—the fact that everything we consider to be psychic refers to an object.

The German phase was dominated by Edmund Husserl (1859-1938), a student of Brentano and Martin Heidegger(1889-1976). Husserl, the father of the Phenomenological Movement' related phenomenology to the question of knowing. He believed that the 'rigor' of philosophy should not only have a 'rigor' but also a new humanism. Husserl emphasized a need of essence, i.e. going beyond the real facts to idealized, logical laws, making generalizations. This is not fundamental to phenomenological research where individual cases are important.

Husserl gave phenomenology the term—'intuiting'. This refers to logical insight based on careful consideration of representative examples; it is not second sight or inspiration. Phenomenological reduction is another influential idea of Husserl and has become a basic procedure of many phenomenological methods. Through 'bracketing' of all judgements about the nature and essence of things, events and so on—putting aside but not denying—and by disregarding their uniqueness, that which is given in cognitive experience is reduced to the 'essentials' of its form (Schultz 1970). Thus, it can be seen as an explanation of consciousness.

Heidegger, a pupil of Husserl, developed a different emphasis in relation to the lifeworld: existential phenomenology—how phenomena present themselves in lived-experience in human existence. Heidegger used phenomenology as a means to a solution, more specifically the search for a solution to 'being'. Heidegger's phenomenology has three essential tenets:

1. Human beings are self interpreting. These interpretations are not just possessions of the self; they are constituents of self.
2. To be human beings means that the kind of being one is is an issue, i.e. the person takes a stand on the kind of being she/he is.
3. The self is not a radically free arbitrator of meaning.

Heidegger believed that a person's meanings were engaged in particular situations (Benner/Wrubel 1989). Though the meanings available to the individual can undergo transformation they are limited by a particular language, culture, and history: self-interpretation is embedded in language, skills, and practice (Benner 1985). No laws or mechanisms can provide a higher meaning to everyday practices and experiences. Heidegger was concerned with what kind of knowing occurs when one does not stand outside the situation but is involved in it. Thus the theory and the practice are intertwined.

This existential phenomenology had a great influence on the French phase of phenomenology. The three prominent philosophers of this phase were: Gabriel Marcel (1889-1961), Jean-Paul Sartre (1905-1980) and Maurice Merleau-Ponty (1908-1961).

Sartre developed a philosophy which became central to existential phenomenology, i.e. to reconcile the object and the subject (Spiegelberg 1965). He believed that a person's behaviour (existence) preceded a person's character (essence), character being the outcome of free acts. Research is guided by examining concrete, real thoughts and behaviour prior to idealized essences or images (Cohen 1987). The practice and theory are intertwined. As Sartre (1963) states, 'concrete thought must be born from praxis and must turn back upon it in order to clarify it, not by chance or without rules, but—as in all scientific methodology—in conformity with principles'. He also reinforces Husserl's intentionality in which the intended object is constituted by consciousness.

Merleau-Ponty, like Sartre, held the proposition that consciousness is of the world and that there is always consciousness of something; such as judging, remembering, dreaming—all of the world, external not internal (Oiler 1986). In this way our body is an access to the world (sensation, language, sexuality). From this perspective pure consciousness 'I am' has no meaning . The meaning comes from 'I am' a nurse, or 'I am' interested in knowing about the nursed.

Merleau-Ponty (1962) developed the idea of perception in his work saying that it is a person's access to the truth, the foundation of all knowledge, and that a person perceives nothing without the world, i.e. the lived-experience. His phenomenology is related to experience, space, time, body, and human relations as we live them (Ray 1990).

Omery (1983) describes Spiegelberg's six steps which are common to all philosophical methods of phenomenology.

1. Descriptive phenomenology (including direct observation, analysis and description, without preconceived expectations and suppositions).
2. Essential or eidetic phenomenology (probing phenomena for typical structures and relationships)
3. Phenomenology of appearances (watching for clarity, seeking appearances in different situations)
4. Constitutive phenomenology (exploring the way in which the phenomena take place in consciousness)
5. Reductive phenomenology (suspending the belief in reality)
6. Hermeneutic phenomenology (interpreting concealed meanings in the phenomena).

By intertwining the being in the world and interpreting the being in the world the phenomenological method attempts to gain access to the world from the human experience through reflection and thematic understanding of the experience. Phenomenological inquiry is a creative attempt to somehow capture a certain phenomenon in life in a linguistic description that is both holistic and analytical, evocative, universal, powerful, and eloquent (van Manen 1984a).

NURSING THEORISTS

Phenomenology has been used as a philosophical approach in the development of some nursing theories.

Watson (1979, 1985) proposes a philosophy of the science of caring stating that caring is central to nursing. Her work has an existential phenomenological perspective being influenced by the work of Heidegger. She describes ten carative factors which each have a dynamic phenomenological component:

1. The formation of a humanistic-altuistic system of values
2. The instillation of faith-hope
3. The cultivation of sensitivity to one's self and to others
4. The development of a helping-trust relationship
5. The promotion and acceptance of the expression of positive and negative feelings
6. The systematic use of the scientific problem-solving method for decision-making
7. The promotion of interpersonal teaching-learning.
8. The provision for supportive, protective and/or corrective mental, physical, socio-cultural and spiritual environment
9. Assistance with the gratification of human needs
10. The allowance for existential-phenomenological forces. (Watson 1979)

These carative factors are centred on psychosocial needs. Biophysical needs appear to form little part of Watson's writing. To the nursed, care can be seen as important in some biophysical sense.

Other nurse theorists who have phenomenology underpinning their descriptions of nursing are Rosemarie Parse, Martha Rogers and Margaret Newman. Parse (1981) builds the assumptions of her Man-Living-Health model of nursing using the tenets of the existential phenomenologists: Sartre, Merleau-Ponty, and Heidegger. Like Watson, in this model of nursing it is difficult to see any reference to the biophysical being which is part of the world of the nursed. Parse also uses concepts of Martha Rogers (1970) whose nursing theory of the unitary human being has a theme open to phenomenological research. Rogers, however, believed that human beings lived in a probablistic universe and were governed by the law of probability. Newman's model of health (1979) seen as the interrelationship between consciousness, space, movement, and time also has similarities to the phenomenological school of thought and would be appropriate for such a research approach.

Paterson & Zderad's (1976) humanistic model of nursing is influenced by existential phenomenologists, particularly Marcel and Merleau-Ponty. Their work is a product of an exploration of their experiences in clinical nursing as they have lived them with psychiatric clients, student nurses, and other health professionals. Assessment and perception of fact are seen as important by these theorists and the biophysical aspects of the phenomena are viewed from the perspectives of nurses and the nursed. Their method of describing the phenomenological approach is more definitive than the other theorists mentioned and will be discussed further.

Heidegger's approach is used extensively by Benner in her investigation of defining the expert nurse (1984). She also uses this philosophical approach with Wrubel (Benner & Wrubel 1989) in their exploration of caring: stress and coping in health and illness.

As can be seen from this discourse, phenomenology is being used in theory building within the world of nursing and, as such, methods need to be explored which both test and extend these theories.

Research methods

When undertaking research using the phenomenological approach some social scientists, such as Morris (1977), discourage the use of a set of steps as determined by specialists. Others will tell novice phenomenologists that one cannot develop steps but rather one must proceed as the direction of the experience indicates without the restrictions that such structure will impose (Swartz & Jacobs 1979). For these researchers phenomenology is an approach rather than a method. However, in order for phenomenology to be recognised as scientific, a definitive method is required. Oiler (1986) states that the phenomenological approach as it relates to nursing research does not offer a well defined set of methods or procedures which establish it as a paradigm and which is not open to criticism. On the other hand Omery (1983) asserts that as long as an experience has meaning the potential is there for the phenomenological approach to be used. The development of phenomenological methods has often been ill-defined and difficult to understand because of the lack of steps. The novice researcher has difficulty knowing where to begin.

The first well defined methodology for phenomenology was developed by van Kaam (1959) in his study of 'really being understood'. The steps in his method include:

1. Preliminary considerations. This is where the reseacher is orientated to the phenomenon. She/he orientates to a particular experience, e.g. giving an intravenous injection.
2. Research question. The question is evoked from the experience, e.g. how does the experience of having an intravenous injection affect the nursed?
3. Awareness phase. This is the stage of the gathering of the data. van Kaam uses written descriptions of the event from independent sources, e.g. the nurse giving the injection, the nursed receiving the injection.
4. Scientific explication. The raw data are listed, expressions are grouped together by labels, vague expressions are eliminated. The researcher

checks the constituents of each case against random cases. van Kaam uses percentage scores in classifying clusters, e.g. if 'having an intravenous injection was painful' was mentioned by 10 of 100 cases he would classify this as a 10% occurrence.

5. Description of the experience. A hypothetical description of the phenomenon is checked against random cases. The reliability of the results are established by checking the descriptions with independent experts, three in van Kaam's research.

Another methodology was used by Giorgi (1971) in his study of child learning. The steps described in his method concentrate on data analysis. Unlike van Kaam the data are collected by extensive interviews which are audiotaped. The interviews are then transcribed into text. His data analysis has five steps. The first step is to read the text to have an understanding of the whole experience. Next the reseacher reads the text again and identifies units (themes) within the whole. The researcher eliminates redundant units, and joins remaining units together. The next step involves reflection on the unit relationships and identification of a concrete language for the subject matter, e.g. using concrete concepts from nursing practice. The researcher then integrates and synthesizes her/his insight and writes a description. The description is sent to experts in the field of study for criticism. The final description of the phenomenon is an integration of descriptions from a number of interviews.

Another method is that by Colaizzi (1978) in which the text of data is collected from a number of sources: interview, nonverbal observation, the researcher's responses to the situation. In some respects the collection appears haphazard. The analysis is similar to Giorgi. The text is read to get a feel for the material. Concrete units (themes) are identified and joined together to form relationships, and then a description is written.

Nursing research

The first definitive method of the phenomenological approach in nursing research is described by Paterson & Zderad (1976). They developed a concept of phenomenological nursing as a method to understand and describe nursing situations. This method seeks to understand the nurse-nursed experience so that the nurse can interact with the nursed in a human way and therefore a healing way. It assumes that there is a perceived health need by the individual who is involved with the health care provider.

Paterson & Zderad describe five steps in their phenomenological nursing.

1. Preparation of the nurse knower to know. By being exposed to a variety of experiences, includng the humanities and clinical nursing, the nurse gains self knowledge.
2. Nurse knowing intuitively. This is self-awareness, getting inside the situation of another's experience. She/he goes into the situation

without any preconceived ideas. It is here the nurse grasps the subtle nuances of the interaction.
3. Nurse knowing scientifically—Separating oneself from what is known. The nurse takes phenomena known intuitively, looks at them, sorts, compares, contrasts, interprets, names, and categorizes them. The challenge of communicating a lived nursing experience reality demands authenticity with the self and rigorous effort in the selection of words, phases, and precise grammar (Paterson & Zderad 1976).
4. Nurse complementarily synthesising known others. This phase is where the nurse relates, compares, contrasts what occurs in the nursing situation to enlarge the understanding of nursing. It is not personal experience alone but an enrichment of the theoretical foundations of nursing.
5. Succession within the nurse from the many to the paradoxical one. This involves the descriptive process of the phenomenon. The truth emerges which, although uniquely personal, has meaning for all—a descriptive theoretical construct of nursing (Paterson & Zderad 1976).

The last three steps of analysis, synthesis, and description involve the comparing, contrasting, and seeking of the characteristics of the phenomena. Clinical experiences can be used to see differences and interrelationships between experiences. They can help to find central chacteristics which are similar or structurally different. Paterson & Zderad (1976) use analogy and metaphor to exemplify what the nurse is not doing. It is important to make this distinction between what is similar and what is different about the phenomena to seek the truth.

Benner (1984, 1985) and Benner & Wrubel (1989), as previously mentioned, use the phenomenological method. The phenomenological approach of Heidegger is used by these researchers in describing a systematic method of the study of text. The text is collected by observation and interview of persons involved in the experience under study. A systematic analysis of the whole text is undertaken together with an analysis of parts (themes), and a comparison of the two for interpretation of conflict and for an understanding of the whole in relation to the parts (Benner 1985). Benner (1985) recommends three strategies in writing the final script to make it adhere to the claim that it is a description of the original text. The first step is to verify the description with paradigm cases. These are full descriptions of particular cases which describe the theme to be established; such as a description of what an expert nurse does in a particular situation compared to a novice nurse in the same type of situation. The second strategy is to use vignettes from cases or exemplars. The last strategy, which is common to most definitive methods, is the description of thematic analysis, i.e. common themes in the text are used to present common meaning. These strategies are used both as a method and as a way of presenting the description of the phenomena from the research.

By using the phenomenological approach Benner (1984) has evolved a definitive work on the world of nursing. Within this she provides a view of nursing which allows for the growth of the individual nurse from novice to expert. Through this work she provides evidence of a model for nursing—an intertwining of theory and practice. Through this conceptualization she opens the way for others to step into the same arena and further the knowledge of what nurses are and what they do.

In their work on caring, Benner & Wrubel (1989) have increased nursing's knowledge base of this concept within the nursing world. In their study they use various lived-experiences of stress and coping to exemplify their definition of caring. They define caring as the person, events, projects, and things that matter to people. They state that caring is essential if a person is to live in a differentiated world where some things are really important and others are not.

The use of phenomenology allows nurse researchers to explore this tenet of caring. Other researchers have explored the perceptions of the person giving the care and the person receiving the care. Brown (1986) allows us to search for caring beyond the untouchable, e.g. the nurse using technology with the patient (client) is caring. This is documented in her study on patients' perceptions of caring. Swanson-Kaufmann (1986a), using this approach to the lived experience, documents four types of caring as seen by women who have just had a miscarriage. These are 'being with' the woman in an engaged manner; 'doing for' the woman by providing comforting and support measures; 'enabling' the woman to grieve for the loss; and 'maintaining the belief' that the woman can bear a child. Others such as Reiman(1986) have identified the non-caring interactions with nurses from the point of view of the nursed.

Ray (1987) uses a modified method developed by van Manen (1984a, b) in her exploration of a model for critical care. Data are collected by interview on audio tape. The interviews are transcribed and the text read. Common themes are extracted from the text of the lifeworld descriptions. Themes are isolated as exemplars and by using the available literature—'unbracketing' the phenomenon—the researcher reflects more deeply and is able to describe the phenomenon. In this method the phenomenological theory is an integration of the participant's description of the experience, the researcher's intuitive grasp of the whole of the experience (unity of meaning), the researcher's use of accumulative knowledge (literature on the phenomenon under study), and the researcher's creativity in the organization and explication of the phenomenon as theory (Ray 1990). van Manen (1984b) tends to use literature more than other phenomenologists.

Sauer (1985) describes her method of using the phenomenological approach to study three couples who had late pregnancies; the women were older than 29 years. Data were collected by interview with some structured questions, as well as by a diary the couples kept for three months after the birth. The researcher used the transcripts and her own log of encounters with the couples to create a context of the experience. She states how she was faced with a mound of data which she reflects was overwhelming. She extracted themes of the experience using exact words and compared these with each couple. She extracted two types of themes; forms, which were typical across couples; and variations, which were unique to an individual couple. From this analysis Sauer found that the central theme of planning stood out in the informants' lived-experiences. From this she describes the transition to parenthood within a framework of 'planned orderly lives'.

Personal research experience

The following is a description of my personal experience using the phenomenological approach in research (Wilkes 1988).

The setting of the study was the educational arena of nursing practice but the approach could easily be applied to the clinical setting to examine phenomena. The study was looking at practice in education. The phenomenon of interest was the Deans of the Nursing Programs in tertiary institutions in New South Wales: their roles.

The study commenced in 1984. I was employed at a tertiary college in New South Wales which was to begin an undergraduate nursing program in 1985. This was a state-wide phenomenon and 14 new programs in nursing were being initiated. In all but two settings, new Deans were to head the programs. Such a unique set of factors allowed for the exploration of the phenomenon of a new person entering a new senior position in a situation which, in most cases, was foreign to that individual. In other words I was becoming orientated to an area of specific interest (van Manen 1984b).

The question posed at the beginning of the investigation was: Does a Dean's perception of role change over time as he/she enters a role in a new institution? Eight of the 12 new Deans in the state were the subjects of the study. The number was selected because of their location close to the metropolitan area of Sydney and this is a limitation of the study.

The main source of data in the project was taken from extensive interviews of the eight subjects. The subjects were interviewed on three occasions over the period of the study. The first interview was early after subjects were appointed to the position of Dean in 1984. The second interview took place at the end of the first semester of the nursing course in 1985 and the final interview was at the end of the third semester of the course in 1986. The interviews were conducted by myself or, in the instance of my own college, by a person employed there but not involved with the nursing program. The questions in the interview schedule had a set format to provide my agenda, but the unstructured comments of the subjects during the interview became an important part of the data.

Data were analyzed in a systematic manner. The taped interviews were transcribed and the text read after each interview to gain an overview of the phenomenon at that time. Three stages of the emerging phenomenon were explored, each interview having the characteristics of one stage. At each stage, elements or themes were abstracted from the manuscripts of each Dean's interview and a description of the Dean's perceived role written. Exemplars from the transcripts were used to verify the written descriptions. For example during the first interview one subject stated: 'I feel fuzzy about the institution and its structure'; at the second interview: 'I am clear on how the institution works. I am developing policies'; and at the last interview: ' I have learnt about the institution, policies are clear'. A theme evolving from these statements was a feeling of clarity for activities of the role and to some extent the Dean's expectation of the institution and the people in it.

Common and contrasting themes were drawn from the 8 descriptions of the Deans' perceptions and a model of a Dean's role at each stage described. Three stages were labelled: newness, awareness, and consolidation.

In the final synthesis, by using accumulated knowledge on the subject of organizational socialization in the literature (van Manen 1984b), and data collected and analyzed, a model of the role transition of the Dean was formulated. The themes were transformed into the context of the subject (Giorgi 1971). Finally the scripts were read and compared to original data by a person experienced in communication for some validation. No extensive cross checking of data was undertaken with outside experts since as with all types of qualitative data (Wilson 1989) the analysis is individual and others will not have the same feel for the data.

In my experience with this method of data collection and analysis I was a novice and as noted by Oiler (1986) few models existed to guide me in my endeavours. At times the lack of prescribed steps was uncomfortable, particularly as I was coming from a natural science research background. However, because of this the exploration of the method was exciting. The benefits of having a co-researcher would have been advantageous in allowing dialogue throughout the research and to provide a counterbalance to my individual bias.

van Manen (1984b) has said that in order to use the phenomenological research method the researcher should be well aware of the phenomenon before starting. The novice may lose the essence of the experience because of lack of knowledge. Both myself, and the Deans, were mostly new to the tertiary sector and I was new to sociological research. This was a disadvantage in one way because of a lack of background knowledge, but having no background in the social sciences could remove some degree of presupposition and subjectivity.

The experience with this form of research has allowed me to reflect on research's real meaning and has allowed a new perspective to be added to my otherwise positivist view of research as encountered in natural science.

Alternatives

Phenomenology is akin to other forms of qualitative research in its concern with the inner and experiential aspects of human behaiour, i.e. how people define events or reality in relation to their beliefs (Chenitz & Swanson 1986).

These methods have their roots in symbolic interactionism. Blummer (1969) suggests that symbolic interactionism rests on three premises:

1. A human being acts towards things on the basis of the meanings that the things have for him.
2. Meaning of such things is derived from or arises out of social interaction that one has with one's fellows.
3. These meanings are handled in and modified through an interpretative process by the person in dealing with the things he encounters.

One of the major differences between phenomenology and symbolic interactionism is that the latter infers that human behaviour is a product of a process. This is common to the other two methods to be discussed and it separates them from phenomenology. These methods are ethnography and grounded theory. These have been used by nurses both in isolation and in a combination with phenomenology to explore the world of nursing.

Ethnography is a systematic process of observing, detailing, describing, documenting, and analyzing lifeways and particular patterns of a culture or subculture in order to grasp the lifeways and patterns of the people in their familiar environment (Leininger 1985b). It is the study of social order and the routines used by people in daily life. The descriptions of the culture are often the perceptions of the researcher rather than of the participants of the culture and are often biased by her/his own culture. This method can be used with the phenomenological method to define culture. Culture is a symbolic interaction in acquired knowledge that people use to interpret experience and general social behaviour (Spradley 1978). Unlike phenomenology the research may start with a theoretical construct. Ethnographic researchers may also use quantitative measures to analyze their data.

Ethnographic research is used extensively by nursing researchers in the United States, particularly by those who are looking at culture and care. Leininger (1978) use this method extensively in the elucidation of a theory of transcultural nursing. She investigated a number of cultures, from the health practices in New Guinea (Leininger 1966) to the comparison of black and white health practices in the southern states of Northern America (Leininger 1985c). Other nurses have studied particular cultures and their health practices, e.g. Boyle (1983) describes the illness experiences of women in Guatamala; Tripp-Reimer (1983) describes the folk healing practices of Greek migrants in Columbia, Ohio.

Another method which has philosophical roots in symbolic interactionism is grounded theory. This method was developed by Glaser & Strauss (1967) and it focuses specifically on the generation of theory from data. The researcher generates constructs (theory) from the data rather than applying a theory constructed by someone else from another data source. It is a highly ordered method in which specific steps are followed to code material (themes), propose relationships (diagramming), and describe the evolving theory. It offers a rigorous, orderly guide to theory development that at each stage is closely integrated with methods of social research. In this sense, generating theory and doing social research is viewed as the same process (Glaser 1978).

Grounded theory is different to phenomenology in that its major aim is theory generation rather than a meaningful description of the phenomenon. It is possible that, unlike phenomenology, preconceptions or sensitization to concepts prior to data collection can occur when using the grounded theory approach. This is because of the ongoing use of available literature on the researched subject during the process of data collection (Omery 1983). Some phenomenologists use literature to help formulate theoretical perspectives; but usually not until after data collection (van Manen 1984b, Ray 1990).

Nurses are using grounded theory to study a number of phenomena in nursing. Wilson (1982) describes a theory of control in a mental institution. Stern (1987) uses the method to study stepfather families and describes the interaction processes within these families. Unlike phenomenology, this method provides a specific structure for the researcher, with steps to follow. Nurses are used to and familiar with structure and when venturing into research seem to seek such a methodology.

A number of nurse researchers combine the three methods described to provide avenues for research sequencing, data collection, and analysis. Swanson-Kaufman (1986b) describes a combined method using these three approaches. In her study of miscarriage and caring, Swanson-Kaufman (1986a) also uses this method. A combination of phenomenology and grounded theory was used by Drew (1986) to investigate patients' experiences with caregivers, particularly in relation to emotional interaction.

All methods discussed are avenues to knowledge and as Speedy (1989) emphasises, a large number of research paradigms need to be explored to determine knowledge about nursing practice.

A future in nursing research

The future of phenomenology as a model of nursing research is worthy of further discourse. Phenomenology has been discussed as a philosophy and a method which allows nurses to better understand their world. It allows nurse researchers to enter the world of the nurse and the nursed to gain meaning for such concepts relating to holism, health, environment, caring, and person which are central to most nurses' ideas of their world. It allows the nurse to see the patients' illnesses and the implications of their illnesses from the patients' points of view (Davis 1978). Phenomenology is a means for helping to break down the practice-theory dichotomy of nursing.

Used alone phenomenology can provide a wealth of knowledge but to investigate the different forms of knowledge, as outlined by Speedy (1989) and Carper (1978), various methods should be combined in research studies of nursing. Both subjective and objective knowledge is important to the world of nursing. Phenomena under investigation can be seen from two perspectives: measurable characteristics, and the situations in which they can be observed. The measurable characteristics are observable, quantifi-able, and stable whilst the situations of the phenomena in human science occur in physical, mental, and intuitive domains. As Wilber (1982) simplis-tically states, there are some data that can only be observed with the 'eye of the flesh' or the 'eye of the Mind' or the 'eye of contemplation'. Therefore phenomena cannot be moulded to the method. The research tradition must be selected to fit the phenomena (Bargaglotti 1983).

Nursing can be seen from many perspectives and as such a variety of research methods should be utilized. Phenomenology is but one side of a multifaceted coin in the search for an explication of the construct of nursing. It provides a baseline to provide ways of elevating nurses to new levels of understanding; for setting parameters for future research in the empirical paradigm; and especially in opening doors to the critical theory paradigm where critical self-awareness is coupled with action, and change. In order to instigate change through action the phenomena need to be understood and have meaning to the humans involved in the experiences. Phenomenology is the window to this world.

REFERENCES

Adams E 1985 Towards more clarity in terminology: frameworks, theorists and models. Journal of Nursing Education 24:151-155
Allen D, Benner P, Diekelmann N L 1986 Three paradigms of nursing research: methodo-logical implications. In: Chin P L (ed) Nursing research methodology: issues and implementation, Aspen, Rockville
Bargaglotti L A 1983 Researchmanship: the scientific method and phenomenology: toward their peaceful coexistance in nursing. Western Journal of Nursing Research 5(4):409-411
Benner P 1984 From novice to expert: excellence and power in clinical nursing practice. Addison Wesley, Menlo Park, California
Benner P 1985 Quality of life: a phenomenological perspective on explanation, prediction and understanding in nursing science. Advances in Nursing Science 8(1): 1-14
Benner P, Wrubel J 1989 The primacy of caring: stress and coping in health and illness. Addison-Wesley, Menlo Park
Blummer H 1969 Symbolic interactionism: perspectives and method. Prentice-Hall, Englewood Cliffs, p 2
Boyle J 1983 Illness experiences and the role of women in Guatamala. In: Uhl J (ed) Proceedings of the 8th annual Transcultural Nursing Conference, Detroit, p 52-71
Brown I 1986 The experience of care—patient perspectives. Topics in Clinical Nursing 8:56-62
Bruni N 1989 Holism: a radical nursing perspective. In: Koch T (ed) Theory and practice: an evolving relationship. Monograph: School of Nursing Studies, Sturt, South Australian College of Advanced Education, Bedford Park p 115-131
Candy P C 1989 Alternative paradigms in educational research. Australian Educational Researcher 16(3):1-10
Carper B A 1978 Fundamental patterns of knowing in nursing. Advances in Nursing Science 1:13-23

Carr W, Kemmis S 1983 Becoming critical: knowing through action research. Deakin University Press, Highton

Chenitz W C, Swanson J M 1986 Qualitative research using grounded theory. In: Chenitz W C, Swanson J M (eds) From practice to grounded theory: qualitative research in nursing. Addison Wesley, Menlo Park, p 4

Cohen L, Manion L 1985 Research methods in education, 2nd edn. Croom Helm, London

Cohen M Z 1987 An historical overview of the phenomenological movement. Image: Journal of Nursing Scholarship 19(1):32-34

Colazzi P 1978 Psychological research as the phenomenologist views it. In: Viale R, King M (eds) Existential phenomenological alternatives for psychology. Oxford University Press, New York, p 48-71

Davis A 1978 The phenomenological approach in nursing research. In: Chaska N l (ed) The nursing profession: views through the mist. McGraw Hill, New York, p 196

Drew N 1986 Exclusion and confirmation: a phenomenology of patients' experiences with caregivers. Image: Journal of Nursing Scholarship 18:39-43

Giorgi A 1971 An application of the phenomenological method in psychology. In: Giorgi A, Fisher C L, Murray E L (eds) Dusquesne studies in phenomenological psychology, Vol. II. Dusquesne University Press, Pittsburgh, p 82-103

Glaser B G 1978 Theoretical sensitivity. Sociology Press, Mill Valley

Glaser B G, Strauss A L 1967 The discovery of grounded theory. Aldine, Chicago

Kramer M K 1990 Holistic nursing. In: Chaska N L (ed) The nursing profession: turning point. C V Mosby, St Louis, p 245-254

Laudan L 1977 Progress and its problems: towards a theory of scientific growth. University of California Press, Berkley

Leininger M 1966 Convergence and divergence of human behaviours: an ethnopsychological comparative study of two Gadsup villages in New Guinea. Unpublished doctoral dissertation. University of Washington, Seattle

Leininger M 1978 Transcultural nursing: concepts, theory and practice. Wiley, New York

Leininger M 1985a Nature, rationale and importance of qualitative research methods in nursing. In: Leininger M (ed) Qualitative research methods in nursing. Grune & Stratton, Orlando, p 1-26

Leininger M 1985b Ethnography and ethnonursing models and modes of qualitative data analysis. In: Leininger M (ed) Qualitative research methods in nursing. Grune and Stratton, Orlando, p 32-72

Leininger M 1985c Southern rural black and white American life ways with focus on care and health phenomena. In: Leininger M (ed) Qualitative research methods in nursing. Grune and Stratton, Orlando, p195-216

Merleau-Ponty M 1962 Phenomenology of perception. The Humanities Press, Atlantic Highlands

Morris M 1977 An excursion into creative sociology. Columbia University Press, New York

Newman M A 1979 Theory development in nursing. F A Davis, Philadelphia

Oiler C 1986 Qualitative methods: phenomenology. In: Moccia P (ed) New approaches to theory development. National League of Nursing, New York, p 75-103

Omery A 1983 Phenomenology: a method for nursing research. Advances in Nursing Science 5: 49-63

Parse R R 1981 Man-living-health: a theory of nursing. Wiley, New York

Paterson J, Zderad L 1976 Humanistic nursing. Wiley, New York

Pearson A 1989 Translating rhetoric into practice: theory in action. In: Koch T (ed) Theory and practice: an evolving relationship. Monograph: School of Nursing Studies, Sturt, South Australian College of Advanced Education, Bedford Park, p 91-103

Ray M 1987 Technological care: a new model of critical care. Dimensions of Critical Care Nursing 6(3):166-173

Ray M 1990 Phenomenological method for nursing research. In: Chaska N L (ed) The nursing profession: turning points. C V Mosby, St Louis, p 173-186

Reiman D 1986 Noncaring and caring in the clinical setting: patients' descriptions. Topics in Clinical Nursing 8:30-36

Rogers M E 1970 An introduction to the theoretical basis of nursing. F A Davis, Philadelphia

Sartre M 1963 Search for a method. Vintage Books, New York

Sauer J L 1985 Using phenomenological research method to study nursing phenomena. In: Leininger M (ed) Qualitative research methods in nursing. Grune & Stratton, Orlando, p 93-108

Schultz A 1970 On phenomenology and social relations. University of Chicago Press, Chicago

Speedy S 1989 Nursing theory and practice: risks and relevance. In: Koch T (ed) Theory and practice: an evolving relationship. Monograph: School of Nursing Studies, Sturt, South Australian College of Advance Education, Bedford Park

Speigelberg H 1965 The phenomenological movement, Vol. I&II. Martinus Nifhoff, The Hague

Spradley E 1978 The ethnographic interview. Holt Rinehart, Winston

Stern P N 1987 Conflicting family culture: an impediment to integration of stepfather families. In: Chenitz W C, Swanson J M (eds) From practice to grounded theory: qualitative research in nursing. Addison Wesley, Menlo Park, California

Swanson-Kaufman J M 1986a Caring in the instance of unexpected early pregnancy loss. Topics in Clinical Nursing 8:37-46

Swanson Knaufman J M 1986b A combination qualitative methodology for nursing research. Advances in Nursing Science 8(3):58-69

Swartz H, Jacobs J 1979 Qualitative sociology: a method to the madness. The Free Press, New York

Tripp-Reimer T 1983 Retention of folk healing practices (Maliasma) among four generations of urban Greek migrants. Nursing Research March-April 32:97-101

van Kaam A 1959 Phenomenological analysis: exemplified by a study of the experience of being really understood. Individual Psychology 15:66-72

van Manen M 1984a 'Doing' phenomenological research and writing. Monograph: Faculty of Education and Public Service, University of Alberta, Alberta

van Manen M 1984b Practicing phenomenological writing. Phenomenology and Pedogogy: A Human Science Journal 2(1):36-69

Watson J 1979 The philosophy and science of caring. Little Brown, Boston

Watson J 1985 Nursing—human science and health care. Appleton-Century-Croft, Norwalk

Wilber K 1982 The problem of proof. Revision 5(10):80-100

Wilkes L M 1988 The work role transition of eight nursing deans. Unpublished Master's Thesis, University of New South Wales, Kensington

Wilson H S 1982 Limiting intrusion; social control in a healing community: an illustration of qualitative comparative analysis. Nursing Research 2(6):103-111

Wilson H S 1989 Research in Nursing, 2nd edn. Addison-Wesley, Menlo Park

12. Phenomenology in clinical practice

Amy Bartjes

I know myself immediately only as an ever-changing sequence of occasions of experience, each of which is the present integration of remembered past and anticipated future into a new whole of significance. My life history continually leads through moments of decision in which I must somehow determine what both I and those to whom I am related are to be. Selecting from the heritage of the already actual and the wealth of possibility awaiting realisation, I freely fashion myself in creative interaction with a universe of others who also are not dead but alive (Ogden 1977).

One of the most vivid and evocative experiences I have had in my years of nursing is that of an interpersonal human interaction between nurse and patient in a hospice ward in England. Two human beings immersed in their world as they communicate in a whisper their messages to one another. The behaviour of the nurse attending to the patient's needs exemplifies tenderness, compassion, and the willingness to bring comfort to her dying patient. Her hands move with sensitivity and gentleness to ease the patient's pain. The gaze of the patient shows implicit trust in her carer. A faint smile forms on the patient's pallid lips as she verbally expresses in a whisper her gratitude for the comfort she experiences. I was touched by the beauty of human interaction I saw captured in a nursing moment. I wondered then whether the meanings that this phenomenon or experience had for me would be the same as those of the persons who enacted the experience. What research method would illuminate the phenomenon beyond the surface structure of this experience to unravel the underlying meanings of the lived-experience of nurse and patient as well as provide meanings for the world of the practice of nursing?

For a moment my attention was suspended in this revealing world of meaningful nursing experience which I have taken for granted so often.

The nursing situation I have observed requires exploration beyond counts and measures of things. It can provide a rich description of human meanings of experiences as lived by nurse and patient (Watson 1988). To unravel the underlying meanings of the lived-experience of both patient and nurse, one has to recognize that human experiences cannot be measured or experimented with—they are simply there and can only be explicated in their givenness (van Kaam 1966).

247

Ideas derived from lived-experience cannot be reduced to quantifiable data because of the multiplicity of coherent and integral meanings of phenomena (Ray 1990). Quantitative method with its abstract categories, general laws, and classification schemas, tends to weaken or diminish the wholeness of the original experience and the meanings constructed and constituted by the person about his or her social world. Too often the fluid richness of the lived-experience is sacrificed to a rigid order of prediction and control from which the person's emotional spontaneity and meaningfulness have disappeared. The clarification of experience demands methods that eliminate the preconceptions that obfuscate objects in the first place (Husserl 1965). That task involves commitment to Husserl's principle of all principles. He said that 'whatever presents itself...is simply to be accepted as it gives itself out to be, though only within the limits in which it then presents itself' (1972).

Nurses can choose methods that allow for the subjective, inner world of personal meanings of the nurse and the other person. Watson (1988) states that we can choose to study the inner world of experiences rather than the outer world of observation. We can choose to be a part of our method and involved in the clinical research process rather than be distant, objectively remote, and primarily concerned with the product of science. We can choose to pursue more of the private, intimate world of human care and inner subjective human experiences, rather than to concentrate on the public world of non-human cure techniques and outer world.

The purpose of this chapter is to present an exploration and brief history of phenomenology, and describe the methodology and its application to nursing practice.

Phenomenology is the study of essence—what makes something what it is (Ray 1990). Its focus is to describe experience as it is lived (Oiler 1982). The central point of phenomenology is the human experience. As a research methodology, it deals in the practical world of concession, compromise, and approximation (Swanson-Kauffman & Schonwald 1988). It differs from quantitative, descriptive, and ethnographic research methodologies in that phenomena are studied from the subjects' unstructured descriptions of lived-experiences. Ray states that the purpose of phenomenology is to seek a fuller understanding through description, reflection, and direct awareness of a phenomenon to reveal the multiplicity of coherent and integral meanings of the phenomenon. It examines a lived-experience as a whole for the purpose of understanding social reality from the context of the person who lived the experience.

Phenomenology is a way of viewing ourselves, of viewing others, and of viewing all else that comes in contact with our lives. In this sense, it is a system of interpretation that helps us perceive and conceive ourselves, our contacts and interchanges with others, and everything within the realm of our experience (Wagner 1983). It purports to be a presuppositionless philosophy. Nothing can be accepted by the inquirer unless he has scrutinized its character and implications and also recognised that it is a feature of experience (Natanson 1973). Its focus is on just that experience, to see and grasp it afresh in order to articulate in full clarity the logic (Kohak 1978) and integral meanings of the phenomenon (Ray 1990).

Phenomenology is a philosophy, an approach, and a method (Oiler 1982). It has been used in many disciplines such as theology, philosophy, physics, psychology, sociology ,and anthropology. As a philosophy, it deals in the realm of the ideal, pure and perfect in search of what is truth.

HISTORICAL MOVEMENT OF PHENOMENOLOGY

Franz Brentano (1838-1917) was the forerunner of the phenomenological movement in the last half of the 19th century (Reeder 1984). His work was further developed in Germany by Edmund Husserl and later refined by Martin Heidegger in the first quarter of the 20th century. It was sustained in France by Jean-Paul Sartre, Gabriel Marcel, and Maurice Merleau-Ponty (Parse et al 1985).

This movement locates its purpose and direction in the theory and praxis called conscious experience, that is, the relationship between a person and the lived-world (Lebenswelt) that he or she inhabits (Zeitgeist). As a theory, phenomenology concerns itself with the nature and function of conscious-ness. As praxis, it operates with an investigation method that explains experience (Lanigan 1988).

As a philosophical movement, Husserl's investigation started as a search for the philosophical foundations of consciousness. In the course of his career, phenomenology then came to mean the study of phenomena, as phenomena appeared through consciousness. Many phenomenologists of this century are still influenced by the Husserlian or transcendental school of phenomenology. This is emphasized in the concepts and ideas which include:

* An analysis of the subject and object as the object appears through consciousness
* An emphasis on bracketing or epoche as a method for suspending naive realist awareness
* Emphasis on describing the full appearance of the object of inquiry' (Speigelberg 1984).

PHENOMENOLOGY AS A FORM OF QUALITATIVE RESEARCH

Quantitative and qualitative research methods are valuable tools in search of true knowledge. They can be complementary to each other. Qualitative research methods tend to generate hypotheses whereas quantitative research methods predict and control the data to test the hypothesis. Dabbs (1982) in his attempt to differentiate between quantitative and qualitative ap-proaches indicated that the notion of quality is essential to the nature of things.

Quantity is elementally an amount of something whereas quality refers to the what, how, when, and where of things—its essence and ambience. Qualitative research thus refers to the meanings, concepts, definitions, characteristics, metaphors, symbols, and descriptions of things (Berg 1989).

One type of research method that deviates from traditionally accepted conceptualizations of research designs and statistics is phenomenology. Ray (1990) states that it is a method of inquiry that is more adequate for the study of human beings wherein the situated meanings of human experience can be understood. It is a method that unfolds the essence of the meaning of what is life and what it means to live, what is nursing and what it means to nurse, what is caring and what it means to care. It addresses one central question which is 'what is the structure and essence of the lived-experience for this person?'. The phenomenon being experienced may be an emotion, relationship, job, and many more. Its defining characteristic is the assumption that there is an essence or essences to shared experience. These essences are the core meanings mutually understood through a phenomenon commonly experienced (Paton 1990). Evidence of growing interest in the phenomenological method is seen in literature and books written by nurses (Paterson & Zderad 1976, Davis 1978, Omery 1983, Reeder 1984, Benner 1985, Parse et al 1985, Ray 1985, Munhall & Oiler 1986, Cohen 1987, Watson 1988, Anderson 1989, Bergum 1989, Morse 1989, Smith 1989, Ray 1990).

PHENOMENOLOGY AS METHODOLOGY FOR NURSING THEORY AND PRACTICE

Paterson & Zderad's method

Paterson & Zderad (1976) proposed a phenomenological methodology relevant to humanistic nursing practice and theory. They referred to it as phenomenological method of nursology. This method aims at the reality of human beings, how they experience their world, or their subjective-objective state. It aims at description of the professional clinical nursing situation which in reality is a subjective-objective world that occurs between subjective-objective beings. There are five phases of phenomenologic nursology. They are presented below.

Phase I: preparation of the nurse knower for coming to know

This phase engaged the investigator as a risk-taker and as a knowing place or a noetic locus. In this phase, the nurse investigator approaches the situation or data openly, letting the structure emerge from it, not deciding what to look for, being willing to be surprised, giving feelings of excitement, fear, and uncertainty. The process of accepting the decision to approach the unknown openly is experienced as an internal struggle and conscious awareness of the rigidity and satisfaction with the status quo of the nursing community to which one belongs. In this phase, the nurse investigator must be aware of her or his own angular view of biases through which she/he regards her/his lived-world.

Phase II: *nurse knowing of the other intuitively*

In this phase, the nurse investigator responds to the uniqueness of the other person with whom she/he interrelates, does not superimpose, maintains a capacity for surprises and questions, and is with the other, as opposed to seeming to be. Therefore, the encounter is personally, responsibly, authentically chosen and invested in by the nurse investigator. This phase requires that the nurse investigator is a part of that which is being studied. Observations interpreted from outside the situation could be classified only as projections.

Phase III: *nurse knowing the other scientifically*

The third phase of the methodology calls for a reflective practice. In this reflective state the nurse investigator analyses, considers relationships between components, synthesises themes and patterns, and then conceptualises or symbolically interprets a sequential view of his/her past lived-experience.

Phase IV: *nurse complimentarily synthesizing known others*

This synthesis allows mutual representation and illumination of one reality by another. The nurse investigator arrives at an expanded view by comparing and synthesising the similarities and differences of like nursing situations.

Phase V: *successsion within the nurse from the many to the paradoxical one*

In this phase, the nurse investigator is able to generate concepts and theories which advance nursing knowledge. This nursing knowledge arises from the multiple communion of nursing situations and arrives at a conception that is meaningful to nursing and is expressed abstractly in units or as a whole, as one.

Since the birth of the phenomenological movement different methods evolved from its philosophy such as those of van Kaam (1966), Van Manen (1984), Giorgi (1970), Colaizzi (1978), Merleau-Ponty (1964) and Spiegelberg (1970) to mention a few.

Spiegelberg's method

Spiegelberg (1970) explains the six steps that are common to all interpretations or modifications of phenomenological philosophy. These steps are as follows:

1. Descriptive phenomenology: direct exploration, analysis, and description of the phenomena under study, as free as possible from unexamined presuppositions aiming at maximum intuitive presentation. It is the turning away from preoccupation with concepts, symbols, theories, and hypotheses. It is the turning toward the concrete referents in experience, i.e. to the uncensored phenomena. It was in the attempt to get at these pure phenomena that Husserl developed the procedure of the so-called phenomenological reduction, the suspension of one's held beliefs in the existence of everyday phenomena.

2. Phenomenology of essences: (essential or eidetic phenomenolgy), probing of the phenomena for typical structures or essences and for relations within and among them. It calls for the constant mobilization of imagination by shuttling back and forth between the concrete and the abstract aspects of the phenomena observed. The natural order of this exercise according to Brockelman (1985) is to go from the familiar to the less familiar, the ordinary to the less special, the concrete and everyday to the more abstract structural relations of the phenomena. Brock (1957) states that what we, the people of the world, need, perhaps most, is to exercise our imaginations, to develop our ability to look at things from outside our accidental area of being. To illustrate the point of view of Brock, there are diverse meanings and values from culture to culture about curing, caring, and healing. The shaman of Africa has as much credence to his tribal people as the doctor in Australia to the clients he or she serves.

Disease and healing perception carry personal and cultural meanings shaped by one's own lived-experience. This in itself presents variation in social construct about health and illness which calls for essential insight. This essential insight according to Spiegelberg (1984) requires that on the basis of such variation we determine what is essential or necessary and what is merely accidental or contingent. To see what is essential is 'seeing life steadily and seeing it as a whole'. But it is no less important to develop the sense for the accidental and the contingent. This sense can effectively counteract one's tendency to take things for granted.

3. Phenomenology of appearances: giving attention to the ways in which such phenomena appear in different perspectives or modes of clarity. It means paying attention not only to the what, but also to the how, to the ways or modes in which the phenomena appear. In the most often taken-for-granted world of clinical nursing practice, the perspectives of caring are inexhaustible. Re-seeing caring in a phenomenological context recognizes and confirms the infinite value of nursing, as 'a discipline of human science and human cares' (Watson 1988).

4. Constitutive phenomenology: studying the processes in which such phenomena become established (constituted) in our consciousness. Spiegelberg (1970) alluded to the work of Husserl. Husserl distinguished constitution into passive and active. In passive constitution, the chaos data take shape against the background of disjointed impressions, whereas active constitution is putting together the pieces of the puzzle by way of constitutive effort. It is a dynamic process of getting to know, of becoming acquainted with the known.

5. Reductive phenomenology: suspending belief in the reality or validity of the phenomena; a process which is basic for phenomenology. It is the bracketing of the natural world, also known as reduction or epoche. Suspending one's belief or rash judgement to knowledge of other people, other groups, and other nations with their different worlds is an expression of simple intellectual humility or open-minded social skepticism.

6. Hermeneutic phenomenology: interpreting the concealed meanings in the phenomena that are not immediately revealed to direct investigation, analysis and description. The steps of the philosophical method put forward by Spiegelberg have inspired some of the researches conducted in the discipline of social sciences (Omery 1983).

Van Manen's method

Van Manen (1984) sees phenomenological research as a dynamic interplay among four procedural activities. They are:

1. Turning to the nature of lived-experience. Lived-experience means not only the sense of awareness but much more. It includes not just happenings in their external aspects—the pain of an injury, the loss of a loved one, the joy of being cared for—but also who you are or who I am now as a person who has had this sensory awareness. It includes all the feelings, memories, and desires which are generated by the awareness of what has happened in the past, what it means at present and the future. Ray (1990) refers to this as the 'eternal now' and alluded to the work of Reeder (1984). It is the unfolding of the lived-experience from the past, the present and the future integrated in one's consciousness or mode of awareness all at once. Reeder refers to it as a domain of 'conscious world'. According to Reeder, it involves an 'unbuilding' process from the everyday way of experiencing the world as possible and intelligible through reflection, intellectual intuition, and imagination.

Van Manen (1984) states that turning to the nature of the lived-experience means that it is a driven commitment of turning to an abiding concern, a quest, a true task, a deep questioning of something which restores an original sense of what it means to be a nurse, or a teacher, a patient, a theorist, or a researcher. At the heart of this quest is the sublime recognition of one's own contribution to humanity—'that which renders fullness or wholeness to life'.

2. *Existential investigation of experience as we live it.* It aims to establish a renewed contact with original experience rather than as we conceptualize it. Brokelman (1985) states that it is a sort of intellectual archaeological investigation. He argues further that it is an attempt of phenomenology to dig deep down into, explore, and to sift out some fundamental aspects of our ordinary lives and experience those which often remain hidden and unavailable to reflective consciousness, because they are covered over with layers of culture, linguistic, and philosophical sedimentation. More specifically, we want to get at and lay out some significant elements of the personal dimension of our lives by means of a careful phenomenological analysis of action and temporality from the point of view of the person who has lived the experience.

3. *Reflecting on essential themes.* Phenomenological research consists of faithful and thoughtful reflective grasping of what it is that gives this or that particular experience its special significance. What is it that makes this reflective experience what it is? It is the application of logos (language and thoughtfulness) to the phenomenon (lived-experience).

4. *Description of phenomenon.* A good description that constitutes the essence of something is construed so that the structure of lived-experience is revealed. The phenomenon of life is captured in a linguistic description that is both holistic and analytical, evocative and precise, unique and universal, powerful and eloquent.

The concerns of phenomenology are a preoccupation with both the concreteness (the ontic) as well as the essential nature (the ontological) of a lived-experience (Van Manen 1984).

Colaizzi's method of analysis of descriptive data

After collecting the informant's descriptive responses, there are analytical steps to consider. Colaizzi (1978) developed a phenomenological method of analysis of the descriptive data based from the lived-experience of the informants. The procedure is outlined using examples from a part of an interview of one of the participants of a phenomenological research study to illustrate the steps. The title of this research is: The meaning of caring based from the lived-experience of hospice nurses.

Step 1:

Read all the subject's descriptions, conventionally termed protocol, to make sense out of them.

Representative original protocol

As a practising nurse in a hospice unit, caring is the object and subject of my nursing practice. I present myself as a human being responding to the call of another human being in need of help or assistance. I respond to this call from the patient all at once as a nurse, a friend and a good Samaritan. Years of experience have taught me to know intuitively when a patient is in pain, anxious, happy, sad or even when death is imminent. I can sense when patients just want my presence or when they want to engage in a conversation. I know when I am expected to just listen. This in itself is a very humbling and yet rewarding experience. I have to be really truly present with the patient. It means that I have to set aside the tasks I have planned to do unless they are very important. It means too that I have to enable the patient to unfold and communicate the remaining pages of the last chapter of his or her life. It means that I have to be very aware not to monopolize the conversation but listen and be present with my whole being authentically. Patients in a hospice unit do not have the luxury of so much time left to live. The nurse does not have the wealth of opportunity to build a long lasting relationship. While patients are still breathing, they deserve the respect of being treated with dignity as a human being alive in the community of the living.

I attended a funeral once and during the eulogy I realized how little I know my patient. If only I had known then what I know now about my patient before he died, it would have made a lot of difference in our nurse-patient relationship.

I remember a patient who (unknown to me) was a wine connoisseur. I was giving him a bed sponge one morning. He was complaining to me how medical science had not done anything to ease his excruiating back pain. Whilst in agony, he expressed his mental, emotional, spiritual and physical suffering. He said that 'death would be a welcome reward to his suffering'. I asked him if there is anything he really wanted beside death which I was powerless to give. He whispered the name of a wine. I asked for more information about this wine and for a quarter of an hour he told me everything I should look for in terms of the qualities of a good wine. In that quarter of an hour he came alive as a person. All of a sudden I saw colour on his pale cheeks, there was excitement and life in his eyes and in his voice. It was a quarter of an hour of pain free 'moment' as he chatted animatedly with all the wisdom he could bring forth to teach a willing listener about the qualities of a good wine. I sensed intuitively then the need to allow time to listen to a very interesting aspect of the life history of my patient.

Caring means that as a nurse I must recognize the importance of the need to find time to listen to what the patient has to say even if it is only a moment...a moment of a life time to a dying patient...a moment that would make a difference in the quality of nursing care.

Step 2:

Returning to each protocol and extracting phrases or sentences that directly pertain to the investigated phenomenon is known as extracting significant statements.

Significant statements

1. Acknowledges intrinsic value system about caring in nursing practice.
2. Presents self as a human being.
3. Acknowledges the patient as another human being.
4. Responds to the call of the patient in need of help or assistance.
5. Knows intuitively how the patient feels.
6. Knows intuitively when the patient's death is imminent.
7. Knows when to listen when the patient needs to talk.
8. Allows time for the patient to talk.
9. Awareness of avoiding monopoly of conversation.
10. Being authentically present with the patient.
11. Recognizes the limited life time of the dying patient.
12. Awareness of the limited opportunity of the nurse to build a longer lasting relationship with the dying patient.
13. Acknowledges the importance of upholding the dignity of the dying patient.
14. Acknowledges the value of knowing the patient as a person and its implication to the quality of the nurse-patient relationship.

Step 3:

Try to spell out the meaning of each significant statement, known as formulating meanings. The formulations must discover and illuminate those meanings hidden in the various contexts and horizons of the investigated phenomenon which are described in the original protocols without severing connection with it.

Step 4:

Repeat the above for each protocol, and organize the aggregate formulated meanings into clusters of themes.

1. Refer these clusters of themes back to the original protocols in order to validate them. If the clusters of themes are not thereby validated, for example if they contain themes which are alien to the original protocols, then the preceding procedures must be re-examined or conducted anew.
2. At this point discrepancies may be noted between the various clusters. The researchers must rely upon their tolerance for ambiguity. They must avoid the temptations of ignoring data or themes which do not fit, or prematurely generating a theory which would merely conceptually-abstractly eliminate the discordance of their findings. Sometimes, there is a tendency for themes to overlap in one or two headings. A summary of clusters of themes is shown below.

Clusters of themes

1. Affirmation of personhood:
   a. Views oneself as a human being
   b. Views the patient as a human being
   c. Acknowledges the upholding of dignity of the dying patient
   d. Acknowledges the importance of knowing the patient as a person.
2. Compassion—sensitivity to the needs of another person:
   a. Responds to the call of the patient for help or assistance
   b. Intuitively knows how the patient feels or what she or he needs
   c. Allows time for the patient to talk
   d. Unpretentious presence with the patient.
3. Competence—knowledge of judgement, skills, experience, and motivation:
   a. Intuitively knows how the patient feels
   b. Knows when to listen
   c. Intuitively knows the needs of the patient
   d. Knows when patient death is imminent
   e. Avoids monopoly of conversation
   f. Recognizes the limited time of the patient
   g. Acknowledges the importance of building a good nurse-patient relationship.

Step 5:

The results of everything so far are integrated into an exhaustive description of the investigated topic.

Exhaustive Description Results
What is taken for granted about the meaning of caring in hospice nursing is now seen in a new light. It brings a new range of possibilities about human caring.

The ordinary lived-experience described by the hospice nurse revealed an ongoing struggle of human experience. Caring entails the capacity to care; the calling forth of this capacity in oneself and others; caring as responsivity to being called by someone who matters; actualization of the capacity to care and caring as manifested in specific, or concrete acts (Roach 1987).

According to Watson (1988) the knowledgeable caring of the nurses presupposed a knowledge base and clinical competence in nursing. She added that compassion and empathy are offered by knowledge of human behaviour and human responses to actual or potential health problems; knowledge of how to respond to others' needs; knowledge of our strenghts and limitations; knowledge of who the other person is, her or his strengths and limitations, the meaning of the situation for her or him; and knowledge of how to comfort.

Knowledgeable caring requires not only an intention, a will, a relationship, and actions which stem from caring as a moral ideal (Watson 1988), it expects of a professional nurse the highest degree of 'competency in clinical nursing practice' (Stiles 1990).

Step 6:

An effort is made to formulate the exhaustive description of the investigated phenomenon in as unequivocal a statement of identification of its fundamental structure as possible.

Step 7:

A final validating step can be achieved by returning to each informant, and, in either a single interview session or a series of interviews, asking the subject about the findings and how they compare with the descriptive results or what has been omitted. Any relevant new data that emerges from these interviews must be worked into the final product of research.

Formulating the phenomenological question

According to Van Manen (1984) when formulating the phenomenological question, one has to be constantly oriented to the experience that makes it possible to ask the question 'what is it like':

• What is the meaning of...?
• What is the nature of this lived-experience?
• What is it like to live a life of...?

For example, my research study addresses the phenomenological question of 'what is it about caring in hospice nursing that gives the experience of caring its pedagogical importance?'. When I ask, 'what is the essence of caring in hospice nursing?', I am searching for the pedagogical ground for caring in hospice nursing. In doing so, I want to come to an in depth understanding of what it is about caring in hospice nursing. Through the lived-experience of being with the dying patients I want to understand the meaning of caring and what is it like to be a caring nurse in a hospice setting.

To truly question something is to interrogate something from the heart of our existence, from the centre of our being (Van Manen 1984). Husserl refers to this as 'to the things themselves' which is the life motive of phenomenological research. Here the concern is that of giving the phenomena a fuller and fairer hearing than traditional empiricism has accorded (Spiegelberg 1984).

In other words, 'to the things themselves' is a procedural admonition to study an object of experience as an object of my experience and to exclude everything that does not belong immediately to that object as directly given

(Rogers 1983). It requires the suspension of all belief in a reality beyond intentionality (Spiegelberg 1984).

IMPLICATIONS OF PHENOMENOLOGY TO CLINICAL NURSING PRACTICE

The continuing quest of nursing involves a search for the meaning of nursing as a 'human caring science and art' (Watson 1988). Nurses have struggled with the questions: What is nursing? Who is a nurse? What is the meaning of health, illness, healing, and caring in the context of nursing? What is the nature of the relationship between nurse-patient, nurse-family and/or significant others, nurse and other members of the health team and their lived world? How can nurses unravel the full range of their human caring potential as healers in order to provide a rich and rewarding service to humanity? In the process of searching and pursuing the answers to the infinite questions about the nature of nursing as a 'human caring science and art' (Watson 1988), new visions of the nature of nursing are beginning to unfold through a variety of research methods utilized by the profession.

One of the perennial problems in understanding the meaning of nursing has been to determine the most appropriate research method for the investigation of the nature of nursing or its essence. Influenced by the empirical-positivist thought, nursing research focused primarily on the reductionist approach. This approach manifested itself even in nursing practice whereby the recipients of nursing care were treated as isolated parts or problems resulting in fragmentation of human beings. In doing so, nurses often lost sight of the patient as a human being. The essential task of phenomenology in nursing practice is to describe, represent, or provide accounts of significant phenomena revealing the essence of nursing.

Nursing is a profession of healing art and science. Its social and scientific responsibility is to provide health and expert human caring service to humanity. Its practice is grounded in a human science context based upon:

- a philosophy of human freedom, choice, responsibility
- a biology and psychology of holism (nonreducible persons interconnected with others and nature)
- an epistemology that allows not only for empirics, but for advancement of aesthetics, ethical values, intuition, and process discovery
- an ontology of time and space
- a context of interhuman events, process, and relationships
- a scientific world view that is open (Watson 1988).

The notion of holistic healing is embedded within the nursing tradition. Its essence is manifested in the sacred wisdom of the art and science of caring. Nurses as healers 'heal with their hands and their words and the deep conviction that they have a knowledge or talent that will help others' (Achterberg 1990). Furthermore, nursing practice involves diagnosing and treating human responses to actual and potential health problems, and since humans respond as whole persons, the knowledge of the lived-experience of health and healing may be an impetus for further theory development, intervention, and social change in nursing (Swanson-Kauffman & Schonwald 1988). For this reason phenomenology becomes essential not only as a research method but also for the actual implementation of holistic, emphatic, individualised delivery of nursing care (Munhall 1989).

In a book developed from the successful radio program broadcast in Australia entitled *The Search For Meaning* hosted by Caroline Jones of the Australian Broadcasting Corporation, Emma Pierce expressed in her interview how she made sense of her lived-experience of mental illness.

I found the treatment in the institutions humiliating. I was consistently patronised, as was everyone else there. I had no compassion for anyone else. As far as I was concerned, all other inmates were really mad but I was just sick. It took me years to discover, after meeting many people who'd spent years in mental institutions, that it's a conviction that first strikes every patient—that everybody else is mad but somehow you're just sick.

By and large the professionals do try to help. I guess what hurts is that they really don't know how to help and I find them now resisting the knowledge that it really is simple—not easy, by no means easy, but definitely simple. The constant diagnosis is that it is a 'physical illness'. I will make a categorical statement and say that even after 500 years of mental illness research, they will never connect it to a physical cause. I'm not talking about epilepsy and actual brain disorders, I am talking about the agonising loss of personal value, of living without a sense of worth and meaning.

When asked about the meaning of the experience and how she made sense of it all, she replied,

I find that it is a growing experience. I don't look at it as a breakdown as much as a breakthrough to better living. It's given me, I suppose, in a sense, a mission in life, which is why I've written *Ordinary Insanity* and I'm still writing.

I hope to give sufferers and healers alike an understanding of what mental illness is and how to deal with it. I want the medical profession to stop and think how would they like to be on the receiving end of the diagnosis. (Jones 1990)

The excerpts from the interview reveal how patients/clients interpret their own lived-experiences and give meaning to them. In the context of phenomenology, human beings, their world, and their experiences of their world are seen as inseparable (Colaizzi 1978). Explication of its inherent phenomena entails an intuitive grasp of the phenomenon, analytic examination of its occurrences, synthesis, and description (Kleiman 1986). The knowledge generated enriches nursing's understanding of health and the human condition (Smith 1989) and conveys that knowledge to others who are at a distance from the situation, event, or location. At the same time, it communicates an important message that calls for social change within the structure of the health care system. The message raises the question of: 'Do nurses see the patients/clients as they really are and know them in their own reality or do nurses see the patients/clients merely as a projection of their own theories of what human beings should be?'

May (1958) argues that without the 'necessary bridge', nurses can only stand on one side of the chasm, forever unable to get to the other side and forever separated from the human being as he or she authentically is.

Nursing practice uses diagnostic and therapeutic interventions to help the sick person towards the healing process. The patient in turn responds as a whole person not as parts, and the part of the whole is the mind and the spirit, as well as the body (Dossey 1984, 1985, Achterberg 1990). Knowledge of the lived-experience of illness, health, and healing are significant points of nursing research which inform practice.

Equally as important in nursing research and practice are the patients and their lived-experience in the health care context within which they experience the nursing services they receive. Patients are recipients of health services and are the reasons for which service structures are designed. They become the central theme of the work and the work place. Unless nurses are conscious of the meaning of human struggle experienced by the patient within the health care system, nursing management will find it impossible to fully achieve those service structures and characteristics necessary to meet the needs of the consumer (O'Grady 1986). It is in this context that phenomenology provides a way of capturing the human meanings of the lived-experience of patients in a language essential for social change shaped according to the values of the recipient of health care.

Another glaring issue within the context of the health care system relates to nurses. It is common knowledge that nurses are the linchpin in the health care delivery system that undermines the values of individuality. The pecking order, so very entrenched within the hierarchical structure of the hospitals, places the nurses' social position at the bottom. The role of the nurse is to carry out medical and administrative orders and in this type of arrangement, clinical nurses often live with the perception of powerlessness. The frustrations that this inhuman situation creates lead to the loss of sense of purpose and meaning in work and in life for nurses. These are vital issues that concern everyone in a society that is increasingly dependent on the diminishing and stringent resources of the health care delivery system. Successful organizations will need to recognise the value of individualism against collectivism. The hidden meanings of the struggle of nurses, their hopes and dreams to be recognized as a profession in their own right calls for an inquiry that examines a lived-experience as a whole for the purpose of understanding social reality from the context of the participants.

Phenomenology endeavours to provide insights into the continuing debate on the role of the nurse as one of the indispensable members of the health team. The crucial dilemma experienced by nurses in the present rigid and highly technocratic health care system can be explicated and communicated to the human world through the use of phenomenological inquiry. Such social reality as lived by nurses, according to Kohak (1978)

Is not material or mental but experiential, the reality of human praxis whose structuring is intentional and teleological. Thus, what we need to explain are not the objects but experiences, and to explain means to grasp the intentional structure of an experience, as a necessary pattern of subject experience, and only secondarily within a particular perspective, to find a cause.

In addition, phenomenological method does not only seek to understand the sensuous matter in the world but all the experienced ideas, facts, behaviours, and aspiration of human beings as they exist in their world.

The greatest gift of the profession to humanity in an age of science and technology is to withstand the forces of technocratic enslavement. The economic and political pressures of organizational gigantism and standardization have found their way to the doorstep of a multi-million dollar health care industry. One of the many adverse effects of this is the depersonalisation of existence.

If the profession of nursing succumbs to these forces, it will have lost its birthright—the practice of holistic healing as a human caring art and science. For it is the function of the profession first and foremost, not to lose sight of the patient as a human being who is an indivisible whole. The accent of the work of nurses is likely to reflect a broad sense of healing that aspires to wholeness or harmony within the self, the family, and the global community (Achterberg 1990).

CONCLUSION

Within the realm of nursing as a human caring art and science, phenomenology offers a different research approach and meanings for use in understanding the healing experience of the individual within the context of her or his lived-experience. Phenomenology communicates the authentic meaning using a language that deepens the understanding of the lived-experience of the person and this understanding of life and healing as it is lived is valuable to the development and growth of nursing knowledge. Clearly, knowledge generated from phenomenological inquiry will strengthen the foundation of nursing practice and contribute to the development of the discipline of nursing.

Acknowledgement

The author wishes to acknowledge the valuable contribution of Lesley Barclay, Associate Professor, School of Nursing Studies, Flinders University of South Australia; Dr Marilyn Ray, Associate Professor in Nursing, Florida Atlantic University; and Professor Jean Watson, Director, Center of Human Caring, University of Colorado.

REFERENCES

Achterberg J 1990 Women as healer. Shamhala, Boston
Anderson J M 1989 The phenomenological perspective. In: Morse J M (ed) Qualitative
    nursing research: a contemporary dialogue. Aspen, Rockville
Benner P 1985 Quality of life: a phenomenological perspective on explanation, prediction,
    and understanding in nursing science. Advances in Nursing Science 8:1-1
Berg B L 1989 Qualitative research methods for the social sciences. Allyn & Bacon, Boston
Bergum V 1989 Being a phenomenological researcher. In: Morse J M (ed) Qualitative
    nursing research: a contemporary dialogue. Aspen, Rockville
Brock G 1957 Prescription for survival. World Health Organization, New York. In: Smith F
    J 1970 (ed) Phenomenology in perspective. Matinus Nijhoff, The Hague
Brockelman P 1985 Time and self. Phenomenological explanations. The Crossroad, New
    York
Cohen M1987 A historical overview of the phenomenological movement. Image 119:31-34
Colaizzi P F 1978 Psychological research as the phenomenologist views it. In: Valle S, King
    M (eds) Existential-phenomenological alternatives for psychology. Oxford University
    Press, New York
Dabbs J M 1982 Making things visible. In: Van Manen J (ed) Varieties of qualitative
    research. Sage, Beverly Hills
Davis A J 1978 The phenomenological approach in nursing research. In: Chaska N L (ed)
    The nursing profession: views through the mist. McGraw Hill, New York p 186-196
Dossey L 1984 Beyond illness. New Science Library, Boulder
Dossey L 1985 Space, time and medicine. New Science Library. Shamhala, Boston
Giorgi A 1970 Psycholgy as a human science: a phenomenologically based approach.
    Harper & Row, New York
Husserl E 1965 Phenomenology and the crisis of philosophy. (Translated by Lauer Q).
    Harper Textbooks, New York
Husserl E 1972 Ideas: general introduction to pure phenomenology. (Translated by Boyce
    W R). Collier, New York
Jones C 1990 The search for meaning. Australian Broadcasting Corporation. Collins Dove,
    Sydney
Kleiman S 1986 Humanistic nursing: the phenomenological theory. Paterson and Zderad.
    In: Winstead-Frog P Case studies in nursing theory. National League for Nursing, New
    York
Kohak E 1978 Idea and experience. Edmund Husserl's project of phenomenology in ideas
    1. The University of Chicago Press, Chicago
Lanigan R L 1988 Phenomenology of communication. Duquesne University Press,
    Pittsburg
May R 1958 The origins and significance of the existential movement in psychology. In:
    May R, Angel E and Ellenberger H F (eds) Existence. Basic Books, New York
Merleau-Ponty M 1964 The primacy of perception. Edie J M (ed) (Translated by Wild J).
    Northwestern University Press, Evanston
Morse J M (ed) 1989 Qualitative nursing research. A contemporary dialogue. Aspen,
    Rockville
Munhall P L, Oiler C J 1986 Nursing research. Appleton-Century-Crofts, Norwalk
Munhall P L 1989 Philosophical ponderings on qualitative research methods in nursing.
    Nursing Science Quarterly 2:20-28
Natanson M 1973 (ed) Phenomenology and the social sciences (2 vols). Northwestern
    University Press, Evanston
Ogden S 1977 The reality of God. Harper & Row, San Francisco
O'Grady P 1986 Creative nursing administration. Aspen, Rockville
Oiler C J 1982 The phenomenological approach in nursing research. Nursing Research
    31:178-181
Omery A 1983 Phenomenology: a method for nursing research. Advances in Nursing
    Science 5:49-63
Parse R R, Coyne A B, Smith M J 1985 Nursing research. Qualitative methods. Prentice-
    Hall, Bowie

Paterson J G, Zderad L T 1976 Humanistic nursing. Wiley, New York

Paton M O 1990 Qualitative education and research method, 2nd edn. Sage Publication, Newbury Park

Ray M 1985 A philosophical analysis of caring within nursing. In: Leininger M (ed) Qualitative research methods in nursing. Grune & Stratton, New York

Ray M 1990 The phenomenological method for nursing research. In: Chaska N L (ed) The nursing profession. Turning points. C V Mosby, St Louis

Reeder F 1984 Nursing research, holism and philosophies of science: points of congruence between E Husserl and M E Rogers nursing science. Doctoral dissertation, New York University, New York. Univeristy Microfilm International, Ann Arbor

Roach M S 1987 The human act of caring. Canadian Hospital Association, Ottawa

Rogers M 1983 Sociology, ethnomethodology and experience. A phenomenological critique. Cambridge University Press, Cambridge

Smith M 1989 Facts about phenomenology in nursing. Nursing Science Quarterly 2:13-16

Spiegelberg H 1970 On some human uses of phenomenology. In: Smith F J (ed) Phenomenology in perspective. Martinus Nijhoff,, The Hague

Spiegelberg H 1984 The phenomenological movement: a historical introduction. 3rd revised enlarged edn. Martin Nijhoff, The Hague

Stiles M K 1990 The shining stranger: a phenomenological investigation of the nurse-family spiritual relationship. Doctoral dissertation, University of Colorado Health Sciences Center, Denver, Colorado. University Microfilm International, Ann Arbor

Swanson-Kauffman K, Schonwald E 1988 Phenomenology. Paths to knowledge. Innovative research methods for nursing. In: Sarter B (ed) The stream of becomings: a study of Martha Roger's theory. National League for Nursing, New York

Wagner H R 1983 Phenomenology of consciousness and sociology of the life world. An introductory study. The University of Alberta Press, Edmonton

Watson J 1988 Nursing: human science and human care. A theory of nursing. National League for Nursing, New York

van Kaam A 1966 Existential foundation of psychology. Duquesne University Press, Pittsburgh

Van Manen M 1984 Doing phenomenological research and writing. An introduction. Monograph 7: The Department of Secondary Education, The University of Alberta, Alberta

13. In support of a scientific basis

Debbie Neyle   Sandra West

Nursing has historically claimed to be both an art and a science. Nightingale, in her *Notes on Nursing* (1859), describes the art of nursing 'to be expressly constituted to unmake what God has made disease to be'. In her prologue, Nightingale laments the tendency of women to misunderstand 'the laws of health' and questions 'Did Nature intend mothers to be always accompanied by doctors?' So it can be said that Nightingale, writing in the late 19th century, clearly saw both an art and a science in nursing.

Social development since Nightingale's era has been predominantly scientifically and technologically based. Nursing, like all other components of society, has felt the effect of this scientifically based knowledge explosion. Chaska (1990), now somewhat cynically, defines the art of nursing as 'intervening between the patient and the technological assault which constitutes modern medicine'.

The layperson's definition of science tends to be significantly confused with the concepts of technology. Nightingale's 'laws of health' can be equated with a science, but she does not direct us to anything which can be equated with a technology. Technology may be a product of scientific knowledge but the growth of technology has different social effects from the growth of science. In evaluating the social value and effects of science, it is important that this distinction between science and technology be understood.

THE SCIENCES OF NURSING

For the purpose of this work science shall be taken to mean 'the advancement of our understanding of the way in which the observable world works, the development of a logical, integrated and self-consistent description of why and how such and such individual events occur: why apples fall from trees; why they are colored red and green; why they are good to eat; irrespective of the immediate utility of these statements' (Ziman, 1984). Applying such a definition to the current conceptualisation of nursing, it can be seen that there are essentially three distinct areas of science involved. These are:

- **The traditional or basic science**—including physics, chemistry, anatomy, physiology and microbiology—from which all health professions borrow. It is these basic sciences which frequently underpin other derived or applied areas of science such as pharmacology and pathophysiology.
- **The behavioural or social sciences**—including psychology, sociology, education and communication—from which the majority of health professions borrow. These behavioural and social sciences within nursing curricula contribute significantly to the practice of nursing.
- **The science of nursing itself**—that is the demonstrated body of knowledge which is uniquely nursing. This is derived from nursing practice itself and is consequently directed towards the improvement of that practice. It is this science which nursing, in its pursuit of professional status, must develop and depend upon.

Whilst not wishing to imply any hierarchical structure to these sciences in their relationship with and to nursing, it is useful to consider them in the order just listed.

Traditional sciences

In relation to the borrowed and established sciences, Doran (1983) states that 'these sciences are genuine intellectual pursuits having their own rules of observation and judgement, and open to criticism and revision...from within the paradigm'. The tenets of scientific methodology which have prevailed in modern civilizations during the industrial and post-industrial phases of development are both stated and implied in Doran's statement.

Scientific methodology and nursing process

Scientific methodology arose from a Baconian tradition of Natural Observation. In Baconian methodology large numbers of precise and extremely detailed descriptions of the natural world were written and suggestions made as to the natural laws or patterns. These descriptions greatly increased the knowledge of natural events. The major revision of Baconian methods can be related to the rise of mathematical knowledge. The experimental-mathematical method which is described in this chapter was originally perfected by Galileo and has become known as the Scientific Method. The steps in Scientific Methodology are:

1. Selection from the phenomena under discussion of specific aspects expressible in quantitative terms
2. Formulation of a hypothesis involving a mathematical relationship (or its equivalent) among the quantities observed
3. Deduction of certain consequences, from this hypothesis, which are within the range of practical verification

4. Observation, followed by change of conditions, followed by further observations, i.e. experimentation embodying, in so far as it is possible, measurement in numerical magnitudes

5. Acceptance or rejection of the hypothesis framed in 2. An accepted hypothesis then serves as the starting point for fresh hypotheses and their submission to test. This step produces gradual but increasingly confident scientific prediction (Needham 1984).

Although the verbiage of such a description is not readily acceptable, nurses should not feel alienated from the scientific method. Indeed, as clearly shown in Table 13.1, the scientific method closely approximates the steps of the nursing process. Thus if a client presents requiring extensive bed rest, the selection of phenomena for examination has largely been predetermined. The nurse is free to make a nursing diagnosis or to hypothesize, for example, that the bedridden client is at a greater risk of developing decubitus ulcers than the ambulant client (note the mathematical form of expression used here). Following the determination of such a nursing diagnosis the nurse makes deductions related to it. The client's risk of any particular consequence is likely to be increased by some actions and decreased by others, but all implementation of action will result in change. In the scientific method all of these change agents are termed variables and a practising nurse must be aware of the existence and importance to her/his client of these variables even without the expressed intention of experimentation.

Table 13.1 The nursing process as a scientific method

Scientific method	Nursing process
Selection from the whole phenomenon of specific, quantifiable aspects	Selection from the whole gamut of nursing aspects those specific to the client
Formulation of an hypothesis	Formulation of a nursing diagnosis i.e. potential and actual problems
Deduction of consequences from the hypothesis	Deduction of consequences from the nursing diagnosis
Observation $\longrightarrow$ Results $\longrightarrow$ Change i.e. the experimental phase	Action $\longrightarrow$ Change i.e. the implementation phase
Acceptance or rejection of the hypothesis with some chance of prediction	Evaluation of actions with consequent potential to generalize and predict

The nurse implements a plan of action and observes the response. The client receiving second hourly repositioning is noted to develop 'red areas' which could be quantified or measured. The use of a ripple mattress is instituted, leading to observed reduction in redness. This same process of actions being undertaken, results observed and appropriate change being made, is the basis of experimentation conducted under the scientific method.

Whilst it is understandable that professional nurses may not be comfortable with the concept that they are experimenting on, and with, their clients, this is in essence what occurs until the establishment of 'the best fit' of the individual client to the available nursing responses. The nurse then evaluates the actions taken in terms of client outcomes and should (but frequently doesn't) allow a moment of self-praise at another successful implementation of the nursing process/scientific method. One argument advanced for including the traditional sciences in nursing curricula, at both pre and post registration levels, is simply to inculcate scientific methodology, as an analogue of the nursing process, and as a method of inquiry that can be used throughout the nurse's entire career. That is not to say, however, that science and scientific methodology is entirely without flaws.

Limitations of scientific methodology

Merton (1957), has identified 'four norms of scientific method' which work to ensure the accurate application of the scientific method within society. These are:

1. Communism (*Communalism*). This refers to the sharing of scientific information freely between members of the scientific community so that any member can pursue a path of study. Communism fails in a social setting requiring unique publications and establishing priority of discovery. The concept of scientific prizes, such as the Nobel prize, discourages communism in scientific practice.

2. Universalism exhorts scientific practitioners to take the world view of research and to make the products of research available equally to all people. Universalism suffers under the assaults of patriotism, military secrecy and bound research funding. If a particular pharmaceutical company has funded a particular research project they may be displeased if, in the spirit of universalism, the results of that research are made freely available to all people of all nations.

3. Detachment. This also suffers in the social context of scientific practice. Detachment requires the scientist to have no vested interest in the outcome of a particular area of research. However, if career status or, perhaps more importantly, patent ownership rights are involved, it would be a very rare scientist , or indeed human being, who remained completely detached.

4. Organised scepticism. In Mertonian terms, this refers to a mind set which questions everything. The outcomes and methods of scientific experiments should always be open to criticism and all scientific data should be capable of replication. Scientists however, like human beings, can be fallible and may criticize on criteria other than science. Replication of experiments is also very rare as it attracts no real benefits for the researcher.

Science performed within a society then may be flawed but the knowledge produced may well retain its relevance. Nurses need to be selective in their use of traditional science and constructively critical of the role of all science both within nursing and the wider community.

The areas of science that are included in the traditional group, also form the basis of medicine and the other mainstream health professions. Hahn and Kleinman (cited by Baer, 1989), when exploring the rise of bio-medicine, state that bio-medicine exhibits a 'primary focus on human biology, or more accurately on physiology, even pathophysiology' and thus tends to divert attention from the social origins of illness. Despite the existence and awareness in many circles of such strong criticism, bio-medicine has been able to establish economic and ideological dominance over alternative medical systems in Western society. Other health related occupations, finding themselves subordinate to doctors in the medically designed division of labour, have tended to absorb some of the philosophical premises, therapeutic approaches and organizational structures of bio-medicine.

Traditional science and nursing

Nursing has also tended to absorb the scientific basis of medicine, altered only by the educational constraints of available time and student entry levels. Akinsanya & Hayward (1980) state 'It is our contention that unless nurses, both educators and clinicians, identify and define the biological basis of nursing education and practice, they cannot claim to contribute to the education of nurses any specialized knowledge derived from these subjects which is distinctive from pure medical knowledge'.

While there is strong evidence to suggest that there is an ideological acceptance of science in the general community (Doran 1983) and indeed amongst nurses (West & Neyle 1990), the challenge to nursing is to borrow only those aspects of the traditional sciences which can be identified as having relevance to the practice of nursing, and to teach science to neophytes in nursing, or to those pursuing a particular nursing specialization, in a manner which ensures the transfer of scientific principles to the actual care of clients. Thus the relevance of traditional science to nursing could be clearly demonstrated during teaching; the curriculum may be slightly lightened; and there ought still to be sufficient content to inculcate the tenets of scientific methodology in students.

The behavioural and social sciences

The humanistic emphasis of the Behavioural Sciences makes a significant contribution to the 'art' of nursing. Nevertheless, these are also sciences in the tradition of scientific enquiry. The knowledge base of these sciences arose from experimentation using scientific methodology in just the same manner as the traditional sciences and suffers from just the same limitations. William Osler (cited by Graver, 1986), writing nearly a century ago, warned his medical colleagues of the danger of too exclusive an association with science, asserting that full-time academic (i.e. research oriented) medicine would isolate the physicians from the public, both physically and emotionally. This warning is echoed by the ambivalence shown by some sections of society, towards both science and scientists, arising no doubt from the perception that science is responsible for many of the world's current ills. Nevertheless, individuals rely on the products of science for a more comfortable existence. Within medicine and nursing, science is often seen as dehumanizing, yet 'society gives greater respect and higher wages to the specialist when compared to the "family doctor" a generalist' (Graver 1986) and 'it is hard to deny that society continues to demonstrate almost a hedonistic need for the products of science' (Shils 1987).

PHENOMENOLOGY

It is into this confused melee that some proponents of the behavioural sciences seek to inject the philosophy and research method of 'phenomenology'. Omery (1983) in proposing this method states that

> For a growing group of nurse researchers, the scientific method has become constraining. The method's inherent nature, which reduces the human being under study to an object with many small quantitative units, has become problematic for many nurse researchers. It gives no clue as to how to fit these small units back into the dynamic whole that is the living human being with whom the nurse interacts in practice.

Before entering into a description of the process of phenomenological research it is interesting to consider the rhetoric both of the above statement and of other similar statements made in support of phenomenology. Carl Cohen (1987) calls such statements 'Heavy Question Arguments', 'so framed as to be either unanswerable yet effective in surrounding the research with an air of catastrophe or to be literally unanswerable, but only upon the supposition of truth of unfounded allegations about the research that are never plainly stated or defended'.

Both aspects of this concept of heavy question arguments are found in Omery's previously quoted statement: 'For a growing group of nurse researchers, the scientific method has become constraining' (1983). This is an irrefutable comment on two levels:

1. Even if the 'growing group of nurse researchers' increases only from one to two, as a circle of personal discontent is formed within an academic institution, the statement is correct. Omery doesn't expand on the defining limits of her briefly described group.

2. The scientific method is constraining on all researchers, requiring as it does definitions of hypotheses, variables and methodologies, and the exposure of the researcher to public scrutiny and possible criticism.

The implication, of course, is that such constraints are damaging to the pursuit of knowledge, yet there is no evidence proffered to support the truth of this assertion. The second focus of Omery's comment is illustrated by the statement 'how to fit these small units back into a dynamic whole'. This is literally unanswerable, unless the contention of a reductionist methodology in all previous science is accepted without any definitive proof. The emotive language, e.g. 'dynamic whole' and 'living human being' is also typical of opponents of traditional and behavioural science who are using heavy question arguments.

Given that the propositions advanced by Omery are unanswerable or only answerable under onerous pre-suppositions there arises the possibility of extended heavy question arguments:

- Why won't proponents of scientific methodology address these simple statements?
- What are they so afraid of?
- Is the silence of the scientific community some admission of guilt for years of reductionist methodology dehumanizing all before it?

The rhetoric and emotion of this level of questioning clearly displays the same aspects of the original heavy question arguments whilst more clearly highlighting the irrationality inherent in such statements. Nurses should be very aware of the potential for anti-science fervour to lead away from the important foundations of our professional knowledge and development, and of the need to be rationally critical of all manner of knowledge and philosophy presented to them.

Phenomenological philosophy and method

To return to the discussion of the phenomenological philosophy and methodology, 'Phenomenology is, in the 20th century, mainly the name for a philosophical movement whose primary objective is the direct investigation and description of phenomena as consciously experienced, without theories about their causal explanations and as free as possible from unexamined preconceptions and presuppositions' (Spielberg 1965). 'Phenomenology also leaves aside all knowledge obtained elsewhere and all the sciences of these objects because it places itself in thought before the beginning of all such science' (Stanage 1987). This process is known as 'bracketing out' and removes from consideration all prior knowledge pertaining to the phenomenon under observation.

If it is possible to allow a philosophy some degree of anthropomorphism, the worst interpretation of these statements presents phenomenology as a supremely egotistical being, blithely dismissing the body of accumulated scientific knowledge gathered over centuries of painstaking observation and experimentation. At best phenomenology appears a little naive. 'The resulting phenomenological method is a solitary, introspective process that aims at seeing the clear apprehension of evident giveness' (Omery 1983). As the meaning of this particular quotation is no doubt not immediately evident, the following is a listing of six approaches to phenomenological method as identified by Spielberg (1965), which may assist in the development of a mind picture of phenomenological method.

1. *Descriptive phenomenology*: description of the phenomena obtained by direct investigation free from preconceptions
2. *Essential (eidetic) phenomenology*: examining the phenomenon for typical structures and relationships within
3. *Phenomenology of appearances*: observing the appearance of the phenomena in different perspectives or modes of clarity
4. *Constitutive phenomenology*: exploring the manner in which the phenomena take shape in consciousness
5. *Reductive phenomenology*: suspending belief in the reality of the phenomena by bracketing 'detaching the phenomena of our everyday experience from the context of our naive or natural living, while preserving the content as fully and purely as possible' (Spielberg 1965)
6. *Hermeneutic phenomenology:* discovering and interpreting the concealed meanings in the phenomena.

Omery (1983) states that phenomenological purists believe that 'for research to be truly of a phenomenological nature, one must not and cannot develop a set of steps but must proceed as the direction of the experience indicates without the restrictions such a structure would impose'. However, for the benefit of beginners Omery tabulates the steps of phenomenological method as suggested by two practitioners Van Kaam and Giorgi. These 'steps' of phenomenological method have been contrasted with the more established steps of the scientific method in Tables 13.2–13.6.

The preliminary step (Table 13.2) in any application of scientific method involves considering all of the phenomena prior to deciding the question to be explored. Giorgi (cited by Omery, 1983) proposes unstructured interviews of subjects as the initial event (Table 13.2). It is important to note that

Table 13.2 A comparison of methodologies—Step 1

Methodology	Process
Scientific	Selection from the whole phenomenon of specific quantifiable aspects
Phenomenological (Van Kaam)	Preliminary consideration of a specific moment of experience
Phenomenological (Giorgi)	Naive description of a phenomenon by interviewing the subject

the subjects do not need to meet specific criteria related to selection and representation of the total population. The group can be simply those interested in a particular phenomenon. From this group naive descriptions are taken without comment or leading by the researcher. Van Kaam's (cited by Omery, 1983) consideration of a specific moment of experience (Table 13.2) is less explicit in its method but would parallel the scientific selection of specific aspects. Deciding the limits of a 'specific moment of experience' is very similar to deciding which aspects of a phenomenon to consider.

Table 13.3 A comparison of methodologies—Step 2

Methodology	Process
Scientific	Formulation of a hypothesis.
Phenomenological (Van Kaam)	Research questions are evoked by the experience. What are the necessary and sufficient constituents of this feeling? What does the existence of this feeling tell me concerning the nature of man?
Phenomenological (Giorgi)	The researcher reads the description to identify individual units, clarifying or elaborating the meanings of the remaining units by relating them to each other and the whole.

Secondly, in the scientific method (Table 13.3), an hypothesis is formulated to state the question which is to be researched in a mathematical format. That is simply to say that the hypothesis expresses some relationship between variables being observed. The hypothesis rises out of the consideration of the whole phenomenon in much the same way as Van Kaam's evocation of research questions (Table 13.3). It is as important to define explicitly the feelings for Van Kaam as it is to state the limits (necessary and sufficient constituents) of a variable in scientific methodology. Giorgi, at this point, is identifying individual units, and clarifying and elaborating units; and at the end of that process understands the units relating together to form a whole. The units may equally be called constituents and thus equated with Van Kaam's method, but Giorgi does not push to the larger world question.

As the scientific hypothesis is expressed mathematically, carefully considered deductions from the hypothesis are possible (Table 13.4). For example an increase in X will result in an increase in Y and all other permutations of

Table 13.4 A comparison of methodologies—Step 3

Methodology	Process
Scientific	Deduction of consequences from the hypothesis.
Phenomenological (Van Kaam)	Awareness phase of explication—Implicit awareness of a complex phase becomes explicit formulated knowledge of its components through the collection of a number of crude scientific explanations made by untrained subjects.
Phenomenological (Giorgi)	The researcher reflects on the given units and transforms them from concrete language into the language and concepts of science.

that relationship will be proportionally affected. The statistical methodologies were devised to assist with complicated situations where multiple factors need to be examined and mathematical relationships established across large groups. Van Kaam returns to the collected descriptions of untrained subjects (Table 13.4). The claim is made by Van Kaam that such collections of explanations constitute formulated knowledge but the relationship is not clearly demonstrated. Giorgi is at this stage transforming the naive language of the subject into the language and concepts of the science involved. The acknowledgement again that the researcher is working within a science is of interest. It is difficult to accept the claim that researchers can transform the language of the units without the description being influenced by their prior knowledge or science.

Van Kaam sets out these latter phases of his phenomenological method very clearly (Table 13.5). He requires random sampling of large numbers of subjects in exactly the same manner as most scientific methods. The researcher is also involved in altering the language of the untrained subjects

Table 13.5 A comparison of methodologies—Step 4

Methodology	Process
Scientific	Observation leading to change, i.e. Experimentation
Phenomenological (Van Kaam)	Scientific explication: - Listing of classifying data into categories - Data come from a large random sample of census taken from the total pool of description - The final testing, a review of various elements and their percentages must be agreed by expert judges - Reduction of concrete, vague, intricate and overlapping descriptions to more precisely descriptive terms by intersubjective agreement of expert judges. Illumination of those elements which are not inherent - Hypothetical identification of categories. Application of hypothetical descriptions to randomly selected cases of the original sample - Careful analysis to determine if new hypothetical categories will appear. If they do, they must be tested against a new random sample of cases
Phenomenological (Giorgi)	The researcher then integrates and synthesizes the insights into a descriptive structure which is communicated to other researchers for confirmation and for criticism

Table 13.6 A comparison of methodologies—Step 5

Methodology	Process
Scientific	Acceptance or rejection of hypothesis with some degree of careful prediction
Phenomenological (Van Kaam)	Final identification and description, validity lasts until other cases are presented which do not correspond to the necessary or sufficient constituents contained in the final listing
Phenomenological (Giorgi)	No corresponding process

and in making decisions about elements which are not inherent. If these elements are included in the untrained descriptions and the researcher is not bound by previous assumptions and knowledge, how can the researcher support the decision to exclude some component of the phenomenon? Both phenomenological methods require the confirmation and objective criticism of other researchers or expert judges, and will suffer the same difficulties in obtaining such criticism as adherents of the scientific method suffer in meeting the norms of detachment and organised scepticism. Van Kaam goes on to identify hypothetical categories encountering all the problems inherent in the derivation of hypotheses and associated categorization. Giorgi at this stage is allowing the researcher to integrate and synthesize descriptions and communicate with other researchers. In this method there is no suggestion of hypothesis formulation or of categorization, and no suggestion of either random sampling or the exclusion of any descriptive data.

For Giorgi (Table 13.6) the final identification is by consensus with other researchers. In scientific methodology acceptance or rejection is based on statistical support. Van Kaam explains description validity in terms which are strongly reminiscent of the nature of Kuhnian revolution (Table 13.6). Kuhnian revolution occurs when sufficient discrepancies are encountered in a scientific theory to require the complete revision of the paradigm. Revolutions are interspersed into normal science and serve to revise and redirect the scientist. Such a revision is possible in Van Kaam's method and the scientific method but does not appear in Giorgi's representation. On initial reading the two methods of phenomenology appear very different from one another. Van Kaam's methodology follows many of the constraints of scientific methodology while Giorgi is more distant from scientific tenets.

The concepts of phenomenological process become more difficult when further terminology and the tenets of Spielberg, another phenomenological philosopher, are introduced. In Spielberg's process of *intuiting phenomena* 'the focus is on the uniqueness of the phenomena themselves as reducible to nothing other or less than what they themselves are' (Stanage 1987). Reduction in scientific methodology is portrayed by Omery as a negative aspect but in phenomenological investigation 'to reduce a given subject matter is to draw it together as constituting a whole, a unity' (Omery 1983). In short, scientific reduction fragments while phenomenological reduction results in unities. A greater degree of explanation than is currently available in literature is required to resolve this dilemma. Spielberg's processes of *particularizing phenomena* by *intersubjective analyzing* and *intersubjective describing* are used prior to *phenomenological description* based on classification. Without even attempting consideration of the complex language used in these statements, it is important to note that classification or categorization has always posed a particular problem in science.

'If my categories of thought determine what I observe, then what I observe provides no independent control over my thought. On the other hand, if my categories of thought do not control what I observe then what I observe must be uncategorized, that is to say formless and nondescript—hence again incapable of providing any test for my thought' (Bulmer, cited by McDonell, 1988).

The process of classification is especially difficult in phenomenology where all previous scientific knowledge and conceptions of the researcher must be bracketed out. Chalmers (1982) supports the view that inductive processes such as used in phenomenological research are not sciences, with the statement that 'science does not start with observation statements, because, theory of some kind precedes all observation and observation statements do not constitute a firm basis on which scientific knowledge can be based'.

• By what criteria do researchers classify if their knowledge base is not available?
• How does the researcher identify constituents, eliminate redundant units, and clarify and elaborate the meaning of the remaining units without any prior concepts?

Outcomes of phenomenology

However, before the discussion slips into exactly the type of argument previously discouraged, an alteration of focus to the outcomes of phenomenology is required. At the end of phenomenological research a descriptive record of the critical constituents of a phenomenon has been produced by consensus.

While such descriptions may be of great benefit, they do not meet the definition of science on which this work is based. These phenomenological descriptions may well alert nurses to problems in client care which had not previously been explicitly identified, but the same description will not explain why these feelings, emotions or events have occurred. More importantly such descriptions will not direct individual nurses or the profession as a whole in the development of methods for the alleviation of such problems. Some proponents of phenomenological method recognize this limitation. Bart O'Brien (1990), cites Reason & Rowan (1981), when commenting at a recent nursing conference that there are obligations over and above simply understanding what is happening. Phenomenological method does not appear to meet those obligations. Stanage (1987), having gone to great lengths to demonstrate the 'fusion of grounds and concepts' between phenomenological and scientific methods states: 'a major claim [of this book] is that phenomenological investigation works the soil of science; that science could not long endure...and surely could not attest spectacular success without the kind of investigation here claimed as 'phenomenological' being undertaken in some degree'. Consideration of both sides of this debate, scientific versus phenomenological method, needs to be brought to bear on the third science—the science of nursing.

THE SCIENCE OF NURSING

The development of the science of nursing, as a unique body of knowledge, has progressed slowly. In 1968, Elliot in her oration to the New South Wales College of Nursing (Elliot 1977), notes that the bulk of research in nursing has, in fact, been directed to external sociometric examination of nurses and to administrative and educational/curriculum aspects. This bias most probably reflects the movement of nurses into these academic areas as part of their personal and professional development. While such studies are important, they are not major contributors to a unique body of nursing knowledge and often have only tangential effects on nursing care itself. In 1986, Batey stated that 'while research conducted in the various biological, physical and social science disciplines may have bearing on questions relevant to nursing practice, the profession of nursing itself must assume the full responsibility for studying those questions which have direct relevance to the conduct of the profession's essence—health services'. As recently as July 1990, Bennett notes, in a conference paper, the continued predominance of non-clinical research. This exhortation for nurses to research nursing is repeated extensively throughout the literature, yet the practice of nursing is little altered. Changes from task allocation to client-centred nursing methods may have occurred (with greater or lesser effectiveness and a strong tendency to fail when pressured by staff shortages) but within the method the individual practices of nursing remain ritualistic and mechanical.

Thus neophytes are taught the steps of 'good dressing technique' without having the chance to explore the adaptability that working from microbiological principles can bring. Daily observations are taken at 10 am because of the convenience to nursing workforce arrangements, when physiological basal measurements could be more accurately obtained on the client's awakening. The wakening of clients at 6 am also has no scientific basis and frequently alters the client's normal sleep/wake pattern. Even the social sciences have fallen prey to this ritualistic approach. Neophytes are instructed to use the SOLAR approach to communication; to Sit with Open posture, Lean toward the patient, Ask open-ended questions and use Reflective listening techniques. The accumulated wisdom of nurses, however, knows that clients frequently feel uncomfortable if they believe they are keeping nurses from their tasks, and excellent communication can be and is achieved while involved in bed-making, attending to client hygiene and other similar client oriented activities. The message, therefore, is that the profession needs to subject the art of nursing to scientific examination and revision; to research even the sacred cows of nursing practice and to be ready, if there is no scientific basis for a particular nursing practice, to remove it from the repertoire of skills required of professional nurses. The corollary of that removal of skills is the need to encourage the development of skills for which a scientific case can be made.

Various reasons can be advanced for why such a body of research does not already exist in nursing. It is only recently that nurses have begun to acquire the necessary research skills. Nursing has suffered as a subordinate to medicine and opportunities have been stifled largely because nursing research does not tend to produce the grand technological advances associated with other medically related fields. Nurses have had difficulty attracting funding for research not only for the reasons already listed but also because nurses are predominantly female, and nursing has not been seen as very different from what all women do for their relatives at home and therefore not worthy of research. Nursing services have been too short-staffed for nurses to participate in research. Nurses have been too busy doing the task to spend time finding out what the task really is! The list can go on and on. All of the above are valid reasons for not conducting research and are either currently applicable or at least have been valid at some time.

NURSING PARADIGM

There are however, other reasons why nursing research faces great difficulties. In Shils' statement regarding genuine intellectual pursuits, proffered at the beginning of this chapter, mention is made of revision and criticism of knowledge produced by research within a paradigm. The Kuhnian notion of a paradigm in science is usefully described by Deets (1990) as including the 'agreement amongst practitioners as to the theory, methods to use in conducting the research and standards for those who conduct research under its rubric. The paradigm also becomes the content taught those aspiring to become members of that scientific community'. The paradigm can be used by researchers to decide what ought to be researched and what ought not. Nursing lacks a cohesive paradigm leading to the dilemma expressed by Eunice Chapman (1985): 'One essential piece of investigation has so far been neglected. Nursing particularly might benefit from research into what needs to be researched'. Nursing theorists, in opinion based works, propose four concepts: environment, nursing, person and health, as the cornerstones of a nursing paradigm (Fawcett 1978, Bush 1979, Flakerid & Halloran 1980, Newman 1983, all cited in Chaska 1990). Without even beginning to address the circular concept that nursing is a cornerstone of a nursing paradigm, the research findings of Deets (1990) lead her to frame two questions:

1. If there have not been data to support the development of the four cornerstone concepts and thus the paradigm (and there have not), what is the rationale of nurse educators who continue to develop curricula and teach nursing as if these concepts are realities?
2. If young nursing scholars have been socialized into a non-existent paradigm and attempt to conduct their research within that paradigm, how greatly will they be distracted and deflected from the much needed scientific research in nursing?

With the elaboration of concerns such as these expressed above it becomes easier to understand why nurse researchers might rapidly retreat to more developed scientific fields.

The lack of a paradigm, however, should not be seen as a terminal event in nursing research. The development of a mature science may reasonably take 50–100 years and nurses should not castigate themselves for having to pass through this developmental phase in their professionalism. Perhaps the expectation of a slightly more rapid transit through this phase can be raised due to the opportunity to learn from the errors of others, but the transition can and will be made.

In the immediate absence of a nursing paradigm, the question of method becomes even more interesting. If we accept, as suggested by Goodwin and Goodwin (1984) that qualitative (e.g. phenomenological) and quantitative (usually considered scientific) research modes have distinct paradigms or world views, then nursing, temporarily without a paradigm, is surely in a position to utilize either or both methods in any combination felt appropriate for the express purpose of advancing nursing knowledge. McMurray (1989) expresses such a conjunction when she states 'qualitative investigations which describe and interpret how nurses actually practice provide rich and meaningful information which complements the body of quantitative research'. The problem inherent in the work of Goodwin & Goodwin (1984) is their sidestepping of the issues underlying the assumptions and purposes of research.

Even without a developed paradigm, it is spurious to say that nursing research is free. Most current nursing research is theory-driven and the bulk of that theory exhibits a basis in scientific methodology. The relationship between theory and practice is described by Carr & Kemmis (1986).

> One view (scientific, positivist) regards theory as a source of principles that can be applied to practice; another regards practice as a matter of professional judgement which can be developed as the wisdom of practitioners and policy matters is developed (phenomenological, interpretive); and a third regards theory and practice as dialectically related with theory being developed and tested by application in and reflection on practice, and practice as a risky enterprise which can never be justified by theoretical principles.

If nursing adopts the suggestion of this work that phenomenology as a pre-science is useful in discovering the problems to be researched by scientific method, then perhaps we have reached the point of practice-to-theory-to-practice exchange. Careful note should be taken, however, that this is a sequential use of research methodologies rather than a combined use.

Combined use of qualitative and quantitative research may have a place. The inclusion of qualitative data (examples or illustrations of phenomena) may render the report of a quantitative research design more readable, thus enhancing transfer to a usage in the clinical setting. Similarly, quantification can assist in qualitative research and indeed is essential in Van Kaam's method of phenomenology either for added description or to underpin projections. If 95% of individuals have feeling X, scientific methodology can then be adopted to elicit why this feeling arises and how to address the resolution of this feeling. This returns to the original definition of science on which this work is based. Powers (1987) states that

> there is an advantage to using the two approaches alternatively over time. The insights derived from qualitative research may well suggest questions best pursued in the quantitative mode. Quantitative findings may alternatively, point to inconsistencies and confusions in the field of enquiry that should be subjected to qualitative analysis. Examples of chains of research studies that effectively use both modes of enquiry would certainly be a landmark of maturity in the conduct of research in this discipline.

The temptation to leave the debate at this happy pass and to allow that nursing, using both methodologies, should proceed flawlessly, if not effortlessly, to a workable paradigm and beyond to a well defined body of knowledge, is very great. Speedy (1990) supports scientific, phenomenological and critical social theories in stating that 'there is a place in nursing for a variety of methodologies underpinned by particular ideologies'. However, it is necessary to return to the purposes of research.

Implications of the use of research methodologies

The choice of research methodology to be used in the continued exploration of nursing's scientific basis needs to be carefully considered for a number of reasons, not least of which is the foundational role of research in investigating the science of nursing. The primary intention of research into such foundational aspects of nursing must be to improve the quality of client care, not withstanding the occasionally achieved secondary intentions related to nursing morale and professionalisation. However, none of these intentions are ever brought to fruition unless the determination of research findings is followed by their appropriate and effective utilization within the realm of professional practice.

Hunt (1981), as cited by Gould (1986), suggests five reasons for the failure of the nursing profession to implement its associated research findings:

1. Nurses do not know about the research findings. If the research findings have at least been effectively communicated to nurses:
2. They do not understand the findings.
3. They do not believe them.
4. They do not know how to apply them.
5. They are not allowed to use them.

While not all these issues are directly related to the research methodology employed, it is possible that the lack of understanding about, and the increasing levels of disbelief with respect to, research findings are consequences of the use/misuse of phenomenological approaches to research which have not provided results that are easily translated to and supported by clinical practice. It is easy to understand rejection of research based change when the research only involves phenomenologically based observation. Gould (1986) when discussing research related to pressure area sores states 'it is sufficient to point out that many more publications have been concerned with case history discussion and loosely-constructed uncontrolled clinical trials than with studies in which a tightly controlled experimental design has been adopted'. Clearly, poorly conducted research employing scientific methodology is seen as an equally ineffective agent for change. In effect, Gould (1986) states 'nurses attempting to make sense of this information cannot be blamed for disillusionment, rejection and a return to their own favourite remedy'. In order to avoid the type of outcome described here the plea must be for well designed and appropriately controlled research to continue the exploration and development of the scientific basis of nursing.

If the outcomes of research into the science of nursing are not translatable to client care then there is little value in pursuing such a difficult process. However, nurses must acknowledge that these client related benefits may not always be obvious in the short-term. Some benefits are indeed accrued by the individual researcher: the development of their own knowledge base manifested in a growing record of publications and associated recognition within the profession, higher qualifications resulting in challenging opportunities and higher pay. However, such professional development of individuals whilst not always directly client related does result in the development of nursing as a discipline, which in the long term can only be viewed as contributing to quality client care.

The continued development of nursing as a profession must also be considered in this examination of the implications of research methodology usage. Bennett (1990) views nursing research as 'embedded in a profession which, although predominantly female, is recognised as such not only by society but all health professionals'. Eventually it is the public that must grant nursing its professional status. The general public is the group who must seek nursing care independent of medical care. It is the general public who must recognize nurses as essential, not for the much dramatised role of 'handmaiden' or from a desire for 'cool hands on a fevered brow' but because of nursing knowledge which is of assistance to the general public themselves. Ultimately it is the role of the public to pressure politicians into providing them with more and better nurses, and to retain these nurses by accepting that the public purse will have to pay for professional service.

Consequently, nurse researchers must be careful to produce nursing science which meets potential criticisms, for the general public is also the group that can most easily be subverted by those, e.g. financial controllers of the 'health dollar', who have something to gain from not encouraging the professionalisation of nursing. These considerations of the broader societal context, of which the nursing profession is only one component, illustrate, we believe, the need for strict adherence to scientific method, with experiential aspects carefully subsumed into the early steps of establishing the research questions to be investigated. It would indeed be counter productive to establish a unique body of nursing knowledge only to see it discounted by other health professionals and the public using arguments such as those now directed at naturopaths and acupuncturists: Where is the proof? Where is the double-blind trial?

A final consideration, which arises because the need for nursing research exists in a competitive financial environment, is the association between research method and funding needs. When competing for research funding nursing has the potential to be disadvantaged by the lack of spectacular consequences attributable to the results of research directed towards the science of nursing. If the research proposes and can deliver a method of better small joint mobilization for some sufferers of arthritis, it is unlikely to be funded by any drug company producing antiarthritic drugs, and will suffer in comparison to most big ticket items such as investigation into the treatment of AIDS. The argument that research dollars should be directed towards doing the most good to the greatest number of people with the least possibility of dire consequences, although attractive, does not yet appear to hold much sway amongst funding bodies.

The research methodology selected as a tool for the exploration of issues related to the science of nursing in these difficult economic circumstances, may well be a significant factor in the research funding decision making process. If under the heading 'research method' in a proposal, a statement similar to 'proceed as the direction of the experience indicates without the restrictions such a structure would impose' (Omery 1983) was found, the reasonably prudent and conservative funding body would in most instances refuse funding. The consequent reduction in the scientific support of nursing practice would be disadvantageous to the client, the community and to nursing as a developing discipline.

CONCLUSION

Nursing needs to develop its scientific base for the benefit of the client, aspirants to the profession and clinical practitioners. From the traditional and behavioural sciences a considered choice must be made of material which clearly augments the more professionally important science of nursing. The science of nursing must evolve from and be directed towards nursing practice.

The intention of this chapter was to explore some of the differing research methodologies which are available to nurses. Phenomenology is presented as a pre-science which is unlikely to find wide acceptance amongst practising nurses in part due to its language and conflicting methodologies. Nevertheless, phenomenology may assist in the definition of problems which become subject to thorough scientific research methodology. While recognizing its limitations, Scientific Methodology is supported not only for its greater acceptability to most nurses but also due to the economic realities of research funding and the professional realities of knowledge production within a developing discipline

REFERENCES

Akinsanya J A, Hayward J C 1980 The biological sciences in nursing education: the contribution of bionursing. Nursing Times, March 6:427-432

Baer H 1989 The American dominative medical society is a reflection of social relations in the larger society. Journal of Social Science in Medicine 28(11):1103-1112

Batey J E 1986 Communicating nursing research. Western Interstate Commission for Higher Education, Boulder Colorado, p 97-101

Bennett M 1990 The tea-bag phenomenon. Conference Proceedings: Dreams, Deliberations & Discoveries: Adelaide: 1-10

Carr W, Kemmis S 1986 Becoming critical: knowing through action research. Deakin University Press, Geelong p 36-40

Chalmers A F 1982 What is this thing called science? University of Queensland Press, St Lucia, p 14-17

Chapman E 1985 Research ? As clear as mud. Nursing Mirror 161(19):43

Chaska N L 1990 The nursing profession: turning points. Mosby, St Louis, p 149

Cohen C 1987 On the dangers of inquiry and the burdens of proof. Southern California Law Review 303-329

Deets R 1990 Nursing's paradigm and a search for its methodology. In: Chaska N L (ed) The nursing profession: turning points. Mosby, St Louis, p 149-156

Doran G A 1983 Scientism versus humanism in medical education. Journal of Social Science in Medicine 17(23):1831-1835

Elliott J E 1977 Research in nursing: its contribution to present and future improvement of health care. Sixteenth Annual Oration. Annual Orations 1953-1977 N.S.W. College of Nursing, Sydney p 143-150

Goodwin L D, Goodwin W L 1984 Qualitative versus quantitative research or qualitative and quantitative research. Nursing Research 33 (Nov/Dec): 378-380

Gould D 1986 Pressure sore prevention and treatment: an example of nurses' failure to implement research findings. Journal of Advanced Nursing 11: 389-394

Graver J L 1986 The primary care crisis: the contribution of antiscientism. Humane Medicine: A Journal of the Art and Science of Medicine 2(2):95-99

McDonell G 1988 On trust. University of NSW, School of Sociology, Seminar Paper

McMurray A 1989 Time to extend the 'process'. Australian Journal of Advanced Nursing 6(4):40-43

Merton R K 1957 The sociology of science: social theory and social structure. Free press of Glencoe, New York, p 456-488

Needham J 1984 The emergence and institutionalization of modern science. In: Wickramasinghe C (ed) Fundamental studies and the future of science. University College Press, Cardiff, p 227-230

Nightingale F 1859 (reprinted 1990) Notes on nursing: what it is, and what it is not. Churchill Livingstone, Edinburgh, p 1-5

O'Brien B 1990 Nursing: craft, science & art. Conference Proceedings: Dreams, Deliberations & Discoveries. Adelaide: 306-312

Omery A 1983 Phenomenology: a method for nursing research. Journal of Advanced Nursing January: 49-62

Powers B A 1987 Taking sides: a response to Goodwin & Goodwin. Nursing Research 36 (2):122-126

Shils L S 1987 Anti-science: Observation on the recent 'crisis' of science. In: Block H (ed) Civilization and Science: in conflict or collaboration? Elsevier, New York, p 137-142

Speedy S 1990 Never mind the width, feel the quality. Conference Proceedings: Dreams, Deliberations & Discoveries: Adelaide: 74-82

Spielberg H 1965 Phenomenology In: Benton W (ed) 1982 Encyclopaedia Britannica, 15th edn. 14: 210-215
Stanage S 1987 Adult education and phenomenological research. R E Kreiger, Florida, p 1-72; 277-305
West S H, Neyle D N 1990 Pilot study (Unpublished)
Ziman, J 1984 The sociology of science: an introduction to science studies: the philosophical and social aspects of science and technology. Cambridge University Press: Cambridge p 106-121

FURTHER READING

Bulmer M 1979 Concepts in the analysis of qualitative data. Sociological Review 27(4):651-677
Kretlow F 1990 A phenomenological view of illness. Australian Journal of Advanced Nursing 7(2):8-10
Price B 1989 The thorny path of nursing research. Nursing Times 85(23):62-63
Rose S, Rose H 1971 Social responsibility: the myth of the neutrality of science. Impact of Science on Society 21(2):137-149
Sandelowski M, Davis D, Harris B 1989 Artful design: Writing the proposal for research in the naturalist paradigm. Research in Nursing and Health 12:77-84

14. Being and nature: an interpretation of person and environment

Judith Parker

INTRODUCTION

This chapter begins with a brief discussion of the development of conceptual frameworks for nursing and their role in crystallizing the concepts described as central to nursing; those of person, environment, health, and nursing. It then moves on to a discussion of the shifts which have taken place in philosophical thinking about nursing. The chapter then explores the influence of the positivistic attitude of Cartesian thought upon the concepts of person and environment from a position which has been informed by hermeneutics and feminist thought. Particular attention is focused upon the concept of person in an attempt to indicate the changing understanding of 'being' in western society under the influence of Cartesianism. The discussion on environment focuses upon the changed understanding of both nature and social life. The chapter concludes with a very brief discussion of the implications of the issues raised for an understanding of health and nursing.

KNOWLEDGE DEVELOPMENT IN NURSING

In examining knowledge development in nursing, the 1960s and 1970s were undoubtedly the era of the burgeoning of conceptual frameworks for nursing practice. The conceptual schema developed by writers such as Rogers (1970), Orem (1980), King (1971), Roy (1980) and Neuman (1982) were utilized widely to provide frameworks for nursing curricula and to guide nursing practice and research. Within these schema nursing phenomena were examined in relation to a range of theoretical formulations which had their origins in disciplines external to nursing such as psychology, sociology, and the human biosciences. However as Chinn & Jacobs (1983) have noted, 'regardless of how the groups or categories of theories are made, the ability to see trends or common traits demonstrates the crystallization of central concepts or images for nursing science' (p. 182). Indeed, within these frameworks four concepts have been identified by a number of writers as central.

In 1975, reporting upon a survey of baccalaureate programs, Yura & Torrens identified the major concepts of nursing as man (sic), society, health and nursing. Subsequently Fawcett (1978) redefined these more fully as person, environment, health ,and nursing. Flaskerud & Halloran (1980) noted that by the late 1970s progress in developing nursing theory had slowed considerably. They expressed concern that theory development was being deterred because nurse theorists were concentrating on differences between their conceptualizations rather than emphasizing areas of agreement. They examined the conceptual frameworks of nursing writers including Levine (1971), Rogers (1970), Roy (1980), Johnson (1980), and Orem (1980), and concluded that there was support within the theories for the centrality of the four concepts. However they noted that Levine and Rogers viewed the concept of person holistically so that the whole was understood to be greater than the sum of the parts. Roy, Johnson ,and Orem on the other hand saw the concept of person in terms of a summation of bio-psycho-socio-cultural parts. Environment was viewed by Levine and Rogers as co-extensive with the person and by Roy and Johnson as interacting with the person. Indeed Brodie (1984) has noted that the various conceptualizations in the literature of the concept of environment make it the most ill defined of all the central concepts. These quite fundamental differences in the conceptualizations of person and environment indicate that there was indeed perhaps less agreement among these writers than Flaskerud & Halloran asserted.

With regard to the two remaining central concepts, health and nursing, Flaskerud & Halloran gave little attention to that of health, other than to note Stevens's (1979) view that 'the concept of health is treated as health–illness because nursing actions occur in this aspect of a person's life' (p.2). However it is clear that the multiplicity of definitions of health found in the nursing literature is an indication that this also is an area of disagreement rather than agreement among nursing scholars (Brodie 1984).

Whether or not nursing was to be regarded as a concept of the same order as the others was a matter of debate in the nursing literature. This debate centred around the issue of whether the science of nursing was separate from the practice of nursing. Fawcett (1978) took the view that the idea of nursing as an activity must be included in any nursing theory in order to explain and predict the relationship between nursing actions and patient outcomes. This view was strongly supported by Flaskerud & Halloran who claimed that all nursing theories incorporate an understanding of nursing as an activity concerned with the management of the patient–environment interaction. Donaldson & Crowley (1978) however pointed out that the failure to differentiate between the existence of the discipline of nursing as a body of knowledge and the activities of practitioners had resulted in confusion about the status of nursing. This view is supported by Conway (1985) who has argued that an appropriate distinction between the science of nursing and its practice must be maintained if nursing is ultimately to acquire a clearly discernible body of knowledge.

In their analysis of the work of the nursing theorists, Flaskerud & Halloran discerned clear differences in the ways that some of the concepts were understood within the various frameworks that had been generated by various nurse theorists. Nonetheless they asserted the need for agreement on concept definition, so as to ensure progress in nursing theory development. They skirted over what were quite fundamentally different philosophical assumptions underpinning the various frameworks. They used a commonsense understanding of philosophy and argued that the way forward lay in agreeing to define the concepts in accordance with generally agreed upon understandings in the American culture about person, environment, and illness and to assert that the concept of nursing was necessary for theory development.

The explicit theorizing about nursing which came into its own over the late 1960s, 1970s and early 1980s appears to have been premised on beliefs about the need to assert continuous development within the theoretical formulations and that nursing theory guides education, research, and practice. It also appears that these theoretical formulations were developed independently of developments in metatheoretical formulations in nursing. This latter body of literature attempted to examine nursing theory development particularly in light of current understandings made available through the philosophy of science. However as Silva & Rothbart (1984) note, 'Several conceptual frameworks published in the early seventies were essentially devoid of any explicit linkage to philosophy of science'. The writings of Dickoff & James (1968), Jacox (1974), and Hardy (1974), concerning nursing theory construction and testing, were particularly influential in the 1960s and 1970s. They developed within the logical positivistic tradition and were influenced by philosophers of science such as Nagel (1961) and Hempel (1966).

POSITIVISTIC ENQUIRY

In positivistic empiricist enquiry, it is assumed that there is a knowable empirical reality to be discovered through the testing of theories, utilizing scientific method based an observation and experiment. Positivism involves a reductionist attitude wherein it is held that all aspects of complex phenomena can be understood by reducing them to their constituent parts (Capra 1982). Attempts are made to explain the whole by reference to those parts and to their external measurable relationships. Instrumentation and tests of reliability and validity are central to empirical testing which is undertaken in the search to establish causal relationships between aspects of phenomena under study.

The philosophy of technique underpinning positivistic enquiry is based on the fundamental idea that the proper application of the right technique will in time yield solutions to any problem (Drengson 1980). The knowledge which is generated via the scientific approach is assumed to be value free, and is expressed as general, abstract laws. Deterministic or mechanistic explanations of causality are sought (Leonard 1989).

The positivistic attitude applied to nursing assumes, as Giddens (1975) might say, that the methodological procedures of natural science may be applied directly to nursing situations, that people can be treated as objects of the natural world and that the outcomes of nursing investigations can be formulated in terms parallel to those of natural science, i.e. in terms of generalizable laws. Furthermore nursing knowledge which is developed through the methods of natural science is understood to be value free. Douglas (1970 p. 250) has described the positivistic approach in terms of the elimination of the human factor through the scientific notion of objectivity.

The positivistic attitude runs counter to many of the intuitions of nurses who are steeped in the practice of their craft. For example nursing takes place in a variety of socio-historical, cultural, and environmental contexts, such as hospitals, home and the community. Nurses recognize that nursing is in part constituted by the cultural practices embedded in the contexts in which it takes place. Yet positivistic science seeks atemporal, ahistorical decontextualized laws.

The heart of nursing lies in the quality of the care which is delivered and which is premised on a recognition of the mutuality of the nurse-patient relationship, on the moral stance of the nurses and on empathy and understanding of the human vulnerabilities and frailties of people cast into patient and client roles. Positivistic science, however, seeks to eliminate human value-laden factors in its search for objectivity.

Nurses attempt to take into account the complexity of the life situation, life history, and life circumstances of people in their care and try to grasp in a holistic way the often complex, contradictory, and uncertain situations in which they find themselves in the planning and delivery of care. But positivistic science seeks to reduce complex phenomena to discrete parts which can be considered in a decontextualized and value-free manner in the search for certainty and general laws.

Additionally, the positivistic attitude is not congruent with many of the early conceptualizations of nursing. Indeed Tinkle & Beaton (1983) have noted wide discrepancies exist between the conceptualizations of nursing by nursing theorists and definitions of positivistic science. Silva & Rothbart (1984) point to the irony that, whilst some nursing theorists revised their conceptual frameworks to bring them more into line with positivist views, at the same time, some of the metatheoreticians themselves, e.g. Hardy (1983) were beginning to move away from their previously espoused position to one more informed by historicist views.

From the early 1980s it was becoming clear to several writers (e.g. Meleis 1985, Moccia 1986) that the positivistic approach seriously limited the scope of investigations of nursing phenomena. It was coming to be recognized that in the search for atemporal causal certainty the integrity of the phenomena under study could not be retained and at the same time be reduced to value-free descriptions. Influenced particularly by the work of Kuhn (1970) and Laudan (1977), a trend towards historicism was becoming apparent in nursing's metatheoretical formulations (Hardy 1983).

HISTORICISM

Historicism arose in part as a reaction to and critique of positivism. Kuhn's work was particularly significant in directing attention away from a focus upon science as product towards the social processes through which inquiry proceeds in science. He showed that the methodological directives that formed part of the tenets of scientific knowledge could not adequately account for what in fact happened in the production of scientific knowledge as a social cultural process. Kuhn came to understand that the actual development of scientific ideas does not take place in a progressive and orderly way, systematically leading to closer approximations of the truth in the way that scientists would have us believe. Rather, he argued that scientific endeavours have been characterized more by crises and discontinuities. Kuhn saw that scientific epochs have been dominated by paradigms which provided a framework for looking at scientific phenomena and within which scientific problems emerged and could be addressed. Kuhn also recognized that what is defined as science at any one time is what the scientific community as a whole chooses to accept as science (Charlesworth 1982 p. 34).

Kuhn stopped short of accepting the relativist implications inherent in his notion of paradigm, i.e. that science and scientific methods are defined relative to a particular historical epoch or culture. Nevertheless he facilitated the understanding of science as a human invention rather than as the method of reaching truth and certainty. His work thus opened the way for studies which provided both naturalistic and critical interpretive accounts of the history and practice of science.

The influence of the work of philosophers such as Kuhn upon nursing thought has been significant. It has provided a philosophical rationale for the scepticism felt by many nursing scholars that nursing knowledge could only be developed through methods which forced enquiry about nursing to be structured in the positivistic mode which meant that issues thought to be relevant and salient to nursing were suppressed.

Historicists such as Dilthey (1960) had long taken the position that an understanding of the human world is not possible when the principles and practices associated with the non-human world are applied to human concerns. That is to say, the methods of enquiry for human sciences have to be necessarily different from those utilized in natural science. This recognition when applied in nursing enquiry has provided a rationale for a move away from the reductionist thought inherent in logical positivism towards more holistic understandings.

Fawcett is one nursing writer who was clearly influenced by the shift towards historicism. In 1984 she made the claim that the discipline of nursing had an identifiable metaparadigm constituted by the four concepts she had previously identified as central to nursing and argued that a range of the conceptual models (e.g. King's, Levine's, Orem's, Roger's, and Roy's) represented disciplinary matrices within the metaparadigm of nursing.

Tinkle & Beaton (1983) contrasted the positivistic view of science with the historicist paradigm and noted: 'Facts and principles are inextricably embedded in a particular historical and cultural setting. All forms of knowledge are historically generated and rooted...Truth...is to be found only in the interactions between persons and concrete sociohistorical settings' (p. 28). They are thus recognizing the relativism inherent in this way of thinking and the implications of a shift in thinking from a search for truth as ahistorical causal certainty established through general laws, to an understanding of multiple truths, context dependent truths, historical truths.

The historicist critique of science facilitated the recognition that logical positivism is a single philosophy of science rather than science itself, which was the first step in recognizing that multiple approaches are appropriate. As Dzurec (1989) has noted: 'the logical positivistic method is now being widely questioned as the ultimate approach for the advancement of the discipline of nursing' (p. 74).

Thus in nursing thought, the influence of the historicist critique of positivistic science has resulted in an understanding of science not as the search for objective truth and certainty but rather in terms of multiple and historically changing research traditions, each of which includes many theories. It provided a rationale for undertaking research in natural settings using various research approaches, including qualitative methods, which appeared to be unblinkered by the constraints of structured scientific methods directed to quantification of relationships. It facilitated exploration of more holistic concerns to do with health and illness in relation to changing socio-cultural contexts and person/environment relationships. It also opened the way for greater recognition to be given to a range of approaches including hermeneutics, critical social theory, post structuralism, and feminism.

However, critics of historicism have noted that historicism shares with positivism a concept of cause inherited from the physical sciences. Within historicism there is a belief in the causality of history. History is thus objectified and turned into something like a general law. Faulconer & Williams (1985) have pointed to this notion of historical causality in Marxist and Freudian thought and in humanistic psychology. They argue that the objectification and reification of history leads inevitably to human events being explained causally. Whether it is the causality of economic/political history, the causality of early experience as a determinant of psychic life, or the causality of psychological states, historicism consists of the objectification of history which is then invoked in causal analysis of behaviour.

TEMPORALITY AND HERMENEUTICS

One key to an understanding of human sciences which is not based in the search for causal explanation lies in Heidegger's profound understanding regarding the nature of time. Heidegger (1962) came to understand that both positivistic and historicist thought are based upon a fundamental misconception about the nature of time. Within historicism, time is understood as an accrual of static events in a world of static entities; that is to say, time is conceived of as linear (Faulconer & Williams 1985). What Heidegger has helped us to understand is that this linear notion of time is, itself, historical. That is to say, it is a construct of our particular historical epoch. Humans have constructed this notion of time as linear and have then used this construct to explain human events in a causal way. Heidegger recognized that time is directional and relational. The now is taken as the point of departure. The past exists as it comes into being for us now. The future also exists only now in terms of our sense of possibilities.

What I am calling a post modern consciousness can be described as one which recognizes linear time as a human construct. Post modernism in these terms may be thought of as the tracing out in various disciplines of the far-reaching implications of this radical yet simple understanding. This understanding of time as a historical cultural interpretation can help us to recognize that as embodied human beings we live bounded by the meanings of the world we live in temporally.

Thus a post modern consciousness starts from an understanding of time as dynamic rather than linear, a belief in the impossibility of objective knowledge and causal certainty and an understanding of the primacy of the ontological question of being, rather than the epistemological question of knowing, in seeking the foundation of knowledge. It recognizes that embodied human beings are born into an already existing world of traditions, cultural practices, artefacts, and shared meanings and relationships. They are thrown into this temporal world, but initially come to an unreflective understanding of themselves and their world because they apprehend the meanings of their world directly through their embodiment.

Further it is recognized that the world sets up possibilities as to who a person can and cannot become and thus the world constrains the ways in which the self constitutes its world. Thus one recognises that as human beings we have situated not radical freedom. Over time persons come to define themselves and to be defined in an ongoing process of self-interpretation.

This position therefore recognizes the historicity of the changing under-standing of being. That is to say, it accepts the position more clearly expressed in Heidegger's later writings, that in different epochs in western culture, different sorts of people, practices,and things have shown up (Magee 1987). It recognizes that most of what we do is not guided by conscious choice or an aware state of mind. However it also recognizes that we can and do engage in consciously directed action and often this happens in the context of something showing up as problematic. We can also imaginatively stand outside the situation and view it in a detached, reflective manner although this is not our everyday mode of being in the world. Such a position acknowledges the importance of self-understanding gleaned from reflection upon one's situation and circumstance. It recognizes the impor-tance of insight and understanding that can be gained from a variety of perspectives. It accepts that truth is an understanding of how things are, and that this truth stems from a moral standpoint constituted in part by one's temporal situation. Such a post modern consciousness if it is developed by nurses can help them to understand that the objectification of scientific method is itself but one way of interpreting nursing.

Taylor (1971) points out that human sciences need to go beyond the bounds of a science based on the traditional epistemology of empiricism to one which studies intersubjective common meanings that are embedded in social reality. He points out that a hermeneutical science does not study raw data; its most primitive data are 'readings of meanings'. Taylor points out that we are bound by temporality and historically situated understandings and interpretations. Because of this, human sciences cannot be value free. A study of human science is inseparable from a study of self. It requires a high degree of self-knowledge, and self understanding. A human science is value based, value directed. It is thus a moral science. Additionally, prediction is not possible in the human sciences because of the recognition that as humans we are self-defining. With changes in self definition come changes in what we are. In defining something we thereby create it. Thus conceptual innovations alter human realities. This is easier to understand after the event than to predict. Human or heremeneutic science thus is largely ex post facto understanding and so conceived, stems from the recognition that there is no Archimedian point for objective knowing because all knowledge emanates from persons already in the world (Leonard 1989).

Human sciences are concerned to render life and the world continually understandable. For Gadamer (1975), who demonstrated the implications of Heidegger's thought for the human sciences, human sciences seek truth. However he does not conceive of truth in the traditional way as correspond-ence of a concept or expression of a thing to the thing itself. Rather he conceives of truth as an understanding of how things are, temporally, in a temporal world.

Faulconer & Williams (1985) point out that this position has been criticized by writers such as Habermas (1970) who claim that Gadamer's position gives no place in which to stand and evaluate and thus a Gadamerian position is inevitably a status quo position. However those who support Gadamer's arguments recognize that 'critique of the status quo does not require that one have a standpoint outside the status quo...because status quo is by definition, itself temporal' (Faulconer & Williams 1985). Furthermore 'denial of an absolute standpoint does not deny the possibility of legitimate criticism. It only denies the possibility of absolute criticism— transcendent, atemporal criticism'. Gadamer, it is noted, insisted on the historical character of any critique of the status quo and demanded that critics have the humility to acknowledge the situatedness of their criticism.

Heidegger's ontology and Gadamer's critique of positivism and historicism have opened the way for approaches to research which question many of the taken-for-granted assumptions in the Western tradition. In particular they have opened the way for approaches which do not seek causal explanation. They have thus provided the philosophical foundation for post modernist formulations, which by definition stem from a position beyond objectivism. A post modernist consciousness goes beyond historicist claims about the inevitable situatedness of human thought within a culture, to focus upon the very criteria by which claims to knowledge are legitimated (Nicholson 1990).

Faulconer & Williams (1985) point out that the alternative to positivism and historicism, a position based on the understanding of temporality, allows us access to human life and a stronger ability to render it intelligible. The goal of such a science must be truth (temporal articulation) not certainty (atemporal objectification).

Drawing upon an understanding of the historical nature of time and recognizing the truth of Taylor's (1979) point that conceptual innovations alter human realities, this chapter now seeks to trace out some of the implications of the influence of positivistic thought upon understandings of person and environment in western society.

CARTESIANISM

Positivistic thought stems in part from Descartes's philosophy, and the historical influence of his thought has been described as Cartesianism (Drengson 1980). This analysis of the influence of Cartesian thought upon the concepts of person and environment draws as well upon historical, anthropological, and feminist thought.

The positivistic attitude associated with Cartesianism had its origins in scientific thinking which began to emerge in Western Europe in about the 15th century. Charlesworth (1982) has pointed out that 'the earliest attempts to define science emphasized the idea of empirical observation of the natural world and the use of experiments both to enlarge our observations and also to test the generalisations about the natural world that we formulate by induction on the basis of those observations'.

Descartes's thinking contributed profoundly to establishing the possibility of science. His dualistic notions of the division between mind and matter, observer and observed, subject and object have become built into the whole of western thought including science. In order to arrive at the foundation of science Descartes sought the foundation of enquiry itself. This led to the famous Cartesian doubt as method. The point at which the doubt stops for Descartes is the reflection that he is himself engaged in thinking. Descartes's fundamental first certainty resulted: 'Cogito ergo sum: I think therefore I exist'. This means that 'I must irreducibly be thought' and the material which is my body is not part of the quintessential me. This leads directly to a view of the world as split between subjects (pure thought) and objects (pure extension) (Magee 1987).

This Cartesian division between mind and matter has had a profound influence on western thought and has resulted in the belief that we are isolated 'egos' inside our bodies. Capra quotes Heisenberg (1961) who stated: 'This partition has penetrated deeply into the human mind during the three centuries following Descartes and it will take a long time for it to be replaced by a really different attitude to the problem of reality' (Capra 1982).

Magee (1987) has pointed out that Descartes's ideas were readily accepted by the educated elite in Western Europe. It seems unlikely however that they would have been embraced so enthusiastically if there had not already been a trend towards this way of thinking in Western Europe. In a classic article in the anthropological literature, Shweder & Bourne (1982) point out that Descartes's formulations reinforced the individualistic and egocentric notion of personhood already deeply rooted in European thought. The concept of the individual appears to be at least as old as Thucydides who wrote 2400 years ago. During the Renaissance and Reformation it was rediscovered and glorified. Thus the scientific positivistic attitude that arose in Europe in the 16th century reinforced the idea of the person as 'a particular incarnation of abstract humanity'. This abstract individual is seen as inviolate, a supreme value in and of itself who is free to choose how to act. This individual is seen to be protected by deeply entwined moral and legal principles. These principles prescribed privacy and proscribed unwanted invasions of person, property, and other extensions of self and thus through these principles, the individual achieves a context-independent recognition.

Descartes's particular contribution to this cultural view of the individual was through the general acceptance in educated (therefore male) European society of the notion that the mind was separate from the material world of objects . The individual thus came to be identified with mind. It is worth noting that the individual identified with mind was a man. Women were conceived of as part of nature. Nature and the human body, as part of the natural world of objects, worked according to mechanical laws and were thought of in terms of the metaphor of the machine. Scientific method provided the means through which the natural world could be brought under the control of individuals. Thus arose the notion of the (male) person whose mind could rationally control external reality.

The separation between mind and matter meant that there was perceived to be a separation also between the observer and that which is observed. The detached self as observer of material reality thus reinforced and perpetuated the notion of decontextualized, generalized, and abstract knowledge which began with Plato and Socrates (Dreyfus & Dreyfus 1986).

As Benner (1989) has pointed out: 'This theoretical formal property aspect of knowledge became privileged in the western tradition so that knowledge came to mean abstract, general, principled, systematic information that can be applied to a wide range of situations...this view of knowledge lent itself easily to Descartes' further privatisation of knowledge in a subject's mind and applied to an objectified world' (1989:5).

Person

Thus in western society a view of person has arisen in which individuals are understood to be separated from their bodies, their world, and those around them. Such individuals are engaged in pursuit of their self-interested aims and are isolated from their own experiences through the value given to decontextualized and abstract knowledge. This is the reductionist image of 'man the machine'. Small wonder that feminists are claiming that this understanding of personhood has by and large not been informed by the everyday life experience of most women!

With the emergence over time of the Cartesian understanding of person, there has also arisen a changed understanding about the meaning of death and time. Clearly our understanding of personal death is closely linked to what we think it means to a person. Aries (1974) had noted the quasi-static nature of traditional attitudes and identifies a prevailing attitude to death which lasted approximately one thousand years in Europe until about 1200AD. In this attitude death was seen as familiar. People accepted death with 'neither fear nor despair, half way between passive resignation and mystical trust'. Time was understood as cyclical and people were part of the cycle of nature as was death. Nature however was embued with a sense of the sacred.

One could thus infer that in this period of European history the fundamental sense of being, i.e. the primary ontology, resided not so sharply in the individual but in the community, which was understood in a holistic organismic way. In such a culture death of the person was not death of a unique individual but rather death of part of a more encompassing totality of the natural sacred world.

However Aries (1974) points out that this attitude became subtly modified in the 13th to 15th century to become more intensely personal. Thus, it is possible to see the beginnings of a changing ontology towards primacy of the individual with the reawakening of Greek thought which occurred at this time. In the 16th century this more personal image of death was associated with a new sense of time. One can begin to recognize how a shift in the understanding of time, from a cyclical understanding towards a linear notion of time as an accrual of events, both constitutes and is constituted by an understanding of person in individualistic terms. With linear time people can construct individual histories and set individual goals and thereby identify themselves as separate from other individuals. Thus in the 16th century we see the emergence of the individual in western society. But all the evidence seems to indicate that the individual was a man. It appears that women were still conceived of as part of the cyclical world of nature.

In the 17th century with the rise of science, Illich (1975) points out that death came to be seen as more natural than sacred. The body was beginning to lose its sacred character, becoming reduced to the status of an object in the natural world. This constitution of the body as a natural object thus in part constituted the understanding of death as natural. As well, the constitution of time as linear provided a way of structuring being in terms of a beginning and an ending and a passage through time. Clearly with the rise of scientific medicine the body was required to be objectified and understood in natural terms. Indeed today most educated people in western society have a conception of their body as an object which can be understood in terms of its structure and function.

Illich has written more recently of the changing interpretations of our bodies that are occurring in western society. He claims that people are now experiencing their bodies as commodities. Scientific medicine particularly, linked to medical technology, has contributed to a shaping of the understanding of the body as a medicalized commodified object. Foucault (1973) describes the 'clinical gaze' wherein patients are viewed as objects of medical scrutiny. Once the body is viewed as a object it can be regarded as a commodity and it can be 'packaged' in a variety of ways. Our understanding of being in this way has been described as a technological self-understanding (Benner & Wrubel 1989). It is worth noting that Descartes upheld the intrinsic value of creatures with souls, but once the conceptions of soul and God are rejected, the view of body as artefact strengthens.

Merleau-Ponty (1962) has pointed out that Descartes's formulation of the body as part of passive nature (res extensa) ignores the dimension of the intentionality of the lived body. Through embodiment meanings are recognized. Indeed, Merleau-Ponty notes that the lived-body constitutes our being in the world. However, the preceding discussion has demonstrated the extent to which concepts can create reality. In a culture wherein the body is conceived of as an object, embodiment comes to be experienced in this way. This understanding is brought into being through everyday practices. Indeed many of our current health practices encourage us to view our bodies as objects and thus contribute to a technological self-understanding.

Shweder & Bourne (1982) refer to studies which show that the western conception of the abstract, decontextualized, disembodied person is rather peculiar within the world's cultures. For other cultures ontological primacy resides in the group rather than in the individual. Such cultures do not separate the individual from the social context or from each other; they are holistic rather than reductionist societies. Shweder & Bourne note that the sociocentric conception of the individual–social relationship lends itself to an organic metaphor. Thus in holistic sociocentric cultures the human body, conceived of not as an artefact but rather as an interdependent system, is frequently taken as a metaphor of society and sometimes as a metaphor for nature. In such cultures, the concept of the autonomous individual who can exercise radical freedom is viewed as alien and indeed bizarre, doomed to a life of isolation and loneliness.

But of particular interest in relation to the abstract decontextualized way of knowing which has become characteristic of western cultures, Shweder & Bourne (1982) found evidence in a comparative study of Oriyas (in India) and Americans and the different modes of thinking between the two groups. The personal accounts of the Oriyas were concrete and relational and differed from the abstract style of the accounts of the Americans. In citing examples of context dependent statements they noted that where Americans might describe a person as 'preoccupied', Oriyas would say: 'he does not disclose secrets'. Rather than describing someone as 'selfish' they would say 'he is hesitant to give money away to his family'.

Shweder & Bourne's study demonstrated that concrete, contextualized, occasion bound thinking in a culture was not a reflection of a deficiency of skills or abstraction. Neither was it a function of education, literacy, socio-economic status or language. Rather, different modes of thinking were explained by them in terms of the holistic sociocentric organic and the egocentric reductionist views of the person which prevailed in the different societies. They were thereby presenting evidence which demonstrated that people in holistic cultures are connected to each other and their sense of interdependence is reinforced both through their group identity and through their language use which remains close to the situated contexts of their everyday lives.

Harding (1986) refers to comparisons which have been drawn between the reductionist individualistic conception of self which is characteristic of Western European or Euro-American culture and an Africanized world view. She cites a paper by a Black American economist (Dixon 1976) who argues that the 'Rational Economic Man' of neoclassical economic theory is a European construct which does not apply to Africans. In an Africanized world view there is no perception of a gap between self and the phenomenal world. One is simply an extension of the other. People live in harmony with nature aiming to maintain balance among the various aspects of the universe. As well, the individual is not separate from the social order, for the community is not viewed as a collection of fundamentally isolated individuals but rather as a unity.

This understanding of the group results in an ethic of responsibility and interdependence with others. In the Africanized world view the knower is not separated from the known. Africans 'know reality predominantly through the interaction of affect and symbolic imagery' (Dixon 1976). What is known is not value free, neither is the process of coming to know either impartial or dispassionate. Harding (1986) describes a process of coming to know which using Rose's (1983) term unites 'hand ,brain and heart'. This can be contrasted with the idea that the separate phenomenal world is regarded as an object to be controlled through 'hand and brain' manipulation and measurement.

Harding (1986) points out many striking similarities between the Africanized world view and the feminine world view within Euro-American society. She contrasts them both with the Euro-American male world view in terms of ontology. In both the Africanized world view and the feminine world view the community rather than the individual is primary; she contrasts them also in terms of epistemology, wherein the knower is inseparable from the known in the Africanized and the feminine world view. The ethical positions of each are also contrasted. In the Africanized and feminine world view responsibility is of a higher order than self-interested rights.

However she also warns against accepting too readily as ahistorical truths, contrast schema which originate in projects of social domination, which are usually constructed by European men and which in many ways are anachronistic. She cautions against 'tendencies to exalt women's different reality when it is also less than the reality we want, is not the only alternative reality and is disappearing' (p..176). One is reminded here of the current tendencies among some feminists to accept Gilligan's (1982) notions of women's different moral voice as an ahistorical truth about women, rather than recognizing it as a function of the socio-cultural and historical situation of women which is changing.

This discussion has indicated that the notion of person which has arisen over the last 300 years within western society is based primarily upon the experiences and conceptualizations of educated European men in the context of changing understandings about ontology and epistemology. These have been associated particularly with the rise of science and the influence of Descartes's philosophy upon everyday understandings. The notion of persons as isolated, individual egos with commodified bodies, subjects in a world of objects, 'spectators, observers, separated by an invisible plate glass window from the world in which we find ourselves' (Magee 1987 p. 258) constitutes a European male view which has contributed to the understanding European male persons have of themselves. It does not appear to reflect the understandings held by persons in mediaeval Europe, in a range of other cultures, or by women in western society at least until recent times.

Environment

This Cartesian consciousness has also profoundly influenced understandings about the environment. It seems that prior to the scientific revolution, the prevailing understanding of nature in Western Europe was as a living, bountiful nurturant mother who could however also render unpredictable violence, storms, and drought (Harding 1986). Womanly earth was understood as God's special creation for man's nurturance and was therefore understood in sacred and respectful terms. Through this nurturant maternal image of nature, people understood themselves as one with nature, interconnected and interrelated, all rendered sacred as God's creations.

However, as Capra (1982) has pointed out, whereas the goal of science in ancient times had been wisdom and understanding, the goal of science since Bacon, has been knowledge that can be used to dominate and control nature. Harding (1986) has pointed to Bacon's view of the relationship between science and nature being modelled on 'rape and torture—on man's most violent and misogynous relationships to women'. Capra (1982) also refers to Bacon's views of nature as a woman who had to be 'hounded in her wanderings', 'put in constraint', made a 'slave' and that the aim of the scientist was to 'torture nature's secrets from her'.

As the understanding of the world was transformed in the 16th and 17th centuries, consistent with Cartesian thinking, the organic view of nature was replaced by the metaphor of nature as a machine. The universe came to be seen as a gigantic machine made up of countless smaller machines. Scientific method divided the world into the smallest building blocks and then tried to build it up again. Nature came to be thought of as mechanical, lifeless, and inert. Nature was desacralized, and became a resource to be mastered, a product of human workmanship.

Drengson (1980) has pointed out that the Cartesian philosophy of technique has resulted in a technocratic understanding of environment aimed at the control of life through so called value-free applied science. Carried to its logical conclusion it seeks to turn the world into a controlled artefact. The environment is simply there to be exploited through the systematic application of technology. Within this mindset governmental and economic policies have growth as their central aim and this is promoted by policies favouring complex high technologies.

The technocratic way of understanding environment is as an object to be exploited in the interests of economic growth linked to technological innovation. There is a dreadful irony, some may say obscenity, in the idea of economic matters being understood in terms of a metaphor of growth, while nature is viewed in lifeless mechanical terms. In the old organismic view the fecundity of nature was understood in terms of both growth and decay. But the economic view of the necessity of growth permits no consideration of decay. Rather technology is developed as an end in its own right to sustain unfettered economic growth. In this understanding all values are then reduced to economic terms.

For some years now increasing concern has been expressed about the notions of unlimited economic growth in the context of a finite planet (Drengson 1980). Basic understanding of population biology helps us recognize that the simpler an ecosystem is, the more unstable it is. However human activity stemming from notions of the scientific aim of controlling nature has resulted in an increasing simplification of complex ecosystems through the destruction of a variety of life forms, thereby making the environment more and more vulnerable. By the 1970s there was unmistakeable evidence of the unprecedented impact of human society on the ecosystem. However the push of environmental exploitation, driven by a powerful global economic system, continues today. It is becoming increasingly clear that the impact of scientific technological innovations is now rendering the environment diseased. Rather than nature being a bountiful source of sustenance, it is now the source of powerful pollutants endangering life as a whole on planet earth.

The Cartesian philosophy of technique associated with applied science and technology aimed at economic growth results also in a reduction of diversity in human, social, and cultural life. 'Lifestyles' become commodities to be marketed. Emphasis is on packaging and reproducibility. Creativity and complexity break down and life becomes plastic, plagiaristic, and imitative. Rather than the richness of diverse multiculturalism we have the monolithic monopoly of McDonalds; Andy Warhol's pop art celebrates or comments ironically and negatively upon the banal, the prepackaged, the disposable. The pervasive sameness of familiar images is found wherever one goes (Parker 1990).

The experience of human social and cultural life in these terms has also been described as post modernism. This is a sensibility characterized by discontinuity, a sense of cultural helplessness and anaesthesia, as the contradictions stemming from the unrelenting impact of Cartesian technique and the technologically driven economy upon everyday life become apparent (Angus & Jhally 1989).

As Drengson (1980) has pointed out, the technocratic mindset, in striving to create uniformity in product and culture, finally fragments human life and lacks any values to sustain life. This post modern experience of fragmentation has thus become characterized in terms of surface impressions and surface values, where every viewpoint has equal validity and there are no generally accepted criteria for judging anything. This can be described as the other side of a post modern consciousness.

This section has indicated how the understandings of nature and environment in terms of a positivistic Cartesian attitude have contributed to a changed understanding of environment from nurturant, but unpredictable mother, to object of scientific technical domination and control. The image of growth has shifted from nature to the economy and the erosion of the environment in the interests of economic growth has resulted in a recognition of the breakdown of diversity both in nature and in everyday life.

Implications for health and nursing

The discussion so far can help us to recognize that the concepts of both health and nursing are constituted in the context of understandings of person and environment and the relationship between the two. Within the cultural context of a positivistic attitude of Cartesianism, isolated individuals are understood as separate and apart from their bodies, from the environment, and from other people. In this cultural context, wherein understandings about scientific medicine have become linked to beliefs about economic growth through technological innovation, it is not surprising that health has come to be viewed as the absence of disease. Attention then focuses upon the search for and cure of disease through high technology diagnostic and therapeutic interventions aimed at cure.

In the traditional classic medical model, as Allen & Hall (1988) have pointed out, disease is treated as a thing in itself, something apart, that attacks the individual. Each disease is assumed to have but one cause. Medical technologies are utilized to diagnose a disease, discover a specific cause and provide a specific cure. The enormous significance of this model in our culture and its reification has resulted in what one writer (Figlio 1977) has described as the 'medicalization of life', whereby complex social and ethical problems have become transformed into a biomedical format and all life processes reduced to these terms.

Capra (1982) has pointed out that the great successes of medical science in this century have all been based on detailed knowledge of cellular and molecular mechanisms which have led to extensive development of drug therapies and have enabled vastly more sophisticated forms of surgery. However, he notes that a serious shortcoming of the biomedical approach is that the phenomenon of healing cannot be dealt with because health is reduced to mechanical functioning. Through concentration upon smaller and smaller fragments of the body, modern medicine loses sight not only of the patient as a human being but also of the broader environmental and sociopolitical context in which disease occurs. At the same time the link between the medical model and advanced technology appears to have resulted in a preoccupation with technology as an end in itself (Taylor 1979). Thus modern medical practice reinforces Cartesianism in everyday life through processes which objectify the body and which result in individuals being treated as if they are independent of social and environment contexts.

It seems to follow that, in a cultural context wherein person and environment are understood as inextricably interrelated and where primary ontology resides in the group rather than the individual, a different understanding of health would arise. It would probably be understood as the wholeness of this integrated unity. Health would be understood as holistic. Such a view of health is however, not consistent with the beliefs, practices, and structures of a culture dominated by Cartesianism.

Understandings of health are thus closely connected to, are constituted by , and help constitute understandings that are held about persons and environment. It is not surprising, within the cultural context of Cartesianism and the dominance of the medical model, that the understanding of health as absence of disease has contributed to an understanding of person in reductionist terms with the body viewed as an artefact and the environment as separate from the person. Neither is it surprising that medical practices have tended to create this view of health. To the extent that nursing practices are medically derived, they too have reinforced this view. However, to the extent that they have been based in traditional female nurturant and healing practices, they have provided a challenge to the dominant medical model of health.

At first glance, it might seem reasonable to describe the practice of medicine as underpinned by a 'medical model' of health and the practice of nursing as underpinned by a 'holistic model' of health. Doctors after all aim for cure through the diagnosis and treatment of disease. Nurses engage in caring practices directed towards ensuring person, family, and community wholeness. However, the sociopolitical and cultural context in which modern professional nursing practice takes place is one far more consistent with reductionist Cartesianism than with socio-cultural holism. There is little structural support for the constitution of holistic understandings about health.

Nevertheless, it is interesting to observe that this notion of health as wholeness and unity does appear to be of central concern in the work of several of the early theorists who formulated conceptualizations of nursing (Levine 1971, Rogers 1970). All of these conceptualizations indicate attempts to encompass more holistic concerns than are found within the medical model, even if these are formulated in reductionist terms (e.g. man (sic) as bio-psycho-socio-cultural-spiritual being).

It is worth noting that while the conceptual models of nursing preceded the positivistically informed metatheoretical formulations within the history of nursing knowledge development, they none the less contained strong threads of positivistic thought. They were a curious mixture of women's traditional concerns about nurturing caring practices cast within the implicit positivistic framework that permeates understandings about health and illness in western society. The medical model of health as an aspect of Cartesianism is, as has been noted, embedded in everyday practices and beliefs and it is reinforced through institutionalized structures of health care, through work practices, and through health legislation. Nurses to a greater or lesser extent have been forced to accommodate their understandings about their caring practices to this meaning system.

A careful reading of the conceptual models of nursing suggests that at least two sets of ideas have underpinned their development. One was the perception that for nursing to be a discipline in its own right, it had to be clearly identified as separate from medicine. Different philosophical as-sumptions needed to underpin nursing knowledge development and nursing practice had to be clearly directed towards different types of practice interventions. Another prevailing view was that in order to be legitimated as a profession, nursing had to be regarded as a science. But as science was understood in terms of Cartesian assumptions, nursing theorists found themselves caught in a trap of logic if they were to accept these assumptions about science and also argue that nursing was different from medicine. Not surprisingly, some nursing writers ignored internal contradictions and tried to assert the unity of nursing formulations in the belief that this was a necessary requirement for science. Thus it was understandable that nursing writers found historicist insights useful in providing a rationale for nursing both as separate from medicine and as a science.

However, when viewed from a position informed by feminist insights such as those found in the work of Harding (1986), the development of nursing conceptual schema based on holistic principles in opposition to the reductionist principles underlying the medical model can be understood as contrast schema articulated within a system of Cartesian dualities. As such, they can be seen to have developed out of understandings about the nature of nursing and nursing work in a medicalized culture strongly influenced and structured by Cartesian thought where nursing work is dominated by medical interests and is undertaken primarily by women. In many ways nursing epitomizes traditional women's work with its emphasis on nurturant caring practices, while medicine has been characterized as an archetypal male profession.

However, the structures and practices of both medicine and nursing are changing. Nurses need to view with caution, therefore, models of nursing based on contrast schema which suggest that holistic, caring (female) nursing models complement the reductionist (male) medical model. It can be argued that such models, like models of women's different reality, originate in schemes of social domination of women and of nurses.

Sarter (1988) has pointed out that the lack of research productivity and the diversity of views flowing from nursing models are indications that the basic foundational work of the discipline is yet to be accomplished. In her view the profession has neglected the development and articulation of a philosophy of nursing. For Sarter the identification of a philosophical foundation for nursing is ideally a precondition for theory development and productive research. While noting that the concepts of person, environment, health/illness, and nursing have been accepted as the backbone of the metaparadigm for nursing, she points out that the underlying assumptions of a discipline are in fact its metaparadigm and these have not been clearly articulated for nursing. Thus in Sarter's view, there is a need to first define the fundamental perspective from which the discipline of nursing ap-proaches reality. This is the domain of metaphysics which deals with questions of ontology and teleology, i.e. the nature of being and its purposes. Issues of epistemology and ethics can then be addressed. That is to say, the study of how we know reality and how we should relate to it follows identification of the basis of the discipline's perspective on life.

This chapter has indicated that the historicist influence upon nursing thought has contributed to a breaking down of implicitly held beliefs and explicitly expressed views that the positivistic search for truth and certainty through scientific method was the only way to proceed in conceptualizations and theory development in nursing. While historicism has opened the way for acceptance of a variety of approaches to research, a major limitation has been identified within historicism. The understanding that linear time is itself historical has led to the recognition that historicism involves causal explanations through a reification of history. The post modern consciousness comes into being through a recognition that understanding stems from one's embodied temporality and openness to possibilities in a meaningful world of language, artefacts, and culture within which one has situated freedom.

A post modernist consciousness recognizes the impossibility of a position outside the status quo because of one's spatiotemporal embeddedness. Nevertheless it can offer a powerful critique of the status quo particularly through examination of assumptions underpinning power structures within the status quo.

This chapter has followed a post modernist approach to critique Cartesianism through exploration of assumptions underpinning Cartesian thought and discussion of the implications for western society of the realities created through belief in Cartesian concepts. Particularly discussion has focused upon the historically changing understanding of being and nature, i.e. of person and environment. This exploration has demonstrated that the Cartesian conceptualization of nature and of human bodies as machines has resulted in each being regarded as if they are passive objects to be shaped by technological processes. Additionally, this view has shaped how people have come to regard themselves. Historical, anthropological, and feminist insights have helped in the understanding that this view of person in terms of mind-body separation has probably been brought into being more in European men than in women or people in general from other cultures. However, this is changing.

Understanding of the consequences for the environment of Cartesianism shows up a ravaged natural environment and an economically driven social environment, wherein the post modern experience is one of surface meanings, purposelessness, and destruction of diversity through the power of packaging and life style production. The widespread acceptance of Cartesian assumptions in regard to issues of health and illness has resulted in an understanding of the body as an object of medical scrutiny and technical intervention and of health as the absence of disease. In this context it is not surprising that conceptualizations of nursing practice have been influenced by Cartesianism and the medical model of health although they have been influenced as well by women's traditional caring practices.

The critique of Cartesianism has thus helped to open the way for addressing foundational philosophical questions for nursing. It has indicated that the question of what it means to be a person can be addressed in terms of a relational ontology which recognizes the boundedness of human being in the world through embodiment, history, and culture, and the inextricable interrelatedness of being and nature. It recognizes that the knower cannot be separated from what is known and that in the process of coming to know, people change. It recognizes also that what it means to be a person in this historic era needs to take account of the influence of Cartesian thought upon understandings of self, body, and environment, and the widespread belief in the medical model of health.

It acknowledges that such understandings have resulted, to a greater or lesser extent, in the human experience of life in terms of separations between mind and body, between self and world, and between persons and environment. It is thus directed towards meanings and actions aimed at enhancing life experiences in terms of wholeness and integration of being and nature.

Epistemological questions about how we know reality stem from a post modernist understanding that there is no objective reliable universal foundation for knowledge. Criteria for truth and falsity are internal to the traditions within which such claims are made and cannot be legitimated outside these traditions. That is to say, in the post modern era, legitimation becomes plural, local, and immanent, i.e. constituted within practice (Fraser & Nicholson 1990). Theory development is seen to be possible for nursing to the extent that it is constituted through practice and claims to be no more than a set of viewpoints at a particular time, justifiable only within its own time.

The ethical question of how we should relate to reality follows from acceptance of assumptions about being and nature in terms of a relational ontology. Ethical decision-making for nurses is then based upon an ethic of responsibility towards oneself and others and towards the natural and socio-cultural environment.

An ethical stance of responsibility to self and others moves beyond the ethic of individual rights linked to Cartesianism. It acknowledges that nurses are not detached neutral observers of the situations and circumstances in which they practise. The practice of nursing as a craft wherein nurses come into a caring, healing, nurturant relationship with troubled, vulnerable, sick, and hurting people requires nurses' involvement, commitment, and insight, as well as their skills and knowledge.

An ethical stance of responsibility towards the natural environment requires ethical decision-making based on life-centred rather than anthropo-centric values. In the post modern world of a devastated and diseased natural environment nurses concerned about health can no longer acritically accept the view that human instrumental and technical concerns and interests must necessarily override those of other forms of life.

An ethical stance of responsibility towards the socio-cultural environment is directed towards scholarly and political activities by nurses which will facilitate the laying open of oppressive structures of meaning that constrain the coming into being of fuller expressions of possibility.

The goal of discipline development and practice in nursing which stems from this philosophical foundation is the achievement of health and wholeness and the resacralizing of being and nature, through a moral stance moved by passions and purposes and a sense of mystery, awe, and wonder.

REFERENCES

Allen J D, Hall B A 1988 Challenging the focus of technology: a critique of the medical model. Advances in Nursing Science 10(3):22-34
Angus J, Jhally S 1989 Cultural politics in contemporary America. Routledge, New York
Aries P 1974 Western attitudes towards death from the middle ages to the present. (Translated P M Ranum) John Hopkins, Baltimore
Benner P 1989 Critical care nursing at the baccalaureate level: strategies for the future. Paper presented at the AACCN Invitational Conference, San Antonio, Texas
Benner P, Wrubel J 1989 The primacy of caring: stress and coping in health and illness. Addison-Wesley, Menlo Park
Brodie J 1984 A response to Dr J Fawcett's paper: the metaparadigm of nursing: present status and future refinements. Image: The Journal of Nursing Scholarship 16:(3):87-89
Capra F 1982 The turning point: science, society and the rising culture. Simon & Schuster, New York
Charlesworth M 1982 Science, non science and pseudoscience. Deakin University Press, Geelong
Chinn P, Jacobs M 1983 Theory and nursing: A systematic approach. C V Mosby, St Louis
Conway M E 1985 Toward greater specificity in defining nursing's metaparadigm. Advances in Nursing Science 7(4):73-81
Dickoff J, James P 1968 A theory of theories: a position paper. Nursing Research. 17 (3):197-203
Dilthey W 1960 Dilthey's philosophy of existence. (Translated W Kluback and M Weinbaum.) Vision Press, London
Dixon V 1976 World views and research methodology. In: King L M, Dixon V, Noble W W (eds) African philosophy: assumptions and paradigms for research on black persons. Farrow Center, Charles R Drew, Postgraduate Medical School, Los Angeles
Donaldson S, Crowley D 1978 The discipline of nursing. Nursing Outlook 26:113-120
Douglas J D (ed) 1970 The impact of sociology. Appleton Century Croft, New York
Drengson A R 1980 Shifting paradigms: from the technocratic to the person-planetary. Environmental Ethics 3:221-240
Dreyfus H L, Dreyfus S E 1986 Mind over machine. The Free Press, New York
Dzurec L C 1989 The necessity for and evolution of multiple paradigms for nursing research: a post structural perspective. Advanced Nursing Science 11 (4):69-77
Faulconer J E, Williams R N 1985 Temporality in human action: an alternative to positivism and historicism. American Psychologist 40:(11):179-1183
Fawcett J 1978 The 'what' of theory development. In: Theory development: what, why and how. National League for Nursing Pub. no 15-1708 New York, p. 17-33
Fawcett J 1984 The metaparadigm of nursing: present status and future refinements. Image: The Journal of Nursing Scholarship 16:84-87
Figlio K 1977 The historiography of scientific medicine: an invitation to the human sciences. Comparative Studies in Social History 19:262-286

Flaskerud J H, Halloran E J 1980 Areas of agreement in nursing theory development. Advances in Nursing Science 3(1):1-7

Foucault M 1973 The birth of the clinic. (Translated S Smith) Tavistock, London

Fraser N, Nicholson L J 1990 Social criticism without philosophy: an encounter between feminism and postmodernism. In: Nicholson L J (ed) Feminism/postmodernism. Routledge, New York, p 19-38

Gadamer H G 1975 Truth and method. Seabury Press, New York

Giddens A (ed) 1975 Positivism and sociology. Heinemann, London

Gilligan C 1982 In a different voice: psychological theory and women's development. Harvard University Press, Cambridge

Habermans J 1970 Toward a rational society: student protest, science and politics. (Translated J Shapiro) Beacon Press, Boston

Harding S 1986 The science question in feminism. Cornell University Press, Ithaca

Hardy M E 1974 Theories: components, development, evaluation. Nursing Research 23: 100-107

Hardy M 1983 Metaparadigms and theory development.In: Chaska N L (ed) The nursing profession: a time to speak. McGraw-Hill, New York p 427-437

Heidegger M 1962 Being and time. Harper & Row, New York

Hempel C 1966 Philosophy of natural science. Prentice-Hall, Englewood Cliffs

Illich I 1975 Medical Nemesis. Pelican Books, London

Jacox A 1974 Theory construction in nursing: an overview. Nursing Research 23 4-13

Johnson D 1980 The behavioural system model for nursing. In: Riehl J, Roy C (eds) Conceptual models for nursing practice, 2nd edn. Appleton-Century-Crofts, New York, pp 207-215

King I M 1971 Toward a theory for nursing: general concepts of human behaviour. Wiley New York

Kuhn T 1970 The structure of scientific revolutions, 2nd edn. University of Chicago Press, Chicago

Laudan L 1977 Progress and its problems: towards a theory of scientific growth. University of California Press, Berkeley

Leonard V W 1989 A Heideggerian phenomenologic perspective on the concept of person. Advances in Nursing Science 11 (4):40-55.

Levine M 1971 Holistic nursing. Nursing Clinics of North America 61:253-263

Magee B 1987 The great philosophers. BBC Books, London

Meleis A 1985 Theoretical nursing, development and progress. Lippincott, Philadelphia

Merleau-Ponty M 1962 Phenomenology of perception. Routledge & Kegan Paul, London

Moccia P (ed) 1986 New approaches to theory development. National League for Nursing, New York

Nagel E 1961 The structure of science: problems in the logic of scientific explanation. Routledge & Kegan Paul, London

Neuman B 1982 The Neuman systems model. Appleton Century Crofts, Norwalk

Nicholson L J (ed) 1990 Feminism/postmodernism. Routledge, New York

Orem D 1980 Nursing, concepts of practice, 2nd edn. McGraw-Hill, New York

Parker J M 1990 Ethics and economics reviewed in economics, ethics and health care outcomes: implications for nursing practice in the 21st century. Royal Melbourne Hospital Nursing Education Centenary Conference Proceedings, Melbourne

Rogers M 1970 Theoretical basis of nursing. F A Davis, Philadelphia

Rose H 1983 Hand, brain and heart: a feminist epistemology for the natural sciences. Signs: Journal of Women in Culture and Society 9(1)

Roy C 1980 The Roy adaptation model. In: Riehl J, Roy C (eds) Conceptual models for nursing practice, 2nd edn.. Appleton-Century-Croft, New York, p 125-143

Sarter B 1988 The stream of becoming: a study of Martha Roger's theory. National League for Nursing, New York

Shweder R A, Bourne E J 1982 Does the concept of person vary cross culturally? In Marsella A J, White G M (eds) Cultural conceptions of mental health and therapy. Dordvecht, Boston, p 97-137

Silva M C, Rothbart D 1984 An analysis of changing trends in philosophies of science on nursing theory development and testing. Advances in Nursing Science 6(2):1-13

Stevens B 1979 Nursing theory. Little Brown, Boston

Taylor C 1971 Interpretation and the sciences of man. The Review of Metaphysics
    25(1): 45-51
Tinkle M, Beaton J 1983 Towards a new view of science. Advances in Nursing Science
    (Jan) 27-36
Yura H, Torrens G 1975 Today's conceptual frameworks within baccalaureate nursing
    programs. National League for Nursing Pub. no 15-1558, New York, p 17-25

15. Professional ethics and reflective practice: a moral analysis

Merilyn Evans

When we conform to a role prescription, we cannot know what is authentically known beyond what is already determined for us

The expectation that nurses will practise ethically and legally alongside other professionals in health care settings, and the recognition that nurses are accountable for their practice (Gray & Pratt 1989), are critical issues for the discipline of nursing. However, whilst there is a subdiscipline of 'nursing ethics' emerging in Australia, the nursing profession here has not yet seriously addressed a question of fundamental concern to professionals and to modern moral philosophers: is there a realm of professional ethics which is separate from the realm of ordinary morality? A central contention of this chapter is that the tensions and dilemmas which arise from this question are a source of 'moral distress' (Jameton 1982) for many nurses in the course of their practice. A further contention is that the concept of a 'professional role' in relation to moral conduct has, in a sense, contributed to the conflict which occurs when professional ethics seems to be at odds with ordinary morality; that is, when it is thought that adherence to one set of moral or ethical prescriptions cannot be achieved without incongruity, and at the expense of another set.

The terms 'autonomy' and 'advocacy' are found throughout the extensive international literature on 'nursing ethics' and are used frequently in the proliferating debates in this field in Australia. Moral autonomy as described by Beauchamp & Childress (1979) is to do with self determination: choosing for oneself, creating one's own moral position, and accepting responsibility for one's own moral views. Moral autonomy is thought to be a prerequisite for morality (Evans 1986, Van Hooft 1990) and is seen as a moral 'good' or 'right' in the context of roles and relationships within health care. The concept has been linked to a newly discovered advocacy role (Gadow 1982, Fry 1987), now claimed as a central and essential one for the professional nurse (ANF 1989, Evans 1992, NHMRC 1991). For nurses, moral autonomy is also thought to be a prerequisite for patient/client advocacy (Becker 1986, Fowler & Levine-Ariff 1987, Evans 1987a).

The view to be put here is that to be an autonomous moral agent and effective patient advocate, an individual must be able to act freely and authentically on moral principles which have been reflected on and given moral weight. A morally autonomous advocate must also have conceptual clarity and the ability and willingness to evaluate critically and present arguments for and against, alternative courses of action. Further, while there are constraints on moral autonomy for nurses (Evans 1986), and just what an advocacy role entails is unclear (Evans 1987a, Johnstone 1989b), at the least, a subjective sense of moral autonomy is necessary for nurses to undertake this function (Evans 1992). It will be suggested further that, in health care settings, sociologically constructed notions of professional roles (and the professional ethic which flows from these), act to constrain the 'authenticity and independence' (Dworkin 1977) of the individual moral agent which are necessary for moral autonomy. Finally, it will be contended here that effective advocacy entails the moral autonomy of both providers and consumers of health care services. As patients or clients, consumers must have sufficient information and understanding to facilitate choices and decisions about their health and welfare which will serve both their present and longer term needs and interests.

This chapter will examine a number of conceptual difficulties in the way terms like autonomy are used in relation to professional ethics, but a major aim is to examine critically the unreflective acceptance of a professional ethic as a guide to nursing practice. The issues are discussed in relation to the surgical procedure of augmentation mammoplasty. The chapter uses information obtained from interviews and correspondence with those involved in elective cosmetic surgery (patients, nurses, surgeons) as well as interested government and consumer organizations. Several scenarios drawn from case studies will be used to illustrate the relationship between moral autonomy, advocacy,and the nature of reflective, ethical nursing practice. The effective implementation of the advocacy function will be referred to briefly. But first, a clarification of terms is necessary.

TERMINOLOGY

Although ethics/ethical and morality/moral are often used interchangeably, certain conceptual distinctions between these terms can be made. For the purpose of this discussion, morals are humanly devised prescriptions or rules to guide day to day human actions, behaviour and aspirations. Ethics is a set of descriptive and analytical tools; essentially a system devised to help us identify 'right conduct' and determine the appropriate behaviour of the moral individual living the 'good life' both privately and publicly. Morality is what we aim for, ethics is a system to help us achieve this aim. Professional ethics as a system of moral rules which prescribes the moral conduct of professionals should be distinguished from 'ordinary morality'. Ordinary morality derives from genuinely reflective moral principles which hold that the rights and interests of all persons are equally worth protecting (Johnstone 1986). This can be contrasted with professional ethics as a set of rules, codes or specified conduct, formulated, operated and enforced by the profession and designed primarily to provide protection for professional interests (Seighart 1982).

The adjectives moral and ethical are also largely interchangeable, but here 'ethical' will refer to the outcome of a process of analytical moral enquiry. At its simplest level, and similar to the problem solving process familiar to nurses, it is an investigation and weighing up of alternatives, which takes account of, but does not rely solely on intuition, convention, or legalism (Johnstone 1987). A individual engaged in analytical moral inquiry is willing and able to provide publicly, a reasoned justification for decisions and actions undertaken (or in some cases, actions omitted).

Whilst conventional notions of morality/morals as rigid prescriptions about the oughts of human conduct (for example with regard to sexual behaviour) have become somewhat dated, ethics in both the public and private domain has become a major topic for debate. The subdisciplines of ethics, medical, nursing, business and legal ethics, and most visibly, that area of applied ethics known as bioethics, have expanded significantly in their scope and concerns. Whilst there is considerable public disenchantment with professionals, a certain respectability is still claimed for the general category of 'professional ethics' as a set of circumscribed rules of conduct derived from the discipline of ethics. A contentious question to be raised here is whether professionals, in adhering to professional codes and rules embodied in a professional ethic, are indeed acting 'ethically' or 'morally'. We should note here that controversy is inherent in any human construct; whether morality 'exists', which set of moral prescriptions are 'right', how ethical analysis should proceed, and the legitimacy of its outcomes, will always be matters for ongoing debate. Although moral rules and ethical codes may conflict and consensus seems improbable, the enormous agreement that does exist about the oughts of human conduct suggests that morality is thought to be an ideal worth striving for, in both the private or personal, and public or professional domains. (As a point of clarification, a moral individual is one who has genuinely reflected on, and attempts to follow certain universalizable moral principles: respect for persons, truth telling, keeping promises and so on). We turn now to the relevance of ethics and bioethical issues in the field of health care, to the ethical practice of professional nursing.

Ethics and medical technology

Ethics in health care, in particular bioethics, now focus largely on the development and implementation of new medical technologies. A useful way of thinking about technology is that it is the application of human skills, techniques, and processes, to practical problem solving in all aspects of human life. Medical technologies defined broadly, can be a range of devices, products or procedures, from pharmaceuticals to life support systems designed to improve, alter or affect our lifestyles and life choices in a multitude of ways. The rapid expansion of medical technology and concerns about its potential for producing both benefits and burdens have generated numerous agencies and processes aimed to better our understanding of, control over, and informed decision making about its development and applications. Statutory bodies like the law reform commission, and health consumer protection agencies like Victoria's Health Services Commissioner regularly develop and revise ethical and legal codes, standards, policy statements and guidelines. Most publicly funded health care institutions have their own institutional ethics committees which, under the direction of professional and research organisations like the National Health and Medical Research Council, set and monitor standards for research on humans protecting their rights to privacy, confidentiality and safe and effective medical care. Legislation and policies are thus constantly under review in response to the many perspectives voiced by various individuals and groups, and the public. However, it could be argued that the greatest pressures come from vested interest groups representative of medical scientists, lawyers and ethicists (both religious and secular) and the commercial sector. Unfortunately the 'benefits' of medical technologies are most often successfully promoted by the more powerful biomedical lobbyists and practitioners, and those who stand to gain financially such as the pharmaceutical companies and manufacturers. Less often are the problematic and unwanted side effects or 'burdens' foreshadowed and avoided, or the voices of consumers and the public heard. Infrequently too, are the dissenting views of nurses heard publicly, even though they are by far the biggest, and therefore a potentially powerful group of health care providers.

NURSES: CONCERNS AND CONTRIBUTIONS

Nurses have a great deal to contribute to biomedical debates and health care ethics generally. Nurses are asking for clarification about restraining and confining patients; about the provision of information about their care and treatment; about the extent and limits of privacy, confidentiality and medical orders; and about nursing responsibilities in these areas. Nurses are also concerned about substandard health care and inhumane and exploitative medical technologies, and doubly so when they find themselves in the role of bystander, colluder, or accomplice in their applications (Jameton 1983, Muyskens 1988). The role of advocate for the patient is the result of calls for consumers and patients to be informed, protected and supported by alert, concerned and effective spokespersons (Russell 1987) through many public advocacy organisations such as the Consumer's Health Forum ACT; the Office of the Public Advocate and the Health Services Commissioner (Health Line) in Victoria; and the Public Interest Advocacy Centre of New South Wales. Advocacy for nurses, which has arisen partly in the process of professionalization (Evans 1987a, Leddy & Pepper 1989), is also a response by the nursing profession to an urgent need to address these issues.

However, some nurses particularly in clinical practice, seem to feel that ethical concerns are nothing new: some have devised their own ways of dealing with problems and dilemmas, either individually ,or at ward or unit level. Some assert that they are simply none of nurses' business. Some nurses also tend to believe that even if answers cannot always be found in legal views of the parameters of practice, there is no need to engage in debate or take the issues further. Others express an often unwarranted fear of legal repercussions for their actions and non actions, or a naive belief that dissatisfied health services consumers can easily obtain acknowledgment of disadvantage or compensation in the law. This situation reflects a poor understanding of the legal system and the nature and complexity of legal and ethical issues, as well as a sense of complacency about the way they are currently handled. But most often it seems to reflect an inability and lack of confidence in expressing one's own or another's moral distress, or defending an ethical position which may, for example, expose and avoid technological applications which have significant potential for harm.

At an academic level, nursing ethics is a rapidly developing area of study, and a vast array of literature is now available, most of it generated from North America. Interest shown by nurses in the ethics of health care is evident in an increasing number of national and international symposia and conferences in which nurses have participated, and the number of new nursing publications in the field. The most recent journal *Ethics in Nursing* was launched in California in July 1990 after an international call for contributions. Late in 1991, the International Council of Nurses will publish a collection of case studies in nursing ethics drawn from many countries.

Australian nurses too have long informally debated their own 'nurse in the middle' dilemmas of multiple conflicting responsibilities and loyalties. They are gradually awakening to the wider debates and finding a voice on multidisciplinary ethics committees, in ethics forums, and as members of political and consumer organisations. Australian nurses have responded to the debates with Bills of Patients' Rights, Revised Codes of Professional Ethics, Standards of Practice, and Policy Statements, for example on euthanasia and conscientious objection (RANF 1989). They have developed ethics resource papers through the Australian Nursing Federation's Professional Development Committee (RANF 1987, ANF 1989b), and ethics courses in university nursing programs, the latter often subsumed under 'Professional Issues in Nursing' (Deakin University 1990), but sometimes standing as discrete units (South Australian College of Advanced Education/Sturt 1990). Continuing education modules in ethics and the law are available through the Royal College of Nursing, Australia (RCNA 1989, 1991), and the NSW Nurses' Association has produced a series of videotapes on ethical and legal issues in nursing for educational and professional development purposes (1989).

Nurses have also contributed to government inquiries, for example the Victorian Government's Inquiry into Options for Dying with Dignity (Gibbs

1986), and in 1987 the Victorian Nursing Council funded a major research study looking at the role of the nurse as patient advocate and autonomous moral agent (Kuhse et al 1988). Nurses in Australia have begun to undertake research in nursing ethics (Evans 1991, McKinley 1986, Slater 1987, Watt 1990), and a nursing focussed text is now available on bioethics (Johnstone 1989b). While two legal texts (Staunton & Whyburn 1989, O'Sullivan 1983), and Amelda Langslow's longstanding series 'The Nurse and the Law' in the Australian Nurses' Journal have been an invaluable resource for nurses, a major absence in the field is a text with a combined approach, incorporating law and nursing ethics.

Australian nursing journals reveal a number of articles on specific topics in the field of nursing ethics. For example, quality vs quantity of life (Johnstone 1988); Not for Resuscitation Orders (Johnstone 1989a); nurse advocacy and womens' health care (Gillette 1988); the ethics of teaching ethics (Lyneham 1988); a nursing ethics literature review (Evans 1986); a commentary on the field of nursing ethics (Evans 1987b); and the research reports referred to above on advocacy (McKinley 1986, Evans 1990b, Watt 1990) and nurses' ethical concerns (Slater 1987).

A number of writers have sought to analyse what it means to be 'ethical' or 'professional', in terms of moral and legal acountability and responsibility (Woodruff 1987, Steele 1988, Chiarella 1990a, Holden 1990), or in relation to moral concepts such as 'caring and commitment' (Van Hooft 1987), 'honesty' in nursing relationships (Chiarella 1990b), and patients 'rights' (Whalley 1990). But reports such as the Marles 'Report on Professional Issues in Nursing' (1988), the Olive Anstey International NursingConference proceedings, 'Professional Promiscuity?' (1988), and the Royal College of Nursing, Australia's 'Nursing in the Nineties' (1990), indicate that, in addition to ethical and legal concerns, for nurses professional matters cover a wide spectrum. Education and clinical practice, gender and ideology, staffing and resources, roles and relationships within health care, as well as a multitude of changes and influences impinging on nursing theory and practice come under the umbrella of professional issues.

It appears too, that despite having laid a firm claim to professional status, many nurses in Australia are still engaged in debates about what is or is not 'a profession' long after others have abandoned it as unfruitful. A glance at the employment section of the newspaper shows that numerous diverse and unlikely occupations are now calling themselves 'professions' and, as alluded to earlier, claims to professional status and many 'professional issues' are to do with establishing and maintaining occupational territory and credibility with the public (as valuable consumers of professional services), whose 'needs' must be confidently served by professionals.

In view of these comments it would seem that the links between nursing ethics and professionalism need to be teased out further. However, whilst awareness of the relationship between these fields has been raised, aside from Johnstone (1986, 1987, 1989b), a substantial body of critical, theoretically informed literature linking them has yet to emerge in Australia. The following moral analysis of professional ethics and ordinary morality aims to contribute to the debate and provide for the discipline of nursing, a perspective on the nature of 'ethical nursing practice', as opposed to 'professional practice'. We now return to the question raised at the beginning of this chapter.

PROFESSIONAL ETHICS AND ORDINARY MORALITY

Is there a realm of professional ethics which is separate from ordinary morality? The literature on professional ethics seems to support a separatist position on this question. Such a position holds that in making ethical decisions, professionals have an overriding duty to follow the norms, values and goals of their chosen profession. But an everyday observation, that laypersons tend to judge professionals by ordinary moral standards, suggests on the contrary, that there is no separate professional ethic, and professionals are bound to follow the principles of an ordinary morality just like all other persons. This view seems a reasonable one, for as children, most of us have learned for example, that it is wrong to act dishonestly. Honesty ideally for most of us then comes to be recognised as a moral principle which guides our daily actions and behaviour. When professionals appear to be deviating from such 'ordinary' principles, they are rightly judged by those who hold them to be acting 'immorally'. It could be suggested for example, that stealing from clients or gross negligence in medical practice is behaviour which may be judged uncontroversially to be morally indefensible. Where it could be shown that a doctor is fraudulently over servicing patients through Medicare, or a nurse is found to be removing narcotics from the patients' drug cupboard for personal use, such behaviour would also be judged by professionals and laypersons alike as dishonest and therefore morally wrong (Callahan 1988).

On the other hand, there are some situations which arise in health care settings where principles of ordinary morality appear to be disregarded by professionals, but it is not so clear that their actions and behaviour are also 'immoral'. Where doctors and nurses appear to be acting dishonestly for example, in not disclosing certain important information to patients by appealing to 'professional ethics', a confusing and distressing ambiguity in what is generally understood to be 'ethical behaviour' can arise. This is in part because 'professional' behaviour is often assumed by its very nature to be 'ethical' or exemplary.

A moral discrepancy arises when professionals consider their behaviour to be beyond reproach, but on examination it is demonstrated to be self serving or immoral by ordinary standards. This can be partially explained (but cannot adequately be defended), in terms of sociological theory (Turner 1974) by the observation that any suggestion of immorality for a professional is both dysfunctional and socially damaging. A doctor or nurse for example, as well being in breach of the law which protects the public from fraudulent, harmful or dishonest actions by any persons, can be disciplined or struck off by professional regulatory bodies. This may mean loss of reputation and livelihood. Further, in view of the status many professionals enjoy in society and the high expectations the public has of them, they are likely to be judged more harshly for immoral behaviour than a layperson, by their peers, the public, and the courts. This would be especially so in the cases cited where professional position has been used for private or personal gain.

As suggested earlier, in anticipation of this, professionals attempt to preserve public confidence and a 'high ethical profile' by adherence to a code of medical or nursing ethics and by setting up special professional norms and standards which are thought to ensure high quality medical and nursing care. Self protection as well as protection of the public interest is therefore the underlying rationale where this special and separate professional ethic is operating. The professional ethic embodies the values, goals and norms of the profession and prescribes behaviour which governs professional relationships. But moral difficulties arise when professional behaviour to protect the public interest becomes blurred with private professional interests. The inadequacy of a narrowly focussed professional ethic as opposed to a broader genuinely reflective morality becomes clear when, for example, surgical procedures which may cause significant harm are performed and it is clear that professionals have not ensured that patients are adequately informed about the risks involved. We should keep all this in mind in the following scenarios where a morally questionable separate professional ethic is appealed to, because of the potential for undermining confidence and trust in the professions in question. Scenarios involving elective aesthetic cosmetic surgery of the female breast have been chosen to illustrate these points. For in this type of elective surgery, moral and legal responsibilities accompanying authorisation or agreement for 'consent' are often foregone, since the patient is requesting the procedure rather than acquiescing in it. In the first scenario, the professional ethic appealed to seems to be in conflict with ordinary morality, and in the second, where the actor (a nurse), is not performing in her professional role, there is no such conflict. It should be noted here that the surgical procedure in question involves the reshaping of body parts to enhance body image, and should be distinguished from those procedures which restore function or relieve pain, or those undertaken to remedy congenital defects, scarring or injury (Shanner 1991).

Aesthetic elective cosmetic surgery

The surgical procedure of augmentation mammaplasty to increase breast size for aesthetic reasons has particular relevance for professional ethics as it involves the application of technology purporting to provide a practical solution to an area of human need. As a relatively simple but lucrative elective operation, performed largely in private hospitals on an increasing number women of all ages (Peacock 1987, Vogue 1989), the aims of the procedure could be questioned on several counts. For example, it might be argued that such cosmetic surgery is unecessary because no significant harm will result if it is not done, and that it is not threatening to health in the same way as non removal of a diseased gall bladder might be. But because it is requested by a woman in the belief that breasts of a larger and more desirable shape and size than she already possesses will enhance her body image and increase self esteem and psychological well being, it is frequently defended as ethically acceptable by a tenuous relationship to 'health'. The argument for 'health' has some plausibility if this is interpreted very broadly. It could be said for example, that the depression caused by negative body image may become a significant threat to physical health. But on reflection, the argument for health is weak, for body image improvement is a psychological not a physical need, and there is evidence to suggest that underlying psychological concerns are rarely appropriately 'dealt with' by surgical means (Wengle 1986, Hollyman et al 1986). Moreover, it is not clear that doctors are the best people to assist with non health matters such as body image which relate to questions of femininity and sexuality (Brownmiller 1984, Wolf 1990). Unfortunately, space will not allow further discussion of that controversy here.

Augmentation mammaplasty is also defended on the grounds that it restores normality. But this argument cannot easily be sustained either since it is often undertaken for breasts which cannot be considered gross enough to be abnormal; they are often quite 'normal' for the age and physique of the woman concerned. Furthermore, the 'pre-existing condition' for which the operation is frequently being performed has effectively been medicalised as 'atrophy', 'hypertrophy', or 'ptosis' (Mitz 1974, Becker 1990). These terms simply refer to small, large or 'droopy' breasts respectively.

It does not follow from these arguments however, that the procedure should not be allowed. We could still insist that women have a right to do what they like with their bodies providing they do not harm others (Draper 1988). Here one might counter with the suggestion that nevertheless, alternatives such as counselling should always be offered to a woman contemplating this sort of remedial surgery whether one believes it to be 'necessary' or not. However, the success of such psychotherapeutic techniques, and how readily acceptable they are as an alternative to surgery to women (or to their doctors), are also controversial questions which can only be alluded to here.

More importantly, one might want to ask whether there is a special duty to obtain 'informed consent' for this type of surgery, in particular consent as understanding or comprehension (of likely benefits, harms and outcomes), as spelled out by bioethicists Beauchamp & Childress (1983) and Faden & Beauchamp (1986). This element seems particularly pertinent in elective aesthetic cosmetic surgery, since the prospective woman patient is assumed to be 'already sold on the idea' (Shanner 1991).

Informed understanding and decision making

Faden & Beauchamp (1986) suggest that informed consent must be solicited whenever a procedure is intrusive, whenever there are significant risks, and whenever the purposes of the procedure may be questionable. We would have no difficulty in agreeing with this statement for the type of surgery under consideration (the risk of harm will be considered at length shortly). But there are problems with an uncritical understanding of some of the elements of consent considered essential for it to be 'valid' (Alberta Association of Registered Nurses 1983, Veatch 1989). For example, voluntariness/non coercion; capacity/competence; information/ disclosure and agreement/authorisation. For while we might conclude that voluntariness and agreement are not in question here (the woman has requested and presented herself for surgery), it may be if we use alternative terminology i.e. 'non coercion' (in that decisions about medical treatment procedures must be freely made). One might reasonably argue that a decision to have aesthetic cosmetic surgery cannot be 'freely made' in that societal expectations of the perfect female body pushed by the popular media, coerce or manipulate women, (see, for example, More 1984, Cleo 1987, Cosmopolitan 1990, Mode 1990). We might want to suggest that women are under pressure from husbands, or partners, or suffer from deficiencies such as 'low self esteem'. While initially plausible, it is important to note that such a view tends to see women as victims (Kenway & Willis 1988) or controlled by others: 'heteronomous' rather than 'autonomous' self determining individuals, in Kantian terms (Dworkin 1977). This is a view we should perhaps reject, since it assumes the woman lacks the capacity to make up her own mind rationally about what she wants, and we would not want to argue that women are incompetent to judge their best interests for themselves. But in taking a conventional view of informed consent, this question of capacity or 'competence' as a further essential element is important. It is clear however, that patients who request augmentation are not 'incompetent' or deficient in their decision making capacities. What they do lack is a reasonable level of knowledge to inform their decisions. While cosmetic surgeons often defend the procedure as if it were a desirable intervention justifiable on the basis of benefits which outweigh the risks, the ethics of informed consent require that as well as benefits (which in the case of elective cosmetic surgery do not need to be persuasive), any substantial risks of harm or untoward outcomes should be disclosed (Beauchamp & Childress 1983). In fact for augmentation mammaplasty as we will see shortly, the benefits are questionable. It will be argued here that many women lack adequate information and have insufficient understanding of predictable and often irremediable adverse outcomes. Thus the element of permission or authorisation for consent and what is consented to should also be critically examined.

A review of the current medical and nursing literature and interviews with cosmetic surgeons and many women who have undergone augmentation mammaplasty, as well as with nurses caring for such women, indicate that a professional ethic is frequently appealed to in defence of the procedure. Further, not only the goal of health (already questioned here), but the professional values and norms of autonomy and confidentiality as used in an absolutist sense (Faden & Beauchamp 1986), are central to the arguments offered. For example, it is claimed that since professionals provide a specialised service which is actively sought by women in the belief that it will improve their 'health', this should be available to all who seek it. But even if we accept that health can be interpreted very broadly to include an operative procedure which may improve psychological well being, a significant pro-portion of women will not be enhanced by the procedure as the following section shows. Rather they will be harmed. It should be noted here that there is some evidence to suggest that general well being is sometimes positively affected, but only if the outcome of the operation is congruent with what the woman expects (Kilmann et al 1987). One medical commentator has warned about the 'mostly positive' results from follow up studies of womens' satisfaction that 'we must be alert to the down side risk that when results do not meet the expectations of patients, they are inordinately furious, even when apparently well informed' (McKinney 1988a).

There is now substantial documented evidence of harms in enough cases to warrant serious re-evaluation of the procedure (De Cholnosksy 1970, Brandt et al 1984, Riddle 1986a, Barton et al 1989, Caffee 1990, Cathcart & Hagerty 1989, Lowerey & Maloney 1990).

Understanding of significant harm

It has been suggested so far that uncritical availability of augmentation mammaplasty is in need of justification on a number of grounds, but we will now focus on significant risk of harm. The procedure involves implanting a prosthetic device made from a variety of materials, (usually silicone gel or saline or a combination of the two) either into a pocket dissected out behind the glandular breast tissue or behind the muscles of the chest wall (Biggs et al 1982, Vasquez 1987). The body reacts predictably to the implant in a highly idiosyncratic way, causing it to become walled off from the surround-ing tissue by a smooth glistening white fibrous capsule. It should be noted here that this physiological response is so predictable that it can be encom-passed by the medical term 'normal sequelae' (McKinney 1988c) and thus can be moved conveniently out of the domain of mandatory disclosure of 'risk or complication' for informed consent. This same medical commenta-tor has further asserted that 'all the implants get hard in time' (McKinney 1988a). This 'hardening' occurs as the non-contractile capsule becomes progressively tighter so that the soft gel or saline filled implant is squeezed into a hard ball-like mass, causing varying degrees of distortion of the breast tissue, and frequently resulting in breasts which are unsightly and unpleas-ant to feel.

The incidence of capsular contracture is variously reported in the literature and manufacturers' advertisements and occurs, it is claimed, in between 4% and 91% of augmented breasts (Rutledge 1982, McGrath & Burkhardt 1984, Burkhardt 1985, Kerrigan 1989). The implant may remain soft and undetectable by sight or feel at first, even for many years, but when contracture does occur, it ruins any initial 'beneficial' effects of the operation. This means that a woman will not only not get an improved soft breast of the size and shape she desires, but it is highly likely that she will need repeated, usually unsuccessful, 'corrective' operations, sometimes over many years, at significant risk, expense and inconvenience. It appears that even the 'new and improved' textured implants have not solved the problem of capsular contracture. Indeed a recent animal study showed that 'texturing of the implant surface resulted in an increase in the contracture problem rather than a reduction' (Caffee 1990).

Data from surveys and reports from consumer health organisations and national and international regulatory bodies have raised serious questions about the safety and efficacy of the implants, for example, rupture, displacement, splitting, and leakage of silicone gel into the body (Theophelis & Stevenson 1986, Moufarrege et al 1987, Schur 1988). 'Minor' complications such as haematoma, infection, and loss of sensation are also common, (Lowerey & Maloney 1990). However, other potentially more serious threats to health such as human adjuvant disease (Sergott et al 1986, Varga et al 1989), and cancer (Deapen et al 1986, Silverstein et al 1988), have been researched and discussed at length but are at present difficult to substantiate.

These assertions are well documented in the medical and pharmaceutical literature (Nelson 1980, McGrath & Burkhardt 1984, Brandt et al 1984, Berrino et al 1986, Barton & Tebbets 1989) and in the nursing literature (Riddle 1986a, 1986b, Walsh 1986). Safety concerns are being addressed following surveys of women by Consumer Health Services in Australia, Health Issues (1990), and investigations by government agencies (Australian Therapeutic Device Bulletin 1990), as well as overseas government bodies (Department of Health and Human Services 1990) and consumer organisations. Many women have contacted government and women's health agencies in Australia reporting dissatisfactions over unfulfilled expectations and the varying degrees of disfigurement and discomforts they live with. Cosmetic surgeons have long been aware of these problems but they nonetheless continue to carry out the procedure (Wengle 1986, Barton & Tebbets 1989, Caffee 1990). These problems are also of current interest to the Department of Community Services and Health; Medical Devices and Dental Products and Therapeutic Devices Branches. Lawyers, implant manufacturers and, of course, women as potential litigants, have concerns in the area of product liability.

Even if these facts could be disputed, we should accept for argument's sake and for the purpose of this discussion, that there is reliable evidence to demonstrate predictable and potential harms for many women. In the light of this evidence, it is clear that women contemplating augmentation mammaplasty should be made aware and more information should be available to them. Anecdotal information and examination of patient information documents such as the Victorian Plastic Surgery Units' Information for patients, family and friends' (undated) or those of the Australian Society of Plastic Surgeons and Society of Aesthetic Plastic Surgery, indicate otherwise. Many women receive minimal information and therefore lack understanding.

The role of the nurse as professional

Now let us consider the situation where a nurse educator coordinating a plastic surgery course for nurses and working in the clinical setting as an instructor, has recently acquired reliable information about the efficacy and safety of the prosthetic devices used to increase breast size and shape in the procedure of augmentation mammaplasty. She has always assumed that women who book into the hospital where she works have been adequately informed about the risks and benefits of the procedure by their doctors before they are admitted. On reflection, she realises that many women who returned for remedial or corrective surgery sometimes three or four times, were clearly not aware of the problems associated with the procedure. She checks the medical and nursing literature (which she uses in her teaching), and realises there are some inconsistencies in recommended post operative nursing care. For example the range of movement allowed and the positioning of patients post-operatively (Conlee 1981, Capozzi 1986), and whether breast implants should be massaged to avoid complications such as contracture (Riddle 1986b, Walsh 1986). She verifies her concerns with colleagues and through research finds that breast implants interfere with effective breast self examination (Cathcart & Hagerty 1989) or mammography (Silverstein et al 1988), or with breast feeding (Neiffert & Seacat 1986, Lawrence 1989). She hears of the need for women to be followed up by their doctors (Cathgart & Hagerty 1989, Caffee 1990), assisted with the management of breast feeding and advised on immediate and long term self care following surgery. She is disconcerted by her findings, but concludes that because the patient is in a private relationship with the doctor, any information that has passed between them is 'none of her business' and she can do nothing. Indeed she considers that it would be both 'unprofessional and unethical' to interfere with this relationship, and jeopardise professional ethics by providing women with any information. Not only that, she can see no way of tackling the doctor about it because her role demands that she confine herself to nursing care only and that 'informed consent is the province of the doctor'.

It would appear that the professional and moral autonomy of the nurse who may become aware of problems of this sort is constrained because she feels powerless to speak with those women who are minimally informed. Professional ethics dictate that what has passed between doctor and patient is a matter of confidential information exchange. The professional norm of confidentiality, it is said, serves to maintain the doctor patient relationship and this facilitates the goals of healing and health. If patients feel they can trust their doctors, they will reveal information essential to achieving therapeutic outcomes. Confidentiality also serves to increase the autonomy of the patient by giving her more control over the information she has disclosed to a health care professional in a therapeutic relationship.

Generally speaking, these are not unreasonable assumptions. However, it is a widely accepted principle of ordinary morality that one should avoid dishonesty. Dishonesty can mean lying, cheating, stealing or deception of any sort. One might wish to argue however, that dishonesty here is not an issue; because there has been no request for information, there is no obligation to disclose. (This question has been discussed in relation to informed consent from an ethical point of view by Buchanan (1983) and Vanderveer (1980) and from a legal perspective by Skene (1990) and others (Law Reform Commissions 1990).)

But now consider the case where a 27-year-old single woman books in to a private hospital late in the afternoon for augmentation mammaplasty the next day. She has no children, and because she has always been 'as flat as a tack' simply wants to improve her breast size and shape. That evening she hears a radio program where the pros and cons of elective surgery of the breast are discussed. She asks the nurse for more information; what ARE the risks and difficulties? This presents a dilemma. What should the nurse do? The answer is usually that she should refer the woman back to her doctor. But what if he or she cannot be contacted (which is frequently the case)? One alternative for the nurse then is to carefully 'suss out' what the doctor has told the woman and reinforce that. In discussing the nurse's role in the care of cosmetic surgery patients, Conlee (1981) says

> Your ECS (Elective Cosmetic Surgery) patient may also try to pump you about the surgeons's competence or ask your opinion about the surgery's outcome. Since at that point your patient's already selected the surgeon and opted for the surgery, just say something like 'Dr Smith's patients all seem happy with the results'

What if the doctor has said 'a very small number of people get a degree of hardening, 1 in 100, but it is highly unlikely that the woman will be one of them'? Should the nurse keep to this misleading and minimal information, or add to it the knowledge she has? She could suggest alternatively that it is not her job to inform or advise patients; she can lie and say she doesn't know; or she can avoid the hard questions altogether, and 'reassure the patient', an important task for nurses performing in their 'professional roles', and in accord with a professional ethic. On the other hand, the nurse who decides to take on the role of patient advocate has a range of options open to her. She may choose to act as reassurer or mother surrogate, as confidante, friend or counsellor, or as advisor, spokesperson or intermediary. She could utilise any one of the many models of advocacy (Abrams 1978, Kohnke 1982, Gadow 1983, Winslow 1984, Curtin 1986), in the nursing ethics literature which have recently been examined by Australian critics (Gillette 1988, Evans 1989, Johnstone 1989b, Chiarella 1990a, Whalley 1990). She is unlikely however, in this case to choose an extended role of advocate as described by Abrams (1978) and Evans (1987a) which goes beyond the 'reasonable bounds' of nursing practice because it is too risky or even 'unethical', for example, watchdog (monitoring the safety and quality of health care services), informant (supplementing gaps in patients' knowledge about care and treatment) or whistleblower (public notification of concerns about unethical or illegal practices).

The nurse as a person

Now consider the following situation. The nurse has a neighbour, a young woman with no children who wants an augmentation to enlarge her small breasts so she feels happier about the way she looks. This woman is unsure about pain, costs, length of stay in hospital, and so on, and her friend recommends she phone the nurse to discuss her concerns. As well as technical questions (what do they actually do?) and nursing questions (will it hurt much?), the nurse is asked 'do many women come back with problems' and could she tell her as much as she knows about the operation including the risks or complications. In a non institutional information sharing 'advisor' capacity (Gillette 1988), the nurse would have no qualms about doing this. She alerts the woman to possible complications without undue alarm, and directs her to the relevant medical and nursing literature. She suggests that she phones both the consumer health service and a womens' health referral centre to get more information. She offers to help the woman with a list of questions for her doctor, and suggests that if she is not satisfied with his replies she seek out another. The nurse then discusses the pros and cons with the prospective patient and explores with her alternatives to surgery. Eventually, given this information, the woman decides not to go ahead with the procedure and instead decides in favour of counselling.

THE MISUSE OF AUTONOMY

Before looking further at these scenarios, we will return to the concept of autonomy, and see how the professional value of maximising autonomy or self determination can operate counterproductively in two ways. First as implied earlier, women as prospective patients are, or should be, treated as if they are autonomous beings who should be able to choose or refuse any surgical procedure. But in truth their ability to make decisions and exercise their autonomy depends on the amount of information they have. In the context of the confidential patient doctor relationship, the doctor is the only one according to professional ethics, who can provide information from which the woman selects and opts for or against. That the women often fail to hear, or decide to ignore the information provided about risks and complications, does not obligate the cosmetic surgeon to go any further than simply offer the minimum and leave it up to the woman to 'choose'.

If it is objected that perhaps the woman may need more information rather than less because the procedure is elective, the professional value of autonomy comes into play in a second sense. It is claimed doctors must be free to make their own judgments about how much information is given to a prospective patient. But in the light of recent discussions on informed consent there is an ethical (Andrews 1985), and indeed a legal responsibility in a duty of care (Law Reform Commissions 1989) to ensure that not only is relevant information given, but that it is understood. In practical terms, this may mean getting the woman to 'feed back' what she understands the outcome of the procedure to be. It may mean showing the woman 'before and after' photographs which include those of hardened and distorted breasts, a suggestion put by one disatisfied augmentation mammaplasty patient. If such means are used to ensure understanding, the incongruity between the doctor's perception of a satisfactory or acceptable outcome and the prospective patient's expectation may be revealed.

It could be further argued that where there is a significant potential risk of harm in the efficacy and safety of the implants the doctor may have a moral obligation to actively dissuade a woman from seeking the surgery. Of course there is always the danger of losing the patient, and the argument usually offered against this view is that the determined patient will go elsewhere. But as previously suggested, in elective surgery there seems to be more of an obligation to ensure that the patient understands what she is consenting to and what she is 'getting', rather than less. To reiterate, a woman who does not have to be persuaded that surgery is necessary for 'health' is in a buyer's market, and the doctor knows she will simply find another to obtain what she wants and what she knows to be available. It is also a seller's market, for the cosmetic surgeon does not atempt to dispel the notion that he has the expertise to offer in a 'technological fix' to solve her 'problems'.

Health care professionals are in a sense correct in recognizing their importance in decision making when women request this procedure. But there are costs in attempting unreflectively to preserve the principle of autonomy. A thoughtful, reflective professional who casts wider than a narrow professional relationship, must recognize sexism as a factor constraining women's autonomy. Sexism is part of social conditioning, and operates in the popular media, and in medically focussed pharmaceutical promotional literature. It could be argued that sexism underlies many personal and professional relationships, including that of male doctor and female patient. It may well influence a professional's perceptions of what body configuration is 'good' for this woman/patient (Jobe 1990).

PROFESSIONAL SELF INTEREST

We now need to return briefly to the professional self interest which a professional ethic sometimes seems to promote. Doctors, it is said, have special permission to do to their patients what would not normally be permitted or would be called 'assault' if carried out by non-doctors. Invasions of the body by surgical means are permitted because of the special rights and duties which doctors have through their professional expertise. This is in part how a professional role is defined. Thus the professional ethic defines the duties inherent in that role and serves an important function. But it must be remembered that this right is only in the context of special permission or 'authorisation' by the patient which cannot simply be assumed. Doctors as professionals also have special benefits and privileges; one is the relatively free exercise of their professional autonomy, which in some cases is too easily abused. It is morally questionable that women should be 'freely' undertaking some sorts of cosmetic surgery when the outcome will not achieve what is claimed for it, and indeed they may be harmed. What seems to be operating here is a form of ethical relativism where morality is a matter between individuals and is not being considered in universalistic terms. Moreover, there seems to be a degree of rationalising self interest, for in contrast to much other elective surgery, a very substantial non refundable 'up front' payment is often required. (Medicare of course does not cover elective cosmetic surgery of this type.) To adhere unequivocally to a narrow professional ethic in such cases is morally indefensible, and professionals who do so must weigh the costs in terms of loss of trust and a devaluing of the professions. If professional practice is to be within the bounds of ordinary morality, as suggested by Ellin (1982) 'a total package of interests must be acknowledged, not just those for which the professional relationship exists'.

SOCIOLOGICALLY DERIVED PROFESSIONAL ROLES

We now turn to look briefly at sociologically derived origins of professional roles and the limitations of social role theory. According to this theory, roles are assigned, ascribed, or in the case of professionals 'chosen', and professionals undergo a socialisation process, learning the norms, conduct and expectations of the chosen profession. The dramaturgical metaphor is often used by sociologists (Turner 1974) describing this process. For example, when a person is fully socialised and becomes a competent and effective professional, she has thoroughly learned a script, she plays to an audience, she performs in a hospital/theatre, and is directed by a doctor/director. Unfortunately the professional is often locked into this rigidly defined role and adheres to a script written by someone else; in this case the script is the professional ethic. This means that in the role of professional, the nurse in the first situation is 'other directed' rather than 'inner directed' (the latter arguably a requirement for any autonomous moral agent attempting to follow the principles of an ordinary morality). Deviations from the script in the form of improvizations (nurses advising or informing patients) can throw the whole play into chaos, particularly if the audience (doctors, patients, other health care professionals) have expectations based on prior experience of how it should be performed. Further, in certain social structures like hospitals, if actors do not perform their roles as expected or if prompts or cues are missing, individuals may find it difficult to restore the flow of the play as these are so interdependent. Rarely is an individual's style or method able to change the script significantly; and actors such as nurses do not have licence to alter it as they think fit or as circumstances demand. This metaphor illustrates well the nurse's dilemma where perceptions of her professional role constrain individual moral agency which is necessary for moral autonomy in ethical decision making. Dilemmas therefore arise because of the way we think about what it means to be a 'professional' and the belief that there is an overriding obligation to adhere to the assigned duties that go with the role. Role prescriptions as suggested earlier, define what we are permitted or obligated to do and allow professionals to provide essential services to society. The professional ethic which governs professional roles reinforces a descriptive professional ethic or 'the way things are'. In one sense then, the separate professional ethic the nurse appealed to provides a guide for action but these rules are not relevant where she steps out of that role. When there is no script or audience, no prompts or cues, and the director is absent, the individual, stripped of the role, must fall back on the prescriptions or oughts of an ordinary morality. It is therefore suggested that a sociological perspective has shaped and continues to direct and inhibit our thinking about the professions, and the meaning of ethical professional practice. We will now return to the earlier scenarios.

THE PROFESSIONAL ETHIC AND NURSING ROLES

In the first scenario the nurse is appealing inappropriately to the professional principle of confidentiality. The rules of professional conduct prevent her from honestly disclosing risks of harm, information which may cause the patient to change her mind. It may be in this case that the only ethical option for the nurse, given the facts, and after having made a genuinely morally reflective judgement, is to advise the woman to defer the operation until she has more information. She could simply advise her of a legal right to sign herself out of the hospital which would be in keeping with a narrow legalistic advocacy function. On the other hand, the nurse may combine strategies. She may advise the woman of her legal rights, and discuss the options of deferring or staying, notifying hospital administration of her actions and concerns. She may insist that the woman speak with her doctor, at the same time documenting her actions and discussions in the patient's records. It is of course, entirely possible that the doctor is not up to date with information which may preclude the procedure, and any nurse claiming a collegial professional relationship should verify this by discussion and by producing documented evidence.

It is true however, that we are describing here an ideal situation, unfettered by a narrow understanding of the professional role, where the nurse acts ethically and legally in the interests of those who may be affected by any decision made. We need now to return briefly to ethical theory to assist us. In the last case it seemed entirely appropriate for the nurse to act as she did because of her different relationship with the woman asking the questions. Since she is unconstrained by a professional role, the same obligation for confidentiality did not apply. Honest disclosure to prevent harm was not a difficulty. It could be argued that the 'professional ettiquette' followed in the first situation is simply a form of rule utilitarianism, more aptly described as 'superstitious rule worship' (Smart 1979). We should consider the implications of unreflectively following any rule in the mistaken belief that in the long run, all will be better off. This reasoning is implicit in the separatist professional ethic in the first case.

It is vital, rather, that in elective procedures like augmentation mammaplasty moral principles and medical facts are carefully weighed. Because of the predictable physiological response to the prosthetic devices, and women's differing psychological needs, each case should be considered individually within the framework of moral autonomy. The woman's ability to make her own decisions is respected and she should be supported when she does so. But, it must be emphasised, only when she has all relevant information. Appeal to a professional ethic by non-disclosure of information where disclosure may prevent an avoidable harm involves deception which violates the rules of ordinary morality. It contravenes the universalisable moral principle of respect for persons as self determining individuals entitled to all the information they need to decide matters which may significantly affect their lives.

The vital question for nurses as advocates is whether the cost to themselves in avoiding such harm is too great. This is an important issue the nursing profession should address. It is suggested here however, that nurses must be educationally prepared to defend an ethical position and have an adequate understanding of the law as it affects their practice. If they are also supported by the 'collective responsibility' of the profession (Muyskens 1988) in their decisions, and in their actions as patient advocates, these difficulties are not insurmountable.

SUMMARY AND CONCLUSIONS

Several issues have been addressed in this chapter. First, that nursing ethics with the focus of nurse in the middle dilemmas cannot be easily separated from ethical and bioethical questions about new medical technologies. Secondly, that behaviour which is within the bounds of ordinary, genuinely reflective morality may not be in accord with professional ethics. Thirdly that there is a need for the nursing profession to question the premise of the argument for a separatist professional ethic, that is, that 'to follow a professional ethic is always to act morally or ethically', and its conclusion that professionals have an overriding duty to follow the dictates of their chosen profession, even at the expense of ordinary morality.

Scenarios where professionals followed a separate ethic or morality foreshadowed possible harms and benefits as these related to individual and public interests. The application of technological knowledge in the research, development and utilisation of prosthetic implants for augmentation mammaplasty with little regard to understanding, informed decision making, or control over outcomes on the part of women whose lives may be significantly affected by their use, formed a focus of moral conflict for nurses as health care providers and as patient advocates. The professional principles of confidentiality, autonomy and the goal of health were critically examined along with the limitations of sociologically based role theory on which a separatist professional ethic seems to rest.

It was suggested that Australian nurses may have relied too heavily on social role theory (and on the North American literature) to promote professional roles such as patient advocate with insufficient thought given to theoretically informed ethical analysis on which to base practice. Nurses need opportunities to contribute to ethical analysis and time to develop and express the thoughtful mirroring of action, and the weighing and balancing needed in problematic situations. Nurses also learn to support and legitimate their advocacy functions by demonstrating an understanding of the relational rights and duties of all persons: patient, nurse, doctor, or employer, as well as those of the broader society beyond health care settings.

The chapter has provided an insight into the process of moral or ethical analysis and the nature of reflective nursing practice as it relates to new technologies and nursing ethics. As there are untoward implications for morality as a reliable guide for action if there are two separate and sometimes conflicting sets of moral rules, this issue should be addressed by the nursing profession. A reconceptualisation of professionalism and professional ethics may be necessary. There is also need for a clear understanding of what the advocacy function entails for nurses, with firm clear protocols for action written into professional practice standards. A first step may be to redefine what is meant by the ethical practice of nursing and teach nurses how to defend effectively a reflective ethical position which is supported by the profession, should nurses' actions come under scrutiny by the law. In this way nurses will be enabled to practice confidently, safely, and effectively with a clear understanding of the ethical and legal parameters of their practice, and the credibility of nursing as a practice discipline will be strengthened.

REFERENCES

Abrams N 1978 A contrary view of the nurse as patient advocate. Nursing Forum 17(3):258-267

Alberta Association of Registered Nurses 1983 Guidelines for registered nurses as client advocates, Edmonton

Andrews K 1985 Informed consent: adrift on a trans-Atlantic crossing. Lawyer 3(6) (Victorian Young Lawyers, Melbourne)

Australian Nursing Federation 1989a Standards for nursing practice, 2nd ed. ANF, Melbourne

Australian Nursing Federation 1989b Ethics: nursing perspectives. ANF, Melbourne, vol 1

Australian Therapeutic Device Bulletin 1990 Safety concerns—breast implants. Australian Therapeutic Device Bulletin 90 (2) (July): 2

Barton F E, Tebbetts J B 1989 Augmentation mammaplasty. Selected Readings in Plastic Surgery 5:28 p 1-26

Beauchamp T L, Childress J F 1979 Principles of biomedical ethics, 1st ed. Oxford University Press, New York p 66-102

Beauchamp T L, Childress J F 1983 Principles of biomedical ethics, 2nd ed. Oxford University Press, New York p 70-93

Becker H 1990 The correction of breast ptosis with the expander mammary prosthesis. Annals of Plastic Surgery: 24(6)489-497

Becker P 1986 Advocacy in nursing: perils and possibilities. Holistic Nursing Practice 1(1) 54-63

Berrino P, Galli A, Raneiro M L, Santi P L 1986 Longlasting complications with the use of polyurethane-covered breast implants. British Journal of Plastic Surgery 39: 549-563

Biggs T M, Cukier J, Worthing L F 1982. Augmentation mammaplasty: a review of 18 years. Plastic and Reconstructive Surgery 69: 445-452

Brandt V, Breitling L, Christensen, Neilsen M, Thompsen J L 1984 Five years of experience of breast augmentation using silicone gel prostheses with emphasis on capsule shrinkage. Scandinavian Journal of Plastic and Reconstructive Surgery 18: 311-316

Brownmiller S 1984 Femininity. Fawcett Columbine, New York, ch 1

Buchanan A 1983 Medical paternalism. In: Gorovitz S, Macklin R, Jameton A, O'Connor J M, Sherwin sS(eds) Moral problems in medicine, 2nd ed. Prentice Hall, New Jersey, p 49-59

Burkhardt B 1985 Fibrous capsular contraction around breast implants: the role of subclinical infection. Infections in Surgery 4:6 (June) 469-474

Caffee H H 1990 Textured silicone and capsule contracture. Annals of Plastic Surgery 24(3):197-199

Callahan J C (ed) 1988 Ethical issues in professional life. Oxford University Press, Oxford, ch 2

Capozzi A 1986 Clinical experience with Heyer-Schulte inflatable implants in breast augmentation. Plastic and Reconstructive Surgery 77:772-778

Cathcart R S, Hagerty R C 1989 Preoperative and postoperative considerations in elective breast operations. Annals of Plastic Surgery, 22(6):533-536

Chiarella M 1990a Trends in expectations of nursing responsibilities- professional and legal perspectives. Nursing in the Nineties Conference Papers. Royal College of Nursing, Australia 12th National Conference, p 69-91

Chiarella M 1990b Honesty in nursing relationships. Bioethics News 9(3):20-26

Cleo 1987 Breast surgery; what it's like...why I had it done. July

Conlee D 1981 Put a new face on your care of cosmetic surgery patients. Nursing 81:42-46

Cosmopolitan 1990 Amazing things doctors can do for you now. September

Culver C M, Gert B 1982 Philosophy in medicine. Oxford University Press, New York, ch 3

Curtin L L 1986 The nurse as advocate: a philosophical foundation for nursing In: Chinn P (ed) Ethical issues in nursing. Aspen systems, Maryland, p 11-20

Deakin University, Department of Nursing 1990 Professional issues in nursing. Deakin University Press, Geelong

Deane D, Campbell J 1985 Developing professional effectiveness in nursing. Reston Publishing, Virginia, ch 1

Deapen D M, Pike M C, Casagrande J T et al 1986 The relationship between breast cancer and augmentation mammaplasty: an epidemiologic study. Plastic and Reconstructive Surgery 77:361-367

De Cholnosksy T 1970 Augmentation mammaplasty. Survey of complications in 10,941 patients by 265 surgeons. Plastic & Reconstructive Surgery 45: p 573

Department of Health and Human Services (US) 1990 Background information on the possible health risks of silicone breast implants. Federal Food and Drug Administration, Rockville 1-3

Draper H 1988 Transexuals and werewolves: the ethical acceptability of the sex-change operation. In: Braine D, Lasser H (eds) Ethics technology and medicine. Gower Publishing, New York, p 114-122

Dworkin G 1977 Autonomy and behaviour control. In: Hunt R, Arras J (eds) Ethical issues in modern medicine. Mayfield, New York, p 363

Ellin J 1982 Special professional morality and the duty of veracity. Business and professional ethics 1(2):84

Evans M 1986 Not free to be moral. The Australian Journal of Advanced Nursing 3(3):35-48

Evans M 1987a The role of the nurse as patient advocate: implications for nursing education. M Ed St thesis, Monash University, Melbourne (unpublished)

Evans M 1987b Entering the ethics arena. The Australian Nurses' Journal 16(8):38-40

Evans M 1989 Patients' rights and nursing roles: Cathy, a case of misplaced advocacy? In: Ethics: nursing perspectives: 2. Professional Development Committee, Australian Nursing Federation, Melbourne

Evans M 1991 Women, elective aesthetic surgery of the breast and the nurse as advocate. Paper presented at the Women and Surgery Conference, University of Melbourne (in press)

Evans M 1992 Advocacy: a role for nurses? In: Gray G, Pratt R (eds) Issues in Australian Nursing 3, Churchill Livingstone, Melbourne (in press)

Faden R R, Beauchamp T L 1986 A history and theory of informed consent. Oxford University Press, New York p 288-336

Fowler D M, Levine-Ariff J 1987 Ethics at the bedside: a sourcebook for the critical care nurse. Lippincott, Philadelphia, p 190

Fry S 1987 Autonomy, advocacy and accountability: ethics at the bedside. In: Fowler M, Levine-Ariff J (eds) Ethics at the bedside.Lippincott, Philadelphia, p 39-49

Gadow S 1982 Philosophical foundations of nursing ethics. Proceedings of a national forum in nursings' encounters with ethics: dilemmas and directions for nursing. Chicago, p20-41

Gadow S 1983 Existential advocacy: philosophical foundation of nursing. In: Murphy C P, Hunter H (eds) Ethical problems in the nurse-patient relationship. Allyn & Bacon Boston, p 40-58

Gibbs J 1986 Dying with dignity: a nurses's viewpoint. Social Development Committee, Parliament of Victoria, First Report into Options for Dying with Dignity. Government Printers, Melbourne p 53-68

Gillette J 1988 Advocacy and nursing care: implications for womens' health care. The Australian Journal of Advanced Nursing 6(1) 4-11

Gray G, Pratt R 1989 Accountability: pivot of professionalism. In: Gray G, Pratt R (eds) Issues in Australian nursing 2. Churchill Livingstone, Melbourne, p 149-161

Health Issues 1990 Breast implant survey. Health Issues 24 (September):4

Holden R 1990 Accountability in autonomous nursing practice: the question of professional responsibility. Royal College of Nursing, Australia. Proceedings of 12th national Conference, p 34-50

Hollyman J A, Lacey J H, Whitfield P J, Wilson J S P 1986 Surgery for the psyche: a logitudinal study of women undergoing reduction mammaplasty. British Journal of Plastic Surgery:39:222-224

Jameton A L 1982 Nurses and moral distress in the hospital. In: Gruzalski B, Nelson C (eds) Value conflicts in health care delivery. Harper & Row, Massachusetts, p 131-149

Jameton A L 1983 The nurse: making hard choices. In: Gorovitz S, Macklin R, Jameton A L, O'Connor J M, Sherwin S (eds) Moral problems in medicine. Prentice Hall, Englewood Cliffs, p 126-136

Jobe J 1990 Plastic surgery. In: Sousa J A (ed) Breast care: get fit self improvement series. Times House Publishing, Kensington, ch 7, p 81-93

Johnstone M 1986 Professional ethics and the problem of conflict with ordinary morality. Unpublished Master's preliminary paper. Monash University, Melbourne

Johnstone M 1987 Professional ethics in nursing: a philosophical analysis. The Australian Journal of Advanced Nursing 4(3):15

Johnstone M 1988 Quality vs quantity of life: who should decide? Australian Journal of Advanced Nursing 6(1):30-37

Johnstone M 1989a The nature and moral implications of 'not for resuscitation' orders. Bioethics News 8(2):26-44

Johnstone M 1989b Bioethics: a nursing perspective. Harcourt Brace Jovanovich, Sydney

Kenway J, Willis S (eds) 1988 Hearts and minds: self esteem and the schooling of girls. Education of Girls Unit of the Department of Employment, Education and Training, Canberra

Kerrigan C L 1989 Report on the Meme breast implant. Prepared for the Minister of Health and Welfare of Canada, McGill University, Montreal

Kohnke M 1982 Advocacy :risk and reality. CV Mosby, St Louis

Kilman P R, Sattler J I, Taylor J, 1987 The impact of augmentation mammaplasty: a follow up study. Journal of Plastic and Reconstructive Surgery 80:374-378

Kilpatrick V 1984 Ethical issues and procedural dilemmas in measuring patient competence. Advances in Nursing Science: p 22-32

Kuhse H, Brumby M, Evans M, Johnstone M, Langslow A 1988 Report on the ethical, legal & social dilemmas in nursing. Centre for Human Bioethics, Monash University, Melbourne

Law Reform Commissions 1990 Informed decisions about medical procedures, joint report. Law Reform Commissions of Australia, Victoria and NSW, Melbourne

Lawrence RA 1989 Breastfeeding: A guide for the medical profession ,3rd edn. CV Mosby, St Louis, p 413-417

Leddy S, Pepper J M 1989 Conceptual bases of professional nursing 2nd edn. Lippincott, Philadelphia, chs 1, 8 & 18

Lowerey P, Maloney D 1990 Breast implants: what are the problems we are learning from consumers? Consumers Health Forum (April/May):36-37

Lyneham J 1988 The ethics of teaching ethics. The Australian Journal of Advanced Nursing 5(4):10-11

McGrath M H, Burkhardt B R 1984 The safety and efficacy of breast implants for augmentation mammaplasty. Plastic and Reconstructive Surgery: 74(4):550-560

MacKinley S 1986 An advocacy role for the critical care nurse. The Australian Journal of Advanced Nursing 4(1):3-12

McKinney P 1988a Editorial comment. Yearbook of Plastic and Reconstructive Surgery. Yearbook Medical Publishers, Chicago, p 181

McKinney P 1988b Editorial comment. Yearbook of Plastic and Reconstructive Surgery. Yearbook Medical Publishers, Chicago, p 182

McKinney P 1988c Editorial comment. Yearbook of Plastic and Reconstructive Surgery. Yearbook Medical Publishers, Chicago, p 185

Marles F 1988 Report of the study of professional issues in nursing. Health Department, Victoria, Melbourne

Mitz V 1974 New data on surgery for mammary hypertrophy and ptosis. Reported in: Yearbook of Plastic & Reconstructive Surgery 1976 p 286

Mode 1990 Bust big boobs bounce back. August:92

More 1984 Sculpting with the scalpel. June:18-24

Moufarrege R, Beauregarde G, Bosse J P et al 1987 Outcome of mammary capsulotomies. Annals of Plastic Surgery: 19:62-63

Muyskens J L 1988 The nurse as a member of a profession. In: Callahan J C (ed) Ethical issues in professional life. Oxford University Press, Oxford, p 290-294

National Health and Medical Research Council 1991 The role of the nurse in Australia. AGPS, Canberra

Neifert M R, Seacat C H A 1986 Medical management of successful breastfeeding. Pediatric Clinics of North America 33(4):743-761

Nelson G 1980 Complications of closed compression after augmentation mammaplasty. Annals of Plastic Surgery 4:460- 463

NSW Nurses' Association 1989 Nurses need help too: introducing an industrial relations education kit for nurses. NSWNA, Camperdown

Olive Anstey International Nursing Conference 1988 Professional promiscuity? (proceedings of the conference) Perth

O'Sullivan J 1983 Law for nurses, 3rd edn. The Law Book Company, Sydney
Peacock E E 1987 Major ambulatory surgery of the plastic surgical patient. Surgical Clinics of North America 67(4):865-879
Riddle L B 1986a Augmentation mammaplasty. Nurse Practitioner 11(3):30-40
Riddle L B 1986b Expansion exercises: modifying contracture of the augmented breast. Research in Nursing & Health 9:341-345
Royal Australian Nursing Federation 1987 Ethics: nursing perspectives.ANF, Melbourne vol 2
Royal Australian Nursing Federation (Victorian Branch) 1989 Policy on conscientious objection, RANF Melbourne
Royal College of Nursing Australia 1989, 1991 Continuing education program for registered nurses: Module 602 Legal concepts and practice of nursing; Module 601E ethics in nursing. RCNA, Melbourne
Royal College of Nursing Australia 1990 Nursing in the Nineties (Conference papers. RCNA, Melbourne
Russell H 1987 What you don't know can hurt. Health Issues 11 (September):17-19:
Rutledge D N 1982 Nurses knowledge of breast reconstruction: a catalyst for earlier treatment of breast cancer? Cancer Nursing (December):469-474
Schur P L 1988 Case of the disappearing breast implants. Journal of Plastic Surgery: 270-271, cited in Breast Implant Clearing House 1990:36
Seighart P 1982 Professional ethics—for whose benefit? Journal of Medical Ethics p 25-32
Sergott T J, Limoli J P, Baldwin C M et al 1986 Human adjuvant disease, possible autoimmune disease after silicone implantation: a review of the literature, case studies and speculation for the future. Plastic and Reconstructive Surgery 78:104-111
Shanner L 1991 The face of prejudice: ethical concerns regarding cosmetic enhancement. Paper presented at the Women and Surgery Conference University of Melbourne (in press)
Silverstein M J, Handel N, Gamagami P et al1988 Breast cancer in women after augmentation mammaplasty. Archives of Plastic Surgery 123:681-685
Skene L 1990 You, your doctor and the law. Oxford University Press, Sydney
Slater P 1987 The good death: registered nurses' concerns about ethical issues. The Australian Journal of Advanced Nursing 4(2)16-28
Smart J J C 1979 Extreme and restricted utilitarianism. In: Foot P (ed) Theories of ethics. Oxford University Press, Oxford, 171-183
South Australian College of Advanced Education/Sturt School of Nursing Studies 1990 Ethics in nursing (ENTO11).
Staunton P, Whyburn B 1989 Nursing and the law, 2nd edn. W B Saunders Balliere Tindall, Sydney
Steele D 1988 Changes in nursing influenced by the legal system. Proceedings of the Olive Anstey International Nursing Conference "Professional Promiscuity?" Perth, p 901
Theophelis L G, Stevenson T R 1986 Radiographic evidence of breast implant rupture. Plastic and Reconstructive Surgery:78:673-675
Turner J H 1974 Role theory: in search of conceptual unity: structure of sociological theory. The Dorsey Press, Illinois, p 160-176
Vandeveer D 1980 The contractual argument for witholding medical information. Philosophy and Public Affairs 9(2):199-205
Van Hooft S 1987 Caring and professional commitment. The Australian Journal of Advanced Nursing 4(4):29-38
Van Hooft S 1990 Moral education for nursing decisions. The Australian Journal of Advanced Nursing 15:210-215
Varga J, Schumacher H R,Jimenez S A 1989 Systemic sclerosis after augmentation mammaplasty with silicone implants. Annals of Internal Medicine 111:337-383
Vazquez B, Given K S, Houston GC 1987 Breast augmentation: A review of subglandular and submuscular implantation. Aesthetic Plastic Surgery 11:101-105
Veatch R 1989 (ed) Medical ethics. Jones & Bartlett, Boston
Vogue 1989 Future Beauty. (October):406
Walsh K C 1986 Breast augmentation: your patient's adjustment to a new body image. Today's Operating Room Nurse 8(9):20-26
Watt E 1990 An exploration of the way in which patient advocacy is perceived by registered nurses working in an acute care ward of a major metropolitan hospital. Masters in Nursing Studies thesis, La Trobe University, Melbourne

Wengle P 1986 The psychology of cosmetic surgery: a critical overview of the literature, 1960-1982 Part 1. Annals of Plastic Surgery: 16(5):435-443
Whalley P F W 1988 Law, ethics and nursing practice. Proceedings of the Olive Anstry International Nursing Conference "Professional Promiscuity?" Perth p 9.06-9.11
Whalley P 1990 Individual rights vs institutional rights: nursing imperatives for the provision of aged care services. Journal of Advanced Nursing 7(3):17-23
Winslow G R 1984 From loyalty to advocacy: a new metaphor for nursing. The Hastings Centre Report 14(3):32-40
Wolf N 1990 The beauty myth. The Weekend Australian Review, (September) 8-9
Woodruff A 1987 Professionalism—ethics- the basis. Professionalism what is it? Conference proceedings College of Nursing Australia, Hobart, p 9-12

FURTHER READING

Argyris C, Schon D A 1987 Theory in practice; increasing professional effectiveness. Jossey-Bass, London
Bok S 1982 Secrets: on the ethics of concealment and revelation. Pantheon Books, New York, p 116-237
Culver C M, Gert B 1982 Philosophy in medicine. Oxford University Press, New York, ch 3
Deane D, Campbell J 1985 Developing professional effectiveness in nursing. Reston Publishing, Virginia, ch 1
Eichler M 1980 The double standard: a feminist critique of feminist social science. Croom Helm, London
Freedman B A 1978-79 Meta-ethics for professional morality. Ethics 89:1-19
Goldman A H 1980 The moral foundations of professional ethics. Rowman & Littlefield, Totowa, New Jersey
Katz J 1984 The silent world of doctor and patient. The Free Press, London
Pence G E 1983 Can compassion be taught? Journal of Medical Ethics 9:189-191
Singer P 1982 Practical ethics. Oxford University Press, Melbourne
Vidovich M 1990 The tragic tale of the feminist nurse. The Australian Nurses' Journal 20(4):12-14
White G 1983 Philosophical ethics and nursing—a word of caution .In: Chinn P L (ed) Advances in nursing theory development. Aspen, Maryland, p 35-47

ADDRESSES

Citizen Health Research Group, Breast Implant Clearing House,
  200 P Street, N.W. Washington D.C. 20036.
  Tel (202) 872-0320
Consumers Health Forum of Australia Inc.
  32 Thesiger Court, Deakin ACT 2600 & P O Box 278, Curtin ACT 2605.
  Tel (062) 81 0811
Ethics in Nursing: An International Journal.
  Fowler D M, Davis A J (eds)
  Editorial Offices: Azusa Pacific University, P O Box APU, Azusa, California.
  Tel (818) 969 3434
Health Line: Office of the Health Services Commissioner,
  440 Collins Street, Melbourne.
  Tel (03) 616 7542, Toll free (008) 13 6066
Health Sharing Women,
  5th floor, 318 Little Bourke Street, Melbourne 3000.
  Tel (03) 663 4457, Toll free (008) 13 3321
Monash University Standing Committee on Research on Humans,
  Clayton 3168.
  Tel (03) 75 2061 or (03) 565 3011

Law Reform Commission of Victoria,
    160 Queen Street, Melbourne 3000.
    Tel (03) 602 4566
Medical Devices and Dental Products Branch,
    Department of Community Services and Health,
    G P O Box 9848, ACT.
    Tel (062) 891 555
Public Interest Advocacy Centre,
    Law Foundation of New South Wales and the Consumers' Health Forum of Australia,
    Level 4, 245 Castlereagh Street, Sydney & P O Box A236, Sydney South 2000.
    Tel (02) 264 5444
Office of the Public Advocate: Advocacy, Guardianship and Administration Board.
    221 Drummond Street, Carlton, Victoria 3053.
    Tel (03) 663 114, Toll free (008) 13 6829
National Health and Medical Research Council Secretariat,
    G P O Box 9848, ACT. 2061.
    Tel (062) 89 6936
The Librarian, NSW Nurses' Association,
    43 Australia Street, Camperdown NSW 2050.
    Tel (02) 550 3244

16. Becoming a reflective practitioner

Carolyn Emden

INTRODUCTION

Reflective practice is of pre-eminent interest to nurses. The topic is related in the nursing literature to discussion about appropriate approaches to inquiry in nursing and in particular to the value of interpretive and critical approaches. The notion of *reflection* as a valid way of knowing arises out of the critical social science paradigm and is currently attracting considerable discussion within nursing courses and professional forums. To be a *reflective practitioner* suggests professional maturity and a strong commitment to improving practice—a reasonable aspiration for every registered nurse.

This chapter describes a strategy of empowerment and emancipation for improving nursing practice. In so doing it leads the reader through a number of interpretive and critical processes which enable discovery, and creation, of personal nursing theory—with a view to influencing the practice of nursing and the generation of nursing knowledge. If you choose to engage in this guided process of reflection, you will be advancing your thinking at a *conceptual level,* and thus better able to effect change within nursing at professional, social, and political levels. The work undertaken is expected to provide an ongoing impetus for socially and politically oriented action—within whatever sphere of nursing you practise. By embarking on the reflective processes described, the potential exists for you to effect change at many points, for example at the point of nurse-client interaction and clinical decision-making; at the level of educational and administrative processes; or within ethical and political debate. Such are the possibilities for you to influence your professional life through reflection as it is described here. It is important to appreciate that the processes can be undertaken on an individual basis or on a group basis. For example, you may wish to work through the processes alone, or to enter into a collaborative arrangement with colleagues in your work setting, or with colleagues across different work settings.

The chapter is structured to provide both theoretical and practical insights: ideas from the fields of critical theory and sociology provide a framework for practical strategies of reflection, as well as examples of others' reflective experiences and the views of nurses on the value of critical social science for nursing. As a result of this approach there is a sense of 'a play within a play' in the chapter which hopefully will prove useful to readers wishing simply to gain an overall impression of the area, as well as those intending to engage in the processes of reflection as a practical experience. Whatever your interest, it is likely you have a sense of anticipation, as if you are embarking on a novel project, and indeed this is so due to the paucity of literature that translates the vision of critical social theory into practical outcomes.

THE KEY PROCESSES: OBSERVATION AND REFLECTION

The project described within this chapter is a highly introspective inquiry involving two complex and overlapping processes: observation and reflection. The ideas surrounding these processes are drawn chiefly from the fields of sociology and critical theory. Sociology offers considerable expertise in relation to strategies for observation and inductive theory development, while critical theory offers valuable insight into reflective techniques. Two key ideas can be drawn from these fields: first that observation occurs under natural conditions; and second that reflection derives from a desire of individuals to free themselves from the constraints of their own conventional thinking.

It is paradoxical that occupants of a 'natural' setting (for example, nurses at work) may be unwittingly 'self-imprisoned'. This latter idea arises from critical theory and work of the contemporary philosopher, Jürgen Habermas (1971) and relates particularly to social and political change. Such notions will be revisited, but meanwhile, more about the practicalities of your personal inquiry into practice and the nature of observation and reflection within this chapter.

The challenge ahead

Observation and reflection within the context of your inquiry mean seeing, hearing, and sensing events within your practice world and pondering their meanings, with a view to action. Both processes are intended to lead to heightened awareness about the practice of nursing and to new courses of action. By engaging in observation and reflection it is possible for all preconceived ideas to be challenged, including principles, theories, policies and 'right' ways of thinking and behaving. The activities themselves will not be new to you. However, their focused application for the purpose of arriving at a personal conceptualization of nursing is likely to be a challenging and possibly unsettling experience. To practise observation and reflection you need access to a clinical venue as a practitioner and an observer, as well as the ability to think creatively.

Creative thought processes

The processes of observation and reflection require creative thought processes and it is pertinent to discuss these briefly now within the contexts of research and learning, both of which are relevant to your inquiry.

In a paper 'Personal construct theory and research method' a psychologist highlights how papers and books on research fail to indicate how the researcher is supposed to think:

> The central issue of how questions are formulated, how we choose, fantasize about, create, uncover, and personally explore the topic of our research is almost totally neglected in literature. The novice research worker must either invent his or her modes of thought, simply copy, with minor amendments, the substance of previous papers, or rely on handy hints and tips from his or her supervisor. (Bannister 1981)

The notion of reflexivity

Bannister (1981) suggests 'reflexivity' is at the heart of personal construct theory. This implies that the questions involved in research have personal meaning and significance for the researcher. It contrasts with traditional research approaches which sharply differentiate the researcher from the subject. Bannister proposes that researchers would be better to 'experiment conjointly *with* their subjects rather than *on* them'. Proponents of reflexivity argue that you are 'free to choose personally relevant issues of research, to draw on and make explicit, personal experience, to enjoy the wisdom and companionship of your "subject"' (Bannister 1981).

New paradigm research methodology

As a researcher engaged in observation and reflection, you are encouraged to take up the concept of reflexivity: recognise the personal significance of the task before you and resist the temptation to view colleagues as 'subjects' when observing them in practice. Regard them, rather, as co-researchers with whom you can freely discuss your project and the purpose of your interest. These ideas represent new paradigm research methodology in which inquiry becomes a collaborative process between researcher and research participants. You may wish to expand your thinking along these lines as you undertake your inquiry.

Boud et al (1985) provide some useful insights about the use of reflection as an aid to learning. They state that reflection comprises 'those intellectual and affective activities in which individuals engage to explore their experiences in order to lead to new understandings and appreciations'.

These authors stress that reflection is purposeful and actively directed toward a goal (it is not 'idle meanderings' or 'daydreaming'); that feelings and cognition are closely interrelated; and that reflection can take place in isolation or in association with others. Importantly, the individual maintains control of the process. No one else can do it for you!

Three phases of reflection

Boud et al (1985) propose that learning from reflection involves three phases which in reality are interrelated and cyclic in nature:

- a preparatory phase in which the individual considers the demands of the experience ahead and the resources required;
- an experiential phase in which practice occurs;
- a processing phase in which the preceding events are reconstructed in order to make sense of them.

Developing a personal approach

While these phases are relevant to your inquiry, the actual processes of reflection and learning remain elusive. These and other mental processes are not fully understood despite the investigative efforts of cognitive psychologists. Hence when you are asked to learn or reflect or observe, there is no one right way for you to proceed, or an ultimate guide to the work you are embarking upon. For this reason a prescriptive approach is carefully avoided in this project. Rather, you are invited to peruse a range of relevant readings in conjunction with this chapter and after reading, develop a course of action and thought that is personally meaningful. The outcomes of your observation and reflection will represent your personal conceptualization, or theory, of nursing and will culminate your inquiry.

FIELDWORK

To participate fully in the processes described, it is necessary to undertake fieldwork and therefore negotiate a clinical placement. The setting should be one where you can participate in the care of clients or patients as a registered nurse and a member of the health care team. The setting may or may not be one in which you regularly work. Realize that familiarity has the potential both to reduce and heighten sensitivity to the setting; the overriding consideration should be that you feel comfortable to practise in the setting you choose.

Three phases of fieldwork

Forty hours of field work are suggested for observation and reflection and these can be allocated into three phases:

1. The preparatory phase—approximately 4 hours
2. The experiential phase—approximately 18 hours
3. The processing phase—approximately 18 hours.

It is reasonable to assume that the inquiry can be undertaken in conjunction with a full time work (employment) commitment.

Negotiation procedures

Your clinical placement should be negotiated as soon as the decision is made to embark on the inquiry. The number of hours required will vary amongst individuals and is likely to depend on how readily you adjust to the setting and the processes involved. Because you are undertaking a clinical placement for the purpose of developing personal nursing theory and insight, it is unlikely you will be required to follow formal research approval procedures within the organization. However, it would be prudent to seek approval to practise, in writing, from the Director of the organization at least two weeks before starting the clinical placement.

Cautionary note

An important point should be appreciated before proceeding further: all three phases involve observation and reflection to some degree. These are closely intertwined *personal* processes: it is simplistic and a potential pitfall to regard observation as an objective viewing of others' behaviour. Observation involves an acute awareness of your own actions, thoughts, and feelings within a complex milieu of people and events. When you comment on others' behaviour it may indeed illuminate as much about yourself as them. This is highly appropriate as the work is directed towards your personal understanding and conceptualization of nursing. It is important to keep this in mind as you seek to extract meaning from your reading and activities in each of the phases. Don't be sidetracked or deterred from the personal purpose of the work!

Phase one: the preparatory phase

This phase essentially requires you to anticipate the experience ahead: the environment (sights, sounds, smells); the people (roles, reactions, conflicts); the climate (social, political); and importantly your role as a participant and observer. Don't overlook your feelings at this stage. Identify your current feelings about nursing and yourself as a nurse embarking upon this personal search for meaning. Think about the historical events and forces that have shaped your views and write a brief statement on your current practice/ theory position. What is your essential, most central, belief about nursing?

Complementary reading

Field & Morse (1985) discuss necessary preliminaries such as gaining access to a formal organization and entry to the study group; establishing rapport and developing relationships; and first days in the field and selecting key informants. (It is unlikely all aspects will be relevant to the way you structure your experience.)

Schatzman &Strauss (1973) discuss many relevant ideas for observation: capitalizing on your sensitivity to a new setting; the value of theoretical leads and personal hypotheses; the distinctions and difficulties of being a participant and non-participant observer; and the effects of the observer in turn being observed. Spradley (1980) discusses several useful aspects including explicit awareness and introspection, and types of participation along a continuum of complete participation to non participation. Discussion about the advantages and disadvantages of the different degrees of participation will be useful in planning your own approach and these readings will assist you to successfully complete Phase One.

Phase two: the experiential phase

During this phase you undertake your field placement as negotiated—the nature of which will be individual. Because your awareness will be heightened by the preparatory work undertaken, you will be susceptible to sensory 'overload' in the clinical setting. Do not attempt long periods of observation and reflection at first—even short periods will yield copious data. You will find that you become increasingly selective about recording experiences and events. For example, be aware of experiences that are 'complete' in terms of beginning, middle, and end (however fleeting) as these are likely to be important for further reflection. When you recognize a complete experience, such as an exchange between yourself and a patient, or between colleagues, try to record your thoughts and feelings before the tide of events carries you on to further experiences. A degree of flexibility will be important, for example, willingness to extend or cut short field work periods or to modify your role according to developing insights.

Writing field notes

Writing will be an important feature of this phase. Some field notes will be recorded at the scene, while others will be completed at varying times after the event. Authors Spradley (1980) and Holly (1984) provide useful advice for both situations.

Spradley identifies three principles:

1. The 'language identification principle' which means the language used for each field note entry should be identified, for example the different uses of language by patients, nurses, doctors, ward clerks, and other team members.
2. The 'verbatim principle' which means you should make a verbatim record of what people say, not restate or summarize in your own words.

3. The 'concrete principle' which means that concrete language should be used when describing observations (for example, what you see, hear, taste, smell, and feel) and not abstract generalizations.

Spradley further discusses different kinds of field notes, including the condensed account, the expanded account, and a field work journal.

Remember, the purpose of this inquiry is to reflect upon your own practice as a nurse, and the practice of others, in order to arrive at a deeper and more significant understanding of nursing. Your reading provides a range of views and strategies from which to create your own approach to reflection. In addition to Spradley's (1980) advice, that of Holly is also highly relevant.

Logs, diaries, and journals

Holly (1984) distinguishes between logs, diaries and journals. Basically, logs are identified as being structured and factual, diaries as being unstructured and personal, and journals as serving the purposes of both. She suggests that keeping a journal is likely to involve several types of writing: *journalistic* where events and circumstances are factually recorded; *analytic* where attention is focused on component parts of the topic; *ethnographic* where writing is grounded in the observer's observation and experience; *creative-therapeutic* which is free-flowing and spontaneous, and often done at the height of feeling; and *introspective* which is the most complex and challenges your own thoughts, sensory experiences, feelings, and behaviour. By writing reflectively, Holly means to write 'thoughtfully, deliberately, and considerately'.

Finding a personal approach to field notes

The various perspectives to be found in your reading are for you to use or reject, according to their perceived usefulness. As mentioned earlier, there is no one right way to observe and reflect, as evidenced by the diversity of ideas in the literature. However you are advised to:

- choose a quiet place to write
- discipline yourself to write regularly
- label your entries as you write (for example, with a date and a heading)
- write essentially for yourself.

By the conclusion of phase two of the reflective process you should have:

- completed your field work according to schedule (which will have been modified as the experience unfolded);
- sensitively closed relationships within the setting (these can become highly significant to all involved) including sending appropriate written communication to the Director of the organization;
- compiled a set of field notes. As indicated above, these are likely to

include several different styles of writing; be handwritten; and suggest emerging themes or common threads. Do not expect your field notes to reach an orderly conclusion—you may have to terminate them 'mid-flight'.

Sample field notes

Two sets of sample field notes are provided for interest. Because field notes are highly individual these sets should not be considered exemplary but rather serve as a source of motivation to pursue a personal approach. The first set comprises entries relating to different incidents on different days; the second comprises a report of one major experience. Both are written by registered nurses.

First set of sample field notes

a. When I arrived three people were in deep conversation at the patient's bedside, one carefully explaining the various intravenous and arterial lines to the other two. It took several minutes for me to realize this person was a registered nurse and the other two were doctors. *I felt elated—a nurse so clearly on top of her topic and the most knowledgeable member of the team!*

b. The young registered nurse bounced in, syringe and kidney dish in hand. 'OK Mr E, roll over'. ('Roll over' I squealed inside, 'Mr E is not on anything intramuscularly and he knows it: how can he be so compliant as to roll over without question!') They burst out laughing simultaneously and Mr E holds out his hand and intravenous canula. *I was completely taken in by their spontaneous 'role play' and enormously impressed by the trust and understanding between them.*

c. One by one the patients hinted, mentioned, complained that the toilet wasn't as clean as it should be. They were sorry, the registered nurses explained, but the contract cleaners only came twice a day. *I felt so frustrated—the patients were distressed and the situation unhygienic—I wanted to clean the toilet myself.*

d. The registered nurses's eyes darted to Mr E's dinner plate: 'Scalloped potato! We'll have to get the dietician to see you—today!' *I felt a flood of anger and agitation:* Why the dietician? Why isn't the registered nurse explaining this? *Where is our holistic care?* Similar feelings swamped me when I heard the social worker explaining the nature and purpose of an angiogram to a patient: surely this is a nursing role?

e. I overheard the conversation at least three times—each a minor modification of the same storyline—on about the third day of admission after all initial treatments and life sustaining measures were passed. 'Mr B I'd like to ask you a few silly questions to complete our records: what time do you normally rise? Are you right or lefthanded? Do you prefer to shower or take a bath?'

It was unmistakeably a nursing history but why, why, why were registered nurses putting these questions so late and so apologetically! Either we believe in nursing history and use it positively as a means to planning care or we judge it inappropriate and don't use it. But this! *It's a charade and violates all we claim to be and do!*

f. She swept in, her cape rustling with authority. 'Good morning everyone...how are we today...any chest pains?' The patients looked up startled. *I turn my head to hide a rush of anger:* what absurd role is this, sweeping in and out of bays asking empty questions; what a shocking waste of training and talent for a senior nurse to be reduced to meaningless encounters with patients and staff.

And then a deeper, more empathic feeling strikes: I have known this meaninglessness—in my own professional life.

Second set of sample field notes

When I walked into the ICU this morning I remember feeling a little bit uncomfortable with what I saw. Three unconscious patients, another being resuscitated, and one conscious but very ill patient with tracheostomy. I got over the feeling as soon as the handover started. My mind became very busy as I sorted out the tasks ahead of me. I was designated the task of looking after Mr L with endarterectomy and tracheostomy.

I was introduced to Mr L by the registered nurse giving the handover report. I noticed his eyes. They were alert but frightened eyes intently scanning the environment. My gut feeling reinforced my observation that he is a very frightened man. Perhaps the scenes in his full view have frightened him. I thought of my own reaction this morning. Initially, I felt taken aback with what I saw happening in the ward. If that was the impact on me then how much more with Mr L who is new to this type of environment. I reached out for his hand to make him feel that I was there with him. I wanted to let him know that he was not alone at this most vulnerable time of his life. I wanted to let him know that I cared. Although I was a little surprised when he wrote on his pad that he knew he could have died the night before, I expect he will inform me about it in due time. Oftentimes patients know what is happening to them.

My instant reaction to what he wrote was to verbalize the old nurse's cliche which goes, 'Oh Mr L, come off it, you will be fine in no time at all' but I knew it would not do him any good. To do so would be underestimating his intelligence. I thought that I owed it to him to be honest since he had trusted me with his feelings. By providing the opportunity to ventilate his fears is in itself a curative measure. My goal initially is to build a trusting relationship between the two of us. Once the trusting relationship is present, I know that our communication will be a reciprocal one. It is only then that I will be able to solicit information from him which will assist me in planning effectively the appropriate intervention for his anxiety.

On reflection, the measures I have provided are basic supportive nursing actions. Helping Mr L to cope with his anxiety, talking to him, giving him the information about his condition and his surroundings, listening, touching, and giving him hope, are nursing tasks which I believe are the essence of nursing tradition and practice. They were behaviours modelled to me by good registered nurses when I was a student; some were taught in theory and often reinforced to me by senior nurses. Patients sometimes compliment me about taking the time to listen to them although I must admit, I still get this funny uneasy feeling when I take time to listen and talk to patients, especially if the Director of Nursing suddenly appears in view. I do not know how she feels about it, but somehow there are registered nurses even now who do not approve of it. If I did not take the time to find out the reason why Mr L is anxious, then how would I know the appropriateness of my intervention. The ghost of the traditional 'appearance of being busy' still haunts me at times because there are still forces in my environment that promote and perpetuate this socialization process.

I believe that my intervention was effective because Mr L was able to communicate his anxiety to me, thereby reducing his fears. I have achieved this because I made the effort and took the time.

I too have gained something from this experience. The environment I am used to, which I often take for granted as a non-threatening one, may not be so to my patients. It is something I have to reckon with all the time.

These sample sets of field notes provide a springboard for the next phase of the reflective process, the processing phase.

Phase three: the processing phase

This is the most reflective and introspective of the three phases: it requires you to go back over your field notes as a whole and derive further meanings from them. At this point you are quite likely to feel overwhelmed by all the data to hand: your field notes, memories, thoughts, and feelings—about yourself as a nurse and others. However, the recorded experiences of others provide a rich source of ideas for the work required. It is expected you will gain various benefits from these experiences and only follow up ideas that are personally significant or useful.

Moustakas (1981) provides a feel for how someone else has come through an experience similar to the one you are facing. Moustakas describes his discovery process in a study of loneliness: his search for self in solitude; an expanding awareness through watching, listening, feeling, discussion; intuitive grasping after patterns of loneliness and further exploration of literature; and finally, creation of a manuscript. He describes the outcomes of the study as being highly significant for himself and many readers.

Glaser & Strauss (1967) believe the source of all significant theorizing is insight, and stress that the theorist should actively cultivate insights up to and beyond the close of a study. In this recommended chapter, the final in their text, they also discuss the value of pitting personal insight against established theory.

Other writers provide more explicit guidance on how to reflect. Boud et al (1985) have developed a model for promoting reflection in learning which is potentially very useful for your purposes. They provide a rationale and context for their model, as well as a discussion on levels of reflectivity. These levels are important in appreciating the scope of the concept. For example the work of Habermas (1971) is referred to as being central to the concept of 'critical reflectivity'.

Further strategies for developing personal theory

Boud and his colleagues then discuss ways of promoting reflection. These are likely to be of particular interest to you and are worthy of careful consideration. They believe three elements are of importance in the reflective process:

* returning to experience
* attending to feelings
* re-evaluating experience (Boud et al 1985).

Further, within the re-evaluating experience stage, they distinguish four aspects that need considering:

* association (relating new data to that known)
* integration (seeking relationships among data)
* validation (determining authenticity of ideas and feelings)
* appropriation (making knowledge one's own).

Assisting one another in the reflective process

Boud et al (1985) further proceed to the outcomes of reflection. For reflection is not an end in itself but a preparation for new experiences—indeed they point out that 'benefits of reflection may be lost if they are not linked to action'. (This facet of reflection will be discussed further.) They also stress the value of assisting one another in the process of reflection. This is useful in terms of working through the suggested strategies yourself, or with a colleague or mentor. Reflection does not occur in isolation, there are many ways we can assist one another.

Walker & Avant (1983) provide another approach to personal theory development that incorporates many of the above features. They describe the process of concept synthesis as one of the most exciting ways of beginning theory building—using clinical experience. Data may also be derived from literature. Essentially the process they propose is one of classifying data into clusters of phenomena or meanings, labelling, and determining if the new concepts fit into existing theory. (The data you will be working with are your field notes.)

Feeling okay about feeling uncertain

It is within this processing phase that you will formulate your personal conceptualization, or theory, of nursing. Possibly you are still uncertain what shape your thinking will take or how to proceed. Such uncertainty reflects the difficulty of the task: the work is intellectually demanding and highly individual.

Developing a structure

Your thoughts will range continually among your field notes, feelings, past and current events, and the task at hand. Your reading should trigger many useful ideas: you may wish to use Boud's et al (1985) model of reflection as a framework for developing your theory, or Walker & Avant's (1983) model, or you may chose to devise your own structure. Diagrammatic representation of your ideas may also be helpful. Discussion of your project with colleagues is encouraged, as is contact with a mentor if you think this may be helpful.

Your personal conceptualization of nursing is likely to include the following elements:

• A brief description of your phase three experience; that is, how you approached the analysis of your field notes.
• Your personal theory of nursing, possibly expressed in terms of key concepts and their relationships; underlying assumptions; and links with existing theory.
• Projected action arising from your observation and reflection.

Comments on sample field notes

First set   These notes were written by an experienced registered nurse after several periods of non-participant observation in a coronary care unit. Several features are worth noting:

• They tend to capture complete incidents, however fleeting.
• The writer's feelings are expressed in each entry.
• The language identification principle, verbatim principle, and concrete principle as proposed by Spradley have been usefully observed in places.
• Some of the features of journals as described by Holly (1984) can be detected. Most entries include journalistic writing: (e) tends towards ethnographic and creative-therapeutic writing, while the most introspective entry is (f) where the writer recognizes the pathos of the scene in her own professional life.

For the purpose of developing a personal theory of nursing from data provided by the field notes, the following remarks are relevant:

• Most entries reveal strong responses in relation to nursing roles and functions;
• Some tentative relationships can be detected with other concepts such as environment (c), person (b), and health (d);

- Underlying assumptions need to be further explored by the writer in the light of her own background and history: these are likely to become increasingly apparent if she becomes an active participant in the situation and hence able to reflect on personal actions as well as thoughts and feelings (speculate how this person may have proceeded to act in entries (c), (d), (e), and (f)—it would be useful if the basis or reasons for feelings were also questioned);
- Exploration of possible links with existing theory that focuses on personal autonomy and humanistic tenets may prove fruitful for this writer, for example, the work of nursing theorists Paterson & Zderad;
- It is interesting to ponder on the projected action that might arise out of this nurse's reflective process (perhaps strategies to define and protect the unique role of the registered nurse).

Second set   These notes differ from the first set in several respects (demonstrating that field notes can take many forms). First, the experienced registered nurse who wrote them was a complete participant in the situation whereas the first registered nurse was a non-participant observer. Second, they were written shortly after the event whereas the first set were written several weeks later. (The further in time field notes are written from the event the more crystallized the meaning of the events tends to become.)

Also, note the highly descriptive and reflective nature of the second set of notes. The writer has incorporated within them both descriptions of events and reflections about those events, whereas the writer of the first sample notes stopped at the point of expressing feelings. (It can be useful to leave each facing page of your field notes blank for further reflective notes.)

Notice that as a result of reflection this registered nurse has clarified the essence of nursing practice as well as the impact of the environment on the patient: critical ideas for developing personal nursing theory.

OUTCOMES OF REFLECTION

Action: a key outcome

Reflection can be viewed as a link between theory and practice. Without action, reflection becomes only an intellectual exercise. Kemmis (1985) describes action as the 'fruit' of reflection and explains how action has meaning and significance in a social world. Hence, in a nursing context, the outcomes of your reflection must be significant not only to you personally, but also to the wider sphere of nursing (and beyond).

So, what are these socially significant fruits resulting from your reflection? The immediate outcome is your personal conceptualisation of nursing. However embryonic or unpolished you may perceive it to be at this stage, it is a significant statement, or set of statements, about your personal practice. Consider the implications of your theory of nursing for your future practice and the practice of others, and the insights that you have gained that motivate you to influence professional practice on a wider scale.

The historical context of action

In discussing the nature of reflection, Kemmis (1985) describes it as being 'historically embedded':

> We do not pause to reflect in a vacuum. We pause to reflect because some issue arises which demands that we stop and take stock or consider before we act. We do so because the situation we are in requires consideration: how we act in it is a matter of some significance. We become aware of ourselves, in some small or large way, as agents of history; we become aware that how we act will influence the course of events, at least for ourselves and usually for others too.

Hence, the outcomes of your reflection need to be understood within their historical context. Your theory of nursing does not exist in a vacuum but in a complex, changing, continuum of time. Consider, for example, the implications of your theory in the light of changes which have occurred within nursing over the past twenty years—and which are projected for the next decade.

The political interests of action

The political nature of reflection is discussed by Kemmis (1985), including the political interests it serves: technical, practical, and emancipatory (or critical).

> Technical reflection aims at problem-solving within a social context of the control of nature; practical reflection aims at wise action in a social context of judgement about what is right; critical reflection aims at recovering and examining the historical and developmental circumstances which shaped our ideas, institutions and modes of action, as a basis for formulating more rational ideas, more just institutions and more fulfilling forms of action.

He suggests that in the most sensitive situations, we need to make a critical response: our aim being 'the conscious and deliberate organization of self reflection as a part of a political struggle towards emancipation from the irrational, unjust, and unfulfilling'. Do you perceive the profession of nursing to be 'irrational, unjust, and unfulfilling'? If so, in what ways? How do the practical consequences of your personal theory address these issues?

Kemmis (1985) goes on to describe reflection as ideological: it is shaped by ideology and in turn shapes ideology.

> In reflection we choose, implicitly or explicitly, what to take for granted and what to treat as problematic in the relationships between our thought and action and the social order we inhabit. In reflection, we have a choice about whether to think and act in conformity with the patterns of communication, decision-making and action in our society, or whether we will intervene at this historical moment on behalf of more rational communication, more just decision-making and more fulfilling human and social action.

These thoughts pose a challenge as you identify the outcomes of your own reflection. Do you wish to act in conformity with, or take for granted, current patterns in the nursing profession? In what ways do you wish to intervene to bring about change?

THE PROMISE OF CRITICAL THEORY FOR NURSING

Nursing traditionally has been swift in grasping schools of thought and theory from other fields that show promise for its own practice. Maslow's hierarchy of human needs is just one classic example. The promise of critical theory has received quickened interest in the nursing literature since the mid 1980s. Thompson (1985) sees nursing at an important stage of 'self-consciousness' in which nurses are looking critically at the traditions that have guided their research. She considers it 'incredibly important' that nurses challenge empiricism, and engage in a process of rational delibera- tion: 'of choosing prejudices that are most productive of knowledge'. Thompson cites Habermas as a post empiricist philosopher who has strug- gled with questions of power and domination in modern society; and proposes that 'the critique of such domination is an important project for intellectuals who are in the process of becoming more self-conscious'. Although this author does not dwell at length on the benefits of the critical paradigm, her paper appears to be one of the first advocating such moves for nursing.

Allen, also writing in 1985, addresses what he considers gaps in the nursing science literature: first, the merits of critical social theory for nursing research; and second, criteria by which researchers may choose between this model and the more widely known empirical and interpretive models of inquiry. He identifies empirical-analytic science as having a fundamental interest in control; interpretive science as having understanding as its key interest; and emancipation as the prime concern of critical science. Bearing these distinctions in mind, he suggests one can immediately sense the significance of critical science for nursing in that one of nursing's central concerns is not imposing values on clients but assisting them make informed choices:

> The advantage of critical social science for nursing and nurses is that it offers an opportunity to shatter the ideological mirror that traps us and our clients in despair and hopelessness. Taken seriously, it forces us to question that status quo at every turn, sifting and winnowing our personal and working lives to enable us to formulate a truly alternative plan.

Perry (1986) is concerned particularly with professional socialization and suggests critical theory adds another dimension to study in this area. Such a perspective enables the researcher to focus on the irrational and oppressive elements which destroy ability to make rational choices, or, the conditions necessary for autonomy. Perry sees critical theory not so much as a body of explanatory theory, but as a form of consciousness which could more accurately be called 'critical theorizing'—an activity she considers has profound implications for nursing education.

Allen et al (1986) propose, in a slightly different vein, a pluralistic vision of research methodology for nursing, incorporating three central philosophical positions, or paradigms: empiricism; phenomenology; and critical social theory. They emphasize that decisions about research methodology need to made in the context of these philosophical positions, and not around disputes about quantitative versus qualitative research. Because critical social theory focuses on meanings and their relationships, it is seen as central to research in nursing education which is a 'primary shaper and conveyor of the meaning of nursing':

> What is essential about experience in nursing education is that students learn to analyze the sources of their own interpretations, to question and resist the predefined meanings we educators encourage them to adopt, and to develop the tools to negotiate a world of nursing in which the twin goals of autonomy and responsibility are achievable. From the point of view of research in nursing education, critical theory reframes the dilemma concerning the value-laden nature of education. Interpretation and values are inseparable, including the interpretation of what it means to be scientific as well as what it means to be a nurse. (Allen et al 1986)

Holter (1988) advocates that critical theory as proposed by Habermas is an increasingly appropriate philosophical and theoretical foundation for the development of nursing theory, instead of the more popular orientations of empiricism and phenomenology. She believes there is a gap between nursing's interest in holism and the philosophies of science that nursing has adopted to date. Unlike some nursing authors, Holter views critical theory as incorporating empirical and phenomenological forms of knowledge and their inquiry processes: 'Critical theory, by synthesizing three processes of inquiry in an essential generic perspective comprehensive enough to apprehend the biological, psychological, and sociological dimensions of the human being, provides a promising alternative for helping to bridge the gap between nursing's emphasis on holism and the knowledge from which nursing theories have been derived' (Holter 1988). Webster (1990), in questioning which traditions in philosophy are most useful for nursing, holds that narrow philosophies of science illuminating only certain physical sciences are a waste of time for nursing, and that nursing needs broad philosophies that reveal differences and relations between sciences. He suggests the work of the Frankfurt School of Philosophy (critical theory) may prove to be quite useful for nursing, but adds that it is difficult work and not for beginners. Webster further suggests that nursing needs richer sources in literature and philosophy than presently exist and that it may be more useful for nursing to support new branches of philosophy, such as that emerging in the caring literature—work that is being largely carried out by nursing scholars.

Interestingly, these authors are writing from the United States, Norway, and New Zealand, indicating the widespread interest by nurses in critical theory. It is nurses in Australia however, who appear to be the world leaders in the development of a critical, reflective, appraisal of nursing practice (Watson 1990). Two important conferences bear evidence to this claim: The National Nursing Theory Conference titled *Theory and practice: an evolving relationship*, held in Adelaide in September 1989; and the conference titled *Embodiment, empowerment, and emancipation: critical theory, reflectivity and nursing practice*, held in Melbourne in January 1990. Papers presented at both gatherings discussed and debated many facets of critical theory and its significance and value to nursing, In Adelaide, Brown presented an argument that critical theory provides a means of bringing nursing theory and practice together through praxis (reflection and action); Master of Nursing students from the South Australian College of Advanced Education, Sturt (now The Flinders University of South Australia) presented personal theories resulting from their own reflective practices within their course; Pearson called for more serious consideration of the critical paradigm and theorizing in action; and Speedy presented a strong argument for nurses to engage in reflective practice and so bridge the gap between theory and practice (Koch 1989). In Melbourne, papers were presented under such titles as 'The promises of critical theory'; 'A critical theory for nursing—exploring possibilities'; 'Critical theory—making it work'; 'Experiencing the deep—what it feels like becoming critical' (Quality Health Forums 1990). Initiatives such as these indicate authors in this country are intent on pursuing the possibilities of contemporary Continental philosophy, particularly critical theory, for nursing. Nursing clearly is a field with a keen ability to draw on philosophy and the history of human ideas for insight into the human condition, and inspiration to pursue its goal of creating a better, and healthier, society. In doing so, nursing in turn contributes to the field of philosophy through its own self-understanding and creation of nursing knowledge, and interpretations of knowledge generated by other fields. Philosophy thus becomes the collective wisdom of humankind, on which all fields can draw and to which all ultimately contribute.

CONCLUSION

The discussion about the promise of critical theory for nursing concludes this guided process of reflection—a process of empowerment and emancipation designed to improve nursing practice. It is suggested the work associated with the process (resulting in a personal conceptualization of nursing) spans at least three months. Time is thus allowed for your thoughts to develop. The purpose of this inquiry has been to provide opportunity for you to advance your thinking about nursing at a conceptual level so that you are better able to act and influence nursing in positive ways at professional, social, and political levels. The inquiry is potentially an important spring-board for further work within your professional life.

The processes and expectations of each of the three phases of reflection described, in briefest terms, are as follows.

Phase one: preparatory

- Negotiation of clinical placement
- Development of observation and reflection schedule
- Anticipation of format of field notes

Phase two: experiential

- Completion of clinical placement
- Collection of field notes
- Closure of field experience and relationships

Phase three: processing

- Report of phase three experience
- Personal theory of nursing developed
- Practical consequences of personal theory identified.

The reflective work you have engaged in has been (and will continue to be) innovative as well as emotionally and intellectually demanding: it is antici-pated the rewards will match these efforts and that you can look forward to a professional life deeply enriched by the fruits of reflection. It is likely your personal theory will continue to occupy you at the most unexpected times, taunting and teasing you for attention and development. You may experi-ence mounting inner pressure to take time out of your work life to pursue the refinement of your ideas, or to extend them within the context of formal study. The outcomes of reflection are so profound, and so personally enlightening, that you are unable to let them go, or to return to former unquestioning ways. Increasingly, you are likely to recognize,and challenge, those political, social, and historical forces which are unjust, irrational, and oppressive in your professional life: together with colleagues and clients, you will wish to create and implement strategies of empowerment that lead to informed choice and fulfilling forms action, for the mutual benefit of all. The significance of how you approach your work and reframe its problems will quickly be noticed by those around you: a ripple effect becomes evident as others seek to understand and emulate your ideas and practices.

By becoming reflective practitioners in this way (whether individually or collectively) we contribute significantly to the development of the discipline of nursing at professional, social and political levels: it is through self-enlightenment that we are able to assist others towards enlightenment; it is through self-empowerment that we are able to assist others towards their empowerment; and it is through the discovery of our undisguised nursing interests that we are able to create knowledge of genuine and ongoing value to nursing—emancipatory knowledge. Central to the creation of knowledge through reflection is open communication and dialogue: this chapter has sought to present an opportunity for personal dialogue with the ideas and practices of reflection; for dialogue between readers of the material on the issues raised; and most importantly, an opportunity for dialogue between individuals, their social world, and its tangled webs of power and illusion. Through direct communication and confrontation with the social world we are able to pull away the potentially suffocating webs and release the constraints that hinder our creation of a more just and enjoyable world of nursing.

Acknowledgements

These ideas have developed from work undertaken in the preparation of the foundation unit of study in the Master of Nursing, The Flinders University of South Australia. Advice from colleagues in the School of Nursing Studies is gratefully acknowledged and thanks are extended to Amy Bartjes for providing the second set of field notes.

REFERENCES

Allen D 1985 Nursing research and social control: alternative models of science that emphasize understanding and emancipation. Image: Journal of Nursing Scholarship XV11(2):58-64
Allen D, Benner P, Diekelmann N 1986 Three paradigms for nursing research: methodological implications. In: Chinn P L (ed) Nursing research methodology: issues and implementation. Aspen, Rockville
Bannister D 1981 Personal construct theory and research method. In: Reason P, Rowan J (eds) Human inquiry: a source book of new paradigm research. John Wiley, Chichester
Boud D, Keogh R, Walker D (eds) 1985 Promoting reflection in learning. In: Reflection: turning experience into learning. Kogan Page, London
Field P, Morse J 1985 Nursing research: the application of qualitative approaches. Aspen, Rockville
Glaser B, Strauss A 1967 The discovery of grounded theory: strategies for qualitative research. Aldine, New York
Habermas J 1971 Knowledge and human interests. Beacon, Boston
Holly M 1984 Keeping a personal-professional journal. Deakin University Press, Geelong
Holter I M 1988 Critical theory: a foundation for the development of nursing theories. Scholarly Inquiry for Nursing Practice: an International Journal 2(3):223-232
Kemmis S 1985 Action research and the politics of reflection. In: Boud D, Keogh R, Walker D (eds) Reflection: turning experience into learning. Kogan Page, London
Koch T (ed) 1989 Theory and practice: an evolving relationship. Monograph, National Nursing Theory Conference,:School of Nursing Studies, Sturt, South Australian College of Advanced Education, Bedford Park
Moustakas C 1981 Heuristic research. In: Reason P, Rowan J (eds) Human inquiry: a source book of new paradigm research. Wiley, Chichester
Perry J 1986 Critical social theory and (nursing) education. Tutor 33:38-45
Quality Health Forums in association with Department of Nursing, La Trobe University 1990 Embodiment empowerment emancipation: critical theory, reflectivity and nursing practice. La Trobe University, Heidelberg

Schatzman L, Strauss A 1973 Field research: strategies for a natural sociology. Prentice-Hall, Englewood Cliffs
Spradley J 1980 Participant observation. Holt, Rinehart & Winston, New York
Thompson J L 1985 Practical discourse in nursing: going beyond empiricism and historicism. Advances in Nursing Science 7(4):59-71
Walker L, Avant K 1983 Strategies for theory construction in nursing. Appleton-Century-Crofts, Norwalk
Watson J 1990 Human science and human care. Two day seminar conducted by School of Nursing Studies, Sturt, South Australian College of Advanced Education, Bedford Park
Webster G A 1990 Nursing and the philosophy of science. In: McCloskey J C, Grace H K (eds) Current issues in nursing, 3rd edn. C V Mosby, St Louis

17. Generating theory from practice: the reflective technique

Joanne Gray   Sally Forsstrom

INTRODUCTION

There is an important role for nurse educators and academics, who can promote the concept of reflective practice and assist student nurses with the development of skills in reflection...What we aim to do is teach nurses how to dialogue with practice; how to 'listen' to practice (Speedy 1989b).

The impetus to write this chapter came from our belief that clinical practice is the primary source of nursing knowledge. As academics involved in teaching student nurses, we felt that the importance of clinical practice was being ignored by academic colleagues and we felt concerned that some colleagues consistently devalued clinical practice as a source of knowledge. The literature (Wald & Leonard 1964, Conant 1967, Speedy 1989a) refers to the theory-practice gap being caused by the fact that academics who developed the theory are divorced from clinical practice. We felt the need to enrich our teaching by returning to the practice area. As academics who practise nursing we felt more able to reduce the perceived theory-practice gap in the minds of our students.

In our lectures we can now demonstrate to the students how our beliefs about nursing have arisen from our practice. By writing this chapter we can demonstrate this belief to all students of nursing as we believe that all nurses who contribute to the discipline are students of that discipline. Few clinicians have been able to contribute to the nursing literature to the same degree as academics largely because of the organization of their work and so we see this chapter as being our way of assisting students of nursing to recognize the primacy of practice and demonstrate how clinical nurses can contribute to nursing knowledge.

Our chapter begins with the discussion of nursing as a discipline and then we look at the practical implications of developing a practice theory of nursing. Exemplars are used from our professional journal to illustrate the reflective technique described by Boud et al (1985) and we also discuss the obstacles that we found in our attempt to develop a practice theory of nursing.

NURSING AS A DISCIPLINE

That there is a unique body of nursing knowledge is still a matter of contention, not only within the Australian community generally, but within the health professions in particular. From our perspective as nursing academics, it is argued that a scholarly evolution is occurring in the development of nursing knowledge, an evolution emanating from a reflection on practice.

Wald & Leonard (1964) predicted a scholarly evolution in nursing knowledge by arguing that 'concepts and hypotheses may come from anywhere, but we are proposing that for the building of nursing practice theory they should come in part from actual nursing experience. Research not geared to improving professional practice may be limited to strictly descriptive propositions, but a practice theory must contain causal hypotheses'.

Benner & Wrubel (1982) argue for the development of nursing knowledge and theory arising from practice. 'Theory and research are generated from the practical world, from the practices of experts in a field. Only from the assumptions and expectations of the clinical practice of experts are questions generated for scientific testing and theory building.'

Whilst one could argue against the need for 'scientific testing', Benner & Wrubel (1982) clearly indicate they believe that theory is generated from practice. They also demonstrate an understanding that practice is much more complex than that which theory alone can define, 'Theory offers what can be made explicit and formalized, but clinical practice is always more complex and presents many more realities than can be captured by theory alone'. It is apparent then, that clinical practice can contribute much more to the development of nursing knowledge than simply in the area of the formation of theories of nursing. Clinical practice is a rich and diverse field and it can provide many opportunities for the nurse to examine the way in which care is provided.

There is much discussion in nursing literature about the need for nursing to develop a unique body of knowledge so that it can become a discipline (Johnson 1968, Carper 1978, Donaldson & Crowley 1978). This discussion requires some examination so that a firm commitment to the need for the development of nursing as a discipline can be made. Armiger (1974) makes her position quite clear in stating that: 'There exists today an unprecedented need for identification of nursing science and practice lest overriding forces in contemporary society lead to disintegration of nursing as a distinct profession'. Donaldson & Crowley (1978) define a discipline in the following manner: 'By definition, however, a discipline is not global; it is characterized by a unique perspective, a distinct way of viewing all phenomena, which ultimately defines the limits and nature of its inquiry'.

When one examines the nature and diversity of nursing practice, it can be seen that there is indeed a distinct body of knowledge embedded within this practice. What needs to occur, therefore, is for nurses to carefully examine their practice and identify what it is that makes nursing such a unique area of knowledge. It is only in the close examination of nursing practice that nursing's uniqueness can be discovered. The time has arrived for the development of theories of nursing that arise from practice. Nurses are becoming increasingly aware of the erosion of their territory in such areas as anaesthetic nursing, midwifery, and intensive care settings. Nurses need to develop nursing theory so that a unique body of knowledge can be identified and a discipline established.

In the past, nurses have 'borrowed' their knowledge from other disciplines such as education and sociology. Wald & Leonard (1974) recognize this borrowing from other disciplines and have stated that nurses have 'consulted with social scientists...as a result, nursing problems are being rephrased as social science questions rather than questions of practice, and nurses are studying nurses. As Henderson (1964) so cogently put it, 'no other discipline studies the workers rather than the work'. Nursing authors such as Beckstrand (1978), have supported this borrowing by suggesting that a separate practice theory for nursing is not necessary, as other disciplines, such as science, have already provided guidelines for nursing practice, 'therefore, it would appear that there is no need for a practice theory distinct from scientific or ethical theory'. Thankfully, however, not all nursing authors take this view. Tinkle & Beaton (1983) find abhorrent this notion of borrowing from other disciplines and feel that this 'may not only retard the development of nursing theory, but will almost certainly dilute its uniqueness as well'.

The role that nurses can play in developing a theory has been undervalued by some nursing authors. Clarke (1986) is one author in particular who devalues the knowledge and skills that the nurse has developed '...practising nurses who carry out routine acts are content with one particular kind of explanation of those acts and see little or no need for more elaborate explanations. It is, of course, also less taxing intellectually to explain acts in terms of routine'. This statement of hers indicates that she feels nurses do not think about the skills that they are utilizing in providing patient care, rather they perform the skills as a matter of routine. It needs to be acknowledged that the skills performed by nurses are done with thought and these skills are part of that knowledge that is unique to nursing. This unique knowledge needs to be captured and explored in the development of a theory of nursing. The attitude that is demonstrated by Clarke is not one that is commensurate with the determination of the need for a discipline of nursing to be developed. It is indeed unfortunate for disciplinary development that such attitudes exist within nursing. With the continued determination and work of nurses toward the development of a unique body of knowledge for nursing, we hope that this type of attitude will change to one of support and acknowledgement of nursing as an important discipline.

The initial discussion of the need for the development of a practice theory began in 1964 by Wald & Leonard, and the fact that this discussion is still continuing today indicates that much more development is required. We would support the work of nurses such as Benner (1984) who define the unique knowledge of nursing and the unique contribution of the nurse to the health care system. Donaldson & Crowley (1978) also take on a positive view of nursing as a discipline and state that it: 'is important to recognize that a discipline emerges as a result of creative thinking related to significant issues. Because of the vital significance of nursing's perspective, its concern with human health and well-being, and its growth through research and scholarly work, nursing will gain full acceptance in time'.

For the development of a body of knowledge representing the unique perspective of nursing the most appropriate research method is the practice-research-theory-research-practice model (Meleis 1985), which states that the development of knowledge must be determined by the issues that arise in practice. As Speedy (1989a) argues: 'As long as nursing theories are too vague and abstract to apply to practice they have little potential to "inform" practice. This functions to create separatism between theorist and practitioner'.

We recognize the extreme importance of practice theory in the development of the discipline of nursing and as academics we decided to return to the practice field on a regular basis to attempt to develop a practice theory. The clinical practice day was incorporated into our academic role as faculty practice, a term used most commonly in the literature for field experience by academics (Lambert & Lambert 1988). The aim of our faculty practice was to be able to develop a practice theory of nursing that did indeed arise from the clinical setting and did not occur by merely reading and developing a theory from our desks.

DEVELOPING A PRACTICE THEORY

How does the practising nurse describe nursing knowledge and place it within a theoretical context? This can be a perplexing question and one that is difficult to answer. This chapter describes our first attempt at working toward a practice theory of nursing by commencing reflective practice.

We were introduced to the technique of reflective practice as part of our study as students in the Master of Nursing degree at the South Australian College of Advanced Education. We found that Boud et al (1985) provide a useful model for reflecting on one's own practice and then developing, from this reflection, a theory. Prior to undertaking faculty practice we determined our belief that the development of nursing theory was essential to enable nursing to become a discipline, and that this theory should arise from practice.

The starting point

The starting point for us was to practise in an area of choice and allow for time to reflect on this practice. As academics teaching in an undergraduate nursing course in a rural university our access to the clinical area was limited. Therefore a first step to developing a practice theory was to negotiate a practice day in an area of our choice. There are a number of faculty practice models described in the literature (Stainton et al 1989) and after examination of these, we selected a practice day per week, as this was best suited to our personal and professional commitments. Our teaching load was divided between internal and external students over the whole semester and therefore it was not possible to plan a block commitment to clinical practice without reorganizing our teaching commitments. Since the practice day would be in addition to our full-time teaching duties, we believed that such a day, in an area of our special interest, would maximize teaching gains from the practice, as well as assist in the main aim of developing theory from practice to advance the discipline of nursing.

We were supported in our negotiation of a practice day by the university and hospital administration, and the nurses in the particular clinical area of our choice. As a midwife, one of the authors negotiated to work in the midwifery unit, to reflect on her practice as a midwife. The other author negotiated to work in an acute medical unit as her practice interests centred on communication between the nurse and the client. The practice day was negotiated three months before the implementation of faculty practice to allow for a thorough consideration of any legal, industrial, and ethical issues by faculty and service staff.

In considering how theory would be generated from practice, we felt it was important to practise in an area of interest, and in an area where we had some level of clinical expertise. This is a point of debate, as some argue that a novice can generate theoretical dialogue from practice (Perry & Moss 1988), while Benner (1984) argues for theory development by expert practitioners. We adopted Benner's view as we considered clinical expertise important to the theoretical development of a practice model. However, in our recommedations for nursing education, we acknowledge that the novice student nurse can be introduced to the process of theory development through reflection on practice providing the educators are practised in this technique. We negotiated to work in a clinical area of choice in order to be able to develop sufficient expertise in our practice to facilitate self reflection. Benner (1984) describes the movement of a practitioner from novice to expert with the development of clinical expertise. The characteristics of a novice might make reflection difficult in that: 'The rule-governed behavior typical of the novice is extremely limited and inflexible. The heart of the difficulty lies in the fact that since novices have no experience of the situation they face, they must be given rules to guide their performance'. Benner goes on to describe novices as being not only those nursing students who enter a clinical area for the first time, but also any nurses who enter a clinical area where they are in a position of having limited or no experience with the client population.

It can be seen, then, that even an experienced registered nurse, who enters an unfamiliar clinical area, may not be able to take on the task of reflection on practice and the subsequent development of a theory of nursing. Therefore the selection of a clinical area of practice was viewed as an important first step in developing a sound technique of reflection on practice.

Reflection

Boud et al (1985) acknowledge that reflection can occur by describing thoughts in a diary or by a debriefing or group discussion process. They also describe several elements that need to be involved in this process. They assert that reflection 'is pursual with intent' and 'is not idle meandering or day-dreaming, but purposive activity directed towards a goal'.

Our goal was to reflect on our practice with a view to not only describing the events of the day, but uncovering the knowledge embedded in practice (Benner 1984). We planned to keep a journal to be recorded daily, as soon as possible after the clinical experience. In the first few days we encountered a major obstacle to reflective practice, that being the enormous volume of experience that could be recorded in relation to just one practice day. We quickly had to refine our journalling technique to focus on just one event, as the time required to write up the experiences of the whole day meant that we did not ever complete our journal. The process of journalling may sound simple and easy to execute, but at times it was extremely difficult. Mostly the incidents recorded where identified because there was an affective component. This may be related to feelings of our own personal inadequacy to cope with the demands of the situation. Alone, it was emotionally painful to journal events that were largely self-critical. For example, if a treatment was omitted or an observation not recorded, self-reflection focused on the shame of it all and it was difficult to proceed further at the time.

Recollection of salient events

Boud et al (1985) describe a number of stages in the process of reflection that lead to the development of theory, and on further to the ultimate goal of theory development. These stages need to be passed through. The first is that of returning to the experience. Boud et al describe this stage as a 'recollection of the salient events'. This can occur during the process of writing about the experience. The salient events within that practice situation come to mind and these are then described. Recollection of the salient events can occur during the process of writing about the experience. It is important to write up the events as soon as possible to recapture the main features. Sometimes the writing process allows the events to be seen more clearly. An example is provided:

Exemplar 1: Sally. On the medical ward there were often people experiencing pain associated with a terminal illness. While making a journal entry, I identified that one Registered Nurse (RN) resisted administering prescribed pain relieving medication stating: 'The morphine was ordered for her cough. I don't hear her coughing.' The RN did not want the woman to receive her pain relieving medication.

This exemplar was discussed at a later date with the palliative care consultant who agreed that pain control for the terminally ill was often poorly managed in the acute care settings and at home. The analgesic protocol that has been developed in this region was not followed, resulting in patients experiencing pain. The question arose: Is the reluctance related to a fear of hurrying death, or a fear of facilitating addiction in the patient? It was a difficult question to answer, and because the nurses were unable to adequately manage the pain and death of a patient, the patient died in pain. It was not until I returned to this event and reflected upon it, that I was able to identify that pain control was an issue on this ward. Having identified this, I was sensitized to the issue on later practice days.

Attending to one's own feelings

The next stage is the need to attend to one's feelings. To merely describe the events does not do justice to the practitioner. Boud et al (1985) describe two aspects of this stage—those of utilizing positive feelings and removing obstructive feelings. They feel that this then allows the practitioner to consider the events rationally and with good feeling, and to be aware that these feelings are important and can affect the reflective process. Boud et al (1985) describe how practitioners can raise a barrier to their reflection by being fixed within one interpretation and that 'when this occurs, the feelings in question need to be discharged or transformed in a way that enables us to regain our flexibility and creativity in responding to the current situation'.

This stage is of particular importance when the nurse practitioner works in any area that is well known. The nurse may automatically take on feelings that are associated with prior events and these will form a barrier to a deeper reflection on their practice. Thus, obstructive feelings need to be removed and positive feelings need to be recognized, explored, and enjoyed. This stage would normally occur at the time of returning to the experience when writing up field notes.

In exemplar one, a destructive feeling would be to make judgements about the action of the nurse reluctant to administer analgesia. Sitting in judgement on the behaviour of others is very obstructive to reflection on practice as the perspective of the practitioners is not explored. A judgemental approach would deflect attention away from the goal of being able to understand the perspective of the nurse, and develop adequate explanatory notes that would, on reflection, lead to an understanding of the behaviour. A positive feeling associated with this incident was that the other nurses were able to argue with the nurse that pain control was a priority need for the patient, despite the nurse's fears of administering analgesia.

The implementation of our faculty practice identified a very powerful obstacle to reflection, that being the need for approval from nursing peers. As nurse academics we were often motivated in our behaviour by an acceptance need; a need to be accepted by the clinical registered nurses, a need to be perceived as a real nurse, not an armchair nurse who had forgotten the challenges and the joys of clinical nursing. When personal illness occurred, there was a felt need to phone the Nursing Unit Manager and explain clearly the reason for illness, even though this was not required or expected. It seemed very important to have the approval of others for our absence. An obstacle to taking 15 minutes in the middle of the day to record a journal entry was the need of the practising academic to be accepted as a 'real' nurse by the clinical staff, and 'real' nurses rarely have the time to reflect and write on their practice during the shift. Clinical nurses welcomed us, as the faculty practice arrangement was organized so that faculty were at all times in the employ of the university, and therefore could not be included in the hospital staffing figures. This meant that we were always extra to normal staffing. This contributed to the success of faculty practice because all nurses on our shift had a lighter workload. It might be expected, then, that since we also had a lighter than normal load, we could find more time for journalling during the shift. In practice this did not occur because of the emotional need of us both to be accepted by the clinical nurses as action oriented, that is practice oriented, despite our main goal of practice being theory construction.

In our clinical experience the acceptance need seems to be very high in clinical nurses. For clinical nurses to be involved in journalling and reflection we would argue that this activity would have to be perceived by the majority as an activity of value in a busy day, otherwise the negative feelings evoked by the activity would lead to its early demise.

Re-evaluating the experience

The third stage described by Boud et al (1985) is that of re-evaluating experience. This is where the analysis of the field notes begins. This stage is further divided into the four elements of association, integration, validation, and appropriation (Boud et al 1985).

Association 'is the connecting of the ideas and feelings which are part of the original experience and those which have occurred during reflection with existing knowledge and attitudes' (Boud et al 1985). This stage allows the reflective practitioner to compare old attitudes to new and judge whether the old are still appropriate. In this way, old attitudes can be discarded if warranted and the new ones can be substituted. An example of this occurred during Joanne's clinical practice.

Exemplar 2: Joanne. During the time that I spent in labour wards, I noticed how often it was the accoucheur who announced the sex of the newborn child to the parents rather than the parents being able to look and see for themselves what sex their new baby was. I had noticed this previously, but had never thought that there was a problem with the way that this occurred. During my reflective process, I re-examined this and determined that it was yet another small way in which nurses and doctors took control from the clients.

Boud et al (1985) describe how the process of association can occur with the group process of brainstorming as this allows for new connections of ideas and thoughts. We were not able to form a discussion group during our three month faculty practice, though we made several attempts to do so. In future planning for reflective practice we would argue for the formation of a discussion group as a priority. A discussion group is essential to the process of association to allow for a thorough examination of the comparison between old attitudes and new.

Exemplar 3: Sally. I had returned from a conference on reflective practice and was feeling elated by the recounting of personal experiences of reflective practice. I was sharing an exemplar with a RN, who listened attentively, and then said, 'So what? The experience assisted the practitioner to understand individual practice in an encounter with a patient, but it has no relevance to me'.

This exemplar clarified an important function of a reference group in association: Do the ideas and feelings raised in the reflective practice have any relevance for the profession as a whole? In comparing old attitudes to new, is the process so individual that it has little meaning for others? A discussion group is essential to keep on target with the aims of reflective practice: to generate new understandings that will have meaning for the profession, not just the individual.

In the absence of a formalized discussion group, we re-evaluated our experience on an ad hoc basis, during coffee breaks, and in short meetings of about 15 minutes. We included other nurse academics, and clinical nurses in these discussions. It is only now in writing this chapter that we have commenced a determined re-evaluation. As six months have passed since our first exemplars, the re-evaluation is proving much more difficult with the passage of time. Integration is the next step after association. Boud et al (1985) state that 'association brings together ideas and feelings in an almost indiscriminate manner; integration begins the process of discrimination'. They further identify two stages in integration, the first being that of 'seeking the nature of the relationships that have been observed through association' and the second is 'drawing conclusions and arriving at insights into the material which we are processing'. In exemplar two, the relationship between the incident described and the nature of how health professionals try to 'control' their clients can be identified and discussed more thoroughly and a conclusion can be made as to whether a relationship does exist and if this is relevant to our practice as nurses. Further examples of association are given under the heading 'Exemplars'.

Exemplars

We have provided a number of exemplars from our clinical practice to show how we used the reflective technique. These exemplars show a personal perspective of our nursing practice and the steps, as described by Boud et al (1985), are used in the explanation of these exemplars.

Exemplar 4: Joanne—maternity unit

Recollection of salient events. Today I was allocated to work in the labour ward. As we came on duty, a mother was in the final stages of labour and the midwife and I assisted her into a squatting position on the bed to facilitate the crowning of the baby's head. Also present was her husband and the doctor who was a resident undertaking the Diploma in Obstetrics and Gynaecology course. The setting was quiet and peaceful as it was early morning and there was a great feeling of expectation and excitement.

As the head crowned, the resident doctor felt the need to perform an episiotomy. She began to cut the perineum and the mother cried out in pain asking what was happening. The doctor continued to cut the perineum, explaining that the baby needed more room and that she was 'sorry'. The mother was obviously feeling a great deal of pain as the noises she made during this procedure of an episiotomy were of quite a different sound to the guttural noises of pushing. The baby was soon delivered much to the parents' joy.

On reflection, the critical part of this incident to me was that the doctor intervened in the delivery in such a manner as to cause the mother pain and anxiety, as the mother did not know what was happening, only that it hurt. There also seemed little point in the doctor saying 'sorry' as she continued to cut the perineum without the use of local anaesthesia. I realized the uselessness of the word 'sorry' when, in fact, the doctor had no intention of stopping what she was doing or of trying to make the procedure less painful.

When returning to this experience, I find that the key element in terms of a theory of nursing is in the nature of the communication. What we say to people in our care and how we say it is of great importance to how we are perceived by the patients. Even though the word 'sorry' is usually sympathetic, it obviously had little meaning to the mother at that time. As nurses, there is a need then to be very careful of what we say and to ensure that our words and actions are congruent in meaning, not conflicting in meaning.

Attending to one's own feelings. The feelings that I had at the time were mixed. I recognized a frustration at the need for the doctor to perform an episiotomy, when one was not clearly indicated or necessary. I felt anger at the doctor's empty words and their lack of meaning, and I felt frustration and impotence as a midwife that I was unable to assist the mother who was feeling this pain.

Re-evaluating the experience—Association. On later reflection on this incident, I remembered an incident that occurred when I was a second year nursing student. I was assisting a young man who had suffered burns to his arm with removing his dressings in the bathtub. As I peeled them off gently, he was obviously feeling some pain and I remember saying 'I'm sorry', but of course I continued to remove the dressings. He looked at me and asked why was I saying sorry when we both knew that the dressings had to be removed and that despite prior analgesia, it was going to hurt him. I am now able to relate this prior event to the one described above and recognize more clearly that communication is the key element here. Even though in both situations, the communication was supposed to be caring, that was not the perception of the client at the receiving end.

Integration. As I was able to see that this experience was not a new one to me, and identify why the interactions were important, I wondered at the nature and importance of communication to people in my care. I have realized that there is little purpose in expressing a sentiment such as 'I'm sorry' when it is going to have little or no meaning. I have also realized that to communicate effectively to patients, means to communicate honestly. In examining my philosophy of nursing as meaning caring, I can see that a caring attitude will not be communicated unless honesty is also communicated.

Exemplar 5: Joanne—maternity unit

Recollection of salient events. Following delivery of the baby, there was much excitement and exclaiming over the mother as she was a primigravida who had arrived in well established labour and had delivered in a semi-squatting position within one hour of arrival to the labour ward. However, the condition of the baby began to deteriorate slowly and so it was necessary to transfer him to the special care nursery. Mother was quickly showered and organised so that she could be with her baby.

When I could leave the labour ward, I went to the nursery to see the parents and to check on the condition of the baby. As I walked into the nursery, the mother was standing by the incubator staring in at her baby. The baby was attached to a number of monitors and was receiving oxygen therapy and had a perspex head box in place. I walked over to the mother and enquired as to her baby's condition. She explained what had happened and I then asked her how much the baby weighed. She began to tell me when the midwife who was working in the special care nursery that day, called out the weight of the baby from across the room. The midwife then came over and proceeded to tell me what was happening with the baby. The mother was left standing there.

On reflection on this incident, I felt very angry that the mother was put in a position where she must have felt that her baby had become, not her own, but the possession of the nursery. She no doubt was already feeling very isolated from her child due to the equipment, and to be further pushed into the background by the midwife ignoring her ability to tell me about her baby, must have been upsetting and frustrating for the mother. We need to be more careful in situations like this and refrain from asserting our own 'rights' and knowledge about the patient's situation. Again, this incident was important in terms of communication but it also caused me to examine the nature of the relationship that we establish with our patients. Perhaps we do not give the patient any autonomy, but automatically assume the right of control over them in our relationship with them. On examination of other incidents it would seem that often, as nurses, we are too busy exerting our control over the patient to allow the patient to establish their own control over their condition. We talk about the need for patients to care for their own health, but as soon as they are in a position where they are vulnerable, nurses often have an unconscious need to automatically assume total responsibility for their care.

Attending to one's own feelings. My immediate feeling was anger. I felt very annoyed that the midwife had interfered in my communication with the mother as I was attempting to give her the feeling that she was in control here. I then recognized a frustration at my inability, again, to intervene on behalf of the mother and restore the information-giving role to the mother. I have recognized previous situations where other nurses have disturbed my communication with a patient and taken control away from them, and I have felt powerless to intervene.

Re-evaluating the experience—associaton. It was easy to associate this experience with many others. Such experiences have occurred many times before. An example that came to my mind immediately is the occasion on which I was sponging a patient and talking to her and another nurse entered the room to assist me and began a conversation with me that excluded the patient. Another example is a situation where I had established good communication with a mother in labour and felt that another midwife who had not appreciated this took over the situation.

Integration. I would feel that there are still two issues here. One is my feeling of the need to assert myself in these situations where I let my relationship with the patient go in deference to another nurse, and the other closely related issue is that of the patient having control over their own situation.

Exemplar 6: Sally—medical unit

Recollection of salient events. It was early morning, just after the handover report from the night staff. Mrs B. was fifty years old with insulin dependent diabetes mellitus admitted two days ago for evaluation of a peripheral ulcer.

Mrs B. was one of four patients allocated to me during handover. As I introduced myself, I asked Mrs B. if she had her glucometer with her so that she could test her capillary blood glucose before preparing and administering her regular mane insulin. Mrs B. responded that the nurses did everything for her in hospital.

This incident was recorded in my journal because I immediately recognized a frequently recurring theme for people in hospital: a person independently monitoring their capillary blood glucose at home, and administering subcutaneous insulin each morning has this responsibility for self-care taken from them on admission to hospital.

Attending to one's feelings. I felt very angry that the person was robbed of their independence by the nursing staff. It was also frustrating because I knew it was the policy of the unit that people with diabetes should remain in charge of their self-monitoring and self-injection of insulin. Often this situation occurs in relation to inadequate staffing: it seems a more efficient use of the nurse's time to do everything for the patient than to assist the patient in self-care. In this particular exemplar, however, the opposite seemed to apply. By taking over an activity that the patient was able to perform unattended the nurse created an increase in nursing activity. A positive feeling arising from the situation was that because I recognized what was happening I was able to make a difference to the patient. The patient was encouraged to regain self-care, instead of relinquishing responsibility for care to the nursing staff. It is a very positive feeling to experience caring as empowering, instead of disempowering.

Re-evaluating the experience—association. This situation has occurred many times in my experience as a nurse. It does not relate only to the particular instance of self care for people with diabetes, but also to all matters of self care. In the 1970s when I first started nursing, it was mooted that patients would continue to self-administer their medication in hospital, just as they do at home. It was planned in one hospital to have a locked medication drawer at each bedside, to facilitate self-administration of prescribed medications. This has not yet occurred in 1990, twenty years later.

As noted in exemplar five, the issue of control is a powerful concept in nursing. Do nurses care for clients in an unequal power relationship? In exemplar six, by disempowering the patient, the nurse blocked the patient's preparation for return to the community. In the community the patient would be expected to be in charge of self care activities. Removing this responsibility in hospital cannot be helpful in preparing the patient for self-care on discharge.

Integration. In this exemplar the power relationship between a nurse and a patient is important to explore. Does the nurse disempower the patient by taking over self-care activities? Or is this action the only way the nurse can control the working environment? Does the nurse disempower the patient because the nurse has no power in deciding minimum staffing levels? It is not common on this medical unit for the nursing staff to be able to refuse admission of a patient in order to maintain adequate staffing for the needs of the inpatients already admitted. Would nurses be able to empower patients in controlling their lives if the nurses felt empowered to control their own working environment?

Validation and appropriation

We felt that we did not progress beyond these first two stages of association and integration and thus the stages of validation and appropriation have not yet occurred. Boud et al (1985) describe validation as a process which involves 'testing for internal consistency between our new appreciations and our existing knowledge and beliefs, for consistency between these and parallel data from others and trying out our new perceptions in new situations'.

They go on to describe how this can occur through 'rehearsal' or 'guided imagery'. We felt that for nursing, the best way to validate new knowledge and attitudes would be to take these back into the clinical area and test them. Appropriation, being the 'taking on' of this new knowledge in a personal way and making it our own, would also best occur in the clinical setting.

Obstacles to re-evaluation

Boud et al (1985) acknowledge that the practitioner may not always wish to reflect on one experience to the same degree as another, and therefore recognize that the practitioner's intent may influence the development of these elements. Our intent here was to reflect on our practice and to re-evaluate the experience in an attempt to formulate a practice theory of nursing. Having only reached the stages of association and integration, we were obviously not ready to begin to formulate a practice theory of nursing. We have identified a number of reasons for this.

The major gain of our experience of faculty practice was our increased understanding of the complexity of the task at hand. In our four months of practice one day per week we did reach the stage of feeling comfortable in the practice setting and so we could begin to reflect on the experience. We also felt that we had increased our understanding of the factors that influence our practice, as has been shown in the preceding exemplars.

The model provided by Boud et al (1985), while extremely useful in the necessary development of key concepts to form a theory, was unable to be fully developed and utilized due to several obstacles. While they provide clear guidelines on how to analyze the experience so that a useful application of the knowledge gained is made, it must be realized by the practitioner that the process of reflection is a lengthy and involved one, and as Boud et al emphasize 'while reflection is itself an experience it is not, of course, an end in itself' (1985).

The factors which would overcome the major obstacles which we have identified are as follows:

A longer time commitment

As Benner (1984) observed, it takes experience to develop expertise in nursing: 'experience, as the word is used here, does not refer to the mere passage of time or longevity. Rather, it is the refinement of preconceived notions and theory through encounters with many actual practical situations that add nuances or shades of differences to theory' (p. 36). Our practice supports this view of Benner's. A longer time period is required to actively interact with practical situations; experience is essential to appreciate the multitudinous factors operating in a given patient care context, and to engage in an analysis of this context. We felt that the time we had in the clinical area was not of sufficient length to enable us to fully utilize the reflective technique and develop a practice theory.

Discussion group

From our experience we would highly recommend a discussion group to engage in this stage of the reflection process. It is difficult to engage in a dialogue with one's journal, as we are a part of the events described. The view of others is helpful to explore the factors in operation in a given setting. In addition, a discussion group would provide that extra motivation to actually complete the journal. We found at the end of a tiring shift, it was easy to write a brief note, and think 'I'll write more detailed notes tomorrow'.

It was difficult to engage in reflection because we were at all times challenging our own practice and questioning 'why?'. For the exhausted practitioner this is an unwanted burden.

Practitioners may ask, 'Exhausted? After one shift?' We found that we were exhausted as our practice was above our normal teaching load. The motivation to write would have been greatly increased by a weekly meeting with peers, faculty and clinical staff, to discuss a journal entry in relation to the development of nursing theory.

Therefore, the practitioner, while realizing more clearly the intent of the reflective process, i.e. to provide a theory from practice that can, in turn, be utilized in practice, must also be aware of the obstacles to this process (Dickoff et al 1968).

RECOMMENDATIONS

Following from our experience with the reflective technique, we make several recommendations.

Nurse academics

To be leaders in the development of the discipline of nursing by developing a practice theory, it is mandatory for nurse academics to be involved in reflective practice. Since this theorizing is a scholarly activity one would argue that a nurse academic engaging in faculty practice with the aim of reflecting on practice must have the support of other faculty. To allow for the time involved in reflection, teaching loads must be allocated with consideration for the amount of time required to make practice reflective. After one semester with full teaching loads, one faculty practice day per week for reflective practice, and two formal research projects we were feeling exhausted by the time commitment and could not continue to engage in reflective practice without a reduction in teaching loads.

Practising nurses

The main implication for practitioners is that theory generation will not just happen. To begin reflecting on practice requires a time commitment on a regular basis over an extended period of time. The process requires not only self-discipline to complete a journal each shift or once a week, but a consideration of organizational factors. To reflect on practice one needs to write a personal journal and discuss the outcome of reflections. If there is not a formal meeting time established, then clinical nurses would need to establish a regular meeting in their off-duty time. Since we were not able to initiate a meeting in our workplace when engaged in clinical practice of one day a week, we would recommend setting up a group and a meeting time and place as a first priority.

Nursing administration

If clinical nurses are to be encouraged to contribute to the development of nursing as a discipline it is important that the activity of reflective practice is seen as an activity that forms part of paid nursing care. Clinical nurses will find it difficult to engage in the practice if it is seen as an activity to perform in one's recreation time, after the real nursing (that being nursing service), is completed.

Inservice educators would appear to have an essential role in promoting reflective practice. Inservice teaching sessions could be planned in paid time, either regular one hour discussion groups to discuss an exemplar in the shift overlap, or a focus for study on inservice education days.

As previously discussed, we adopt the view of Benner (1984) that the nurse needs to have clinical expertise in an area in order to be able to develop a practice theory. The implication here for nursing administration is that Registered Nurses must be able to remain in a clinical area for long enough periods of time to enable them to gain expertise in that area.

Nursing education

For undergraduate nurses to be involved in reflective practice requires an involvement at all stages of the nursing course. If students are to be encouraged to reflect on practice with the aim of developing a practice theory, they will require the time commitment from the teachers who plan their course. All teaching situations would require a commitment to this form of learning about the discipline: from the classroom to the clinical area. We predict that it would be very difficult for a teacher to incorporate reflective practice as a strategy in the implementation of a curriculum without tried skills in the activity of reflective practice.

CONCLUSION

We remain committed to our belief in the primacy of practice as the source of nursing knowledge. It can be seen from our personal experiences of reflective practice that this technique provides a rich source of data for nurses wishing to contribute to the theoretical development of the discipline. We felt that it was important to describe the practical implications of reflective practice and provide some guidelines for the implementation of this technique into the practice of clinical nurses. We would like to see that all practitioners of nursing are able to gain encouragement from sharing in our experiences of reflective practice. This chapter has demonstrated that all clinical nurses are able to theorize given a supportive work environment. This chapter has also demonstrated the diversity and richness of the clinical area as a source of unique nursing knowledge.

Our goal to develop a practice theory of nursing has not been achieved in one semester of activity. This chapter has been a means of recording our experience of the reflective technique. Our experience supports the effectiveness of the technique developed by Boud et al (1985) in focusing practice experiences for knowledge development even though the technique was completed in part only. The technique allows for obstacles to the development of the disciplines to be clearly identified. Writing this chapter allows for the complexity of theorizing to be acknowledged: an ongoing activity requiring a time commitment of years, not months.

Writing of our experiences is an effective means of sharing with other nurses our experience of implementing the reflective technique. It is hoped that this sharing will help other nurses in the practice setting to structure their working environment so that a commitment to the development of a practice theory of nursing is established. The diversity and richness of experience in the clinical setting must be analyzed by the practitioners using a reflective technique to promote the disciplinary development of nursing. By implementing an effective technique such as that developed by Boud et al all nurses in a practice setting can contribute to the development of the discipline and patient care will then reflect caring in practice. The resulting growth of a discipline of nursing will lead to changes in patient care that reflect the experience and the theorizing of the practitioner.

REFERENCES

Armiger B 1974 Scholarship in nursing. Nursing Outlook 22:160-164

Beckstrand J 1978 The notion of a practice theory and the relationship of scientific and ethical knowledge to practice. Research in Nursing and Health 1:131-136

Benner P 1984 From novice to expert: excellence and power in clinical nursing practice. Addison-Wesley, Menlo Park

Benner P, Wrubel J 1982 Skilled clinical knowledge: the value of perceptual awareness, part 2. Journal of Nursing Administration (June:) 28-33

Boud D, Keogh R, Walker D 1985 Reflection: turning experience into learning. Keagan Page, London

Carper B A 1978 Fundamental patterns of knowing in nursing. Advances in Nursing Science 1(1):13-24

Clarke M 1986 Action and reflection: practice and theory in nursing. Journal of Advanced Nursing 11(1):3-11

Conant L 1967 Closing the theory-practice gap. Nursing Outlook 15 (11):37-39

Dickoff J, James P, Wiedenbach E 1968 Theory in a practice discipline Part II: practice oriented research. Nursing Research 17(6):545-554

Donaldson S K, Crowley D M 1978 The discipline of nursing. Nursing Outlook 26(2):113-120

Henderson V (1964) The nature of nursing. American Journal of Nursing 64:62-65

Johnson D E 1968 Theory in nursing: borrowed and unique. Nursing Research 17(3):206-209

Lambert C E, Lambert V A 1988 A review and synthesis of the research on role conflict and its impact on nurses involved in faculty practice programmes. Journal of Nursing Education 27(2):54-60

Meleis A 1985 Theoretical nursing: development and progress. Lippincott, Philadelphia

Perry J, Moss C 1988 Generating alternatives in nursing: turning curriculum into a living process. Australian Journal of Advanced Nursing 6 (2):35-40

Speedy S 1989a Theory-practice debate: setting the scene. The Australian Journal of Advanced Nursing 6(3):12-19

Speedy S 1989b Nursing theory and practice: risks and rewards. In: Koch T (ed) Theory and practice—an evolving relationship. Monograph: National Nursing Theory Conference. School of Nursing Studies, Sturt, South Australian College of Advanced Education, Bedford Park

Stainton M C, Rankin J A, Calkin J D 1989 The development of a practising nursing faculty. Journal of Advanced Nursing 14(1):20-26

Tinkle M, Beaton J 1983 Toward a new view of science: implications for nursing research. Advances in Nursing Science 5 (2):27-36

Wald, F S, Leonard, R C 1964 Toward a development of nursing practice theory. Nursing Research 13 (4):309-313

18. Exploring reflection: knowing and constructing practice

Helen Cox   Pat Hickson   Bev Taylor

Maree's journal, 14 May 1989

What a day. My feet are so sore! I feel like I've run non stop all day. Day stays in a ward like mine increase the pace so much. This place is just like a production line: they come in, hello, clothes off, prep, premed, off you go...next!

Bloody Mr Jones, 'Surgeon Most High', marched in in the middle of handover; ripped off all the dressings, upset everyone and marched out. God knows if there was an order change. Then along came Dave Rogers; he's such a caring Doctor, but he still wants my time. Everyone wants my time! That's the lot of a charge nurse I suppose.

I keep thinking when is there going to be time for Robyn? Ah Robyn! The biopsy report came back today. She hasn't got a clue—or has she? She's so quiet, but sometimes I get the sense that she is almost about to ask me a question but can't. I think she knows.

Mr Jones read the report and grunted, went in to her just when I was caught up and couldn't go with him, I've got no idea what he told her; I'm going to have to make my way really carefully with her now.

Why do I feel so intimidated by Mr Jones? I know his footsteps, I just have to hear him coming and I start to feel tense.

Why does someone like Robyn get so little of our time? We put her in a single room, why? Are we looking after her interests? Is it because we are already shutting her away? Have we given up on her? Isn't it funny how not curing is somehow failing.

I've just read over what I've written—'When is there going to be time for Robyn?' When will there ever be time unless I create it? Am I avoiding her? I will watch out for that tomorrow!

Isn't it interesting how nurses who are engaged in the world of everyday practice are theorizers of their own practice. It seems that nursing is never atheoretical.

The intent of this chapter is to explore the theoretical nature of practice through the perspective of a nurse's journal within a broad discussion of the nature of reflective practice.

Nursing is careful people-orientated work, which is energised by knowledge. The combination of work for practical purposes with knowledge for understanding the nature of nursing, create for nursing the label of 'practice discipline'. Nursing as a practice discipline conveys the idea that nursing is concerned with the pursuit of knowledge for practical purposes. The practice of nursing relates to professional issues of how, when, why, and with whom nursing is actualized.

The discipline of nursing can be conveyed through theory which depicts in words the nature of the phenomena constituting the concerns of nursing. Donaldson & Crowley (1978) define a discipline as a 'unique perspective, a distinct way of viewing all phenomena, which ultimately defines the limits and nature of its enquiry.' Given this definition and based on the premise that nursing is about 'hands-on' work with people, it would seem that the central business of nursing is practice and that the nature of nursing will be revealed by illuminating and articulating nursing practice.

The tendency in nursing literature has been to polarize and keep distanced, professional and disciplinary endeavours. Such polarization finds its expression in arguments that the concerns of practice and theory are separate; nursing is an applied science; nurses with the mandate to research nursing should be kept apart from practice; and that practice informs practitioners, but not the disciplinary content of nursing (Beckstrand 1978, Donaldson & Crowley 1978, Gortner 1983). In this chapter we seek to present a different perspective, by claiming that theory and practice can be considered as mutually synergistic (Pearson 1988); that nursing is known in a variety of ways (Carper 1978); that nurses, who are practitioners, can be theorisers of their own work (Smyth 1986); and that the practice of nursing can inform the discipline of nursing, by virtue of its nature and location as the central business of nursing (Tilden & Tilden 1985, Visinstainer 1986). Rather than continuing to see professional work and disciplinary theory as being two separate dimensions in nursing, an alternate view would be to see them as creating a dialogue with one another to reconcile their apparent contradictions (Moccia 1986).

Barricading theory off from practice, from fear of tainting the purity of concept constructions performed by nurse academics with the work concerns of nursing performed by clinical nurses (Gortner 1983), has controlled interaction and understanding between communities of nurses. Permitted to mix, tussle a little, and exchange ideas to set up a continuing dialogue, professional issues of practice and disciplinary concerns of theory can be mutually synergistic. The dialogue is between equal partners, if one agrees with Pearson (1988) that nursing practice is 'a sophisticated intellectual pursuit which incorporates a variety of patterns of knowing'. When the two meet and confront each other to sort out similarities and inconsistencies, the synergistic effect can begin to illuminate and interpret the complexities of nursing.

The tendency to label nursing as an 'applied science', based on the contributions other disciplines make to nursing, is shared by some nurses who agree with Beckstrand (1978) that all knowledge necessary for nursing is borrowed, leaving nursing without its own unique identity and practice theory. Counter to this view is the claim that nursing is known in a variety of ways (Carper 1978) and that the generation of knowledge from borrowed, as well as original sources in the practice of nursing, creates the substance of a practice discipline.

The polarized positions of professional and disciplinary concerns have been maintained by nurses, who work with the assumption that the people best able to research nursing are those nurses who are able to remain aloof from the nurses who 'roll up their sleeves' in the daily grind of practice (Donaldson & Crowley 1978). Such a stance sets theoretical pursuits operationalized in research projects as separate and superior, as activities for nurses who are intellectually superior somehow to nurses who are entrusted with the everyday care of people. A contrasting view would be that professional and disciplinary issues can create a dialogue between practice and theory, when nurses, who are practitioners, are encouraged to become theorizers of their own work (Smyth 1986).

Arguing that science seeks universal truths and that practical knowledge and clinical wisdom in practice cannot move from the particular, Gortner (1983) contends that practice informs practitioners on local levels, but that it cannot inform the disciplinary content of nursing in general. This view places immense faith in the tenets of scientific knowledge or empirics, whilst underestimating the equal contributions made to nursing theories by aesthetics, personal knowledge, and ethical patterns of knowing (Carper 1978). The tensions may be reconciled here by the recognition that practice can inform the discipline of nursing, by virtue of its nature and location, as the central business of nursing (Tilden & Tilden 1985, Visinstainer 1986). The nature of nursing is to nurse; it is what practitioners do. To impose theories on practice generated aloof from the context of practice is tantamount to a penguin telling airborne birds how to fly. Practitioners know themselves and they can be encouraged to find ways to uncover and express the sophisticated knowledge they embody in their day to day nursing interactions.

It can be seen, therefore, that when the so-called opposing views of professional and disciplinary concerns are brought together, the dialogue can be exceedingly valuable to the profession and the discipline of nursing. The separation of the two has been maintained, much as the separation of practice and theory has been perpetuated, by creating diametrically opposed identities which serve to rob each of the value of the other. Rather than deplete the generative sources of each other by separation, a reconciliation of the perspectives in terms of a critique of their similarities and differences, can fortify nursing as a practice discipline.

THEORY INFORMING PRACTICE IS PROBLEMATIC

Continuing to talk about something often serves to maintain its existence. Comparisons drawn between disciplinary and professional knowledge and the so called 'theory practice gap,' suggest that the conceptualization of a gap maintains the separation between theory and practice. Theory is often seen as somehow more edifying intellectually than the work of practice, just as the distinctions made between disciplinary and professional knowledge draw much the same conclusion. Smyth (1986) contests the widespread view that theory and practice are entirely different, by asserting that there is 'an interpenetration of the two, that is to say, elements of each exist in the other'. If this is so, even at the most fundamental level, it means that assumptions about the sources of the most informative knowledge for nursing become obsolete, because opposition and competition cease to exist in a climate of mutuality in which one adds to and is added to by the other.

If it were so that there was a unilateral flow from theory formulated by outside sources to practice arenas, with no reciprocal processes within and between each, the value of that knowledge to clinicians is questionable. Benner (1983, 1984) claims that the practice experience of practitioners is vast and accessible and is loaded with meaning for each nurse and nursing, when it is uncovered and articulated in a practice discipline. This view is supported by Tilden & Tilden (1985) citing Fawcett (1980) who insists that 'research questions must originate in the empirical reality of the practice arena', and Christman & Johnson (1981) who warn that 'in order to be self-directing, professionals must acquire knowledge relevant to the decisions they make about actions to be taken'. Smith (1984) extends this view to remind nurses that the 'problems of nursing practice reside in the concrete instances of persons in a situation of being nurses and patients'.

Without negating the value of some knowledge applied from other disciplines to nursing, it is interesting to wonder about what knowledge practitioners value in terms of their own practice. Chinn & Jacobs (1983) caution that whilst other disciplines make a contribution to nursing, they cannot adequately reflect the real conditions of practice. They assert that 'theories and knowledge from other disciplines have proved useful, but they have not been sufficient to provide a complete, comprehensive body of knowledge for nursing practice, nor have they adequately explained the nature of phenomena encountered in nursing'.

The apparent contradictions between professional and disciplinary knowledge resurface when the argument is pursued. If the issues of practice and theory are seen as separate, the suitability of knowledge from other disciplines is beyond doubt. Proponents of the applied science model of nursing, would see as totally legitimate the claim that only scientifically validated knowledge can be included in a discipline. Following on from this, they claim that in as much as professional knowledge is by its nature particularistic, it is unable to provide such knowledge. Thus, they argue, disciplinary knowledge must be adopted which fulfils the tenets of scientific knowledge. In this view, a comprehensive body of knowledge for nursing practice is not the main aim of a discipline and the relative contentment of practitioners in their work understandings is of little consequence.

When the issues of professional and disciplinary knowledge coalesce, however, the outcomes can be mutually synergistic and instructive. When practice is given equal footing with theory, both are able to stand firm. In an egalitarian context of dialogue in which differences are constantly being reconciled, practice is embedded in theory and theory is embedded in practice, so that the interface becomes relatively imperceptible and an unnecessary delineation. This being so, the activities of day to day nursing practice house within them the intricacies of nursing and thus, the seeds of disciplinary knowledge, if indeed nursing is to make claims of having unique knowledge. If nursing is about being with people in nursing contexts, the central business of nursing is clearly spotlighted in practice settings, in which the work of nursing is done. Given that nursing is careful people-orientated work, energized by knowledge, it stands to reason that the knowledge embedded in practice is sophisticated and highly informative to a practice discipline and that cycle upon cycle of professional and disciplinary knowledge growth will result in an expanded practice discipline. When nurses are encouraged to become theorizers of their practice, knowledge contributions from practice can be explored and valued.

Whenever we talk about the nature of knowledge, we are bound by the constraints of language. When we convey ideas it is through language which may become jargonistic even when that is not the intention. It is especially difficult when we try to talk about theory to practitioners who become disillusioned with the complex and abstract nature of the words. All nurses think and talk in everyday language but that language is culturally specific. For practitioners the language of academics may be remote from their experience.

Schön (1987) describes professional practice in topographical terminology. First there is the high hard ground, where manageable problems are resolved by applying research based theory and technique. Scholars live in the high country. Then there are the swampy lowlands, where problems are messy, confused, and chaotic. Clinicians live in the swampy lowlands. The High Land Dwellers have long been recognized for their expertise, but the Low Land Dwellers develop high levels of knowledge also, and must do so if they are to cope successfully with contextual realities of practice. Nursing has been slow to recognize the expertise of its clinicians. Schön (1983) calls the knowledge held by practitioners 'knowledge-in-action'. He describes this as a type of problem setting which, rather than following a technical rationality where theory guides practice, discovers the boundaries of problems and works out what will be considered as relevant to the problem. The practitioner does not operate from a defined method of problem solving but decides the process according to the demands of the particular situation.

Reflection *in* and *on* action are processes which nurse practitioners can use to help them make sense of the situations in which they are required to act. The conflicts, the confusion, the unpredictability, and the uniqueness of each situation are somehow absorbed into a normal day for nurses. The very nature of practice precludes the use of standard rules for solving problems. Thus the knowledge used by practitioners is sophisticated indeed. Street argues that nurse practitioners rely on 'knowledge, experience, improvisation, invention and new strategies relevant to the given situation' (1990). Nurses constantly choose from a number of options, which are often embedded in a range of beliefs, attitudes and value stances. What is selected as a solution in one instance may be rejected as inappropriate in another.

Uncovering the nature of knowing and the beliefs that underpin choice in clinical practice can occur as a result of reflective processes. One form of reflection that may be useful to nurses in theorizing their practice is that which contributes to a process of critical theorizing. Reconstruction of nursing practice and the practice worlds of nurses may occur through this process. Such theorizing allows us to expose nursing practice (theories of and in practice), to scrutiny and to understand our practice in terms of its historical and social construction, to begin to find explanations as to why we are what we are and why our practice is as it is.

Hickson (1990) writes of three ways by which we can understand and act in our worlds.

1. First we can understand our worlds uncritically, prereflectively, not questioning the legitimacy of the existing social organization, relationships, practices, and beliefs
2. Second we can achieve an 'enlightened' understanding of our worlds, becoming aware of elements of our social worlds which are unjust, contradictory or frustrating, of the mechanisms by which they may have come to be that way, and of the factors that serve to maintain them
3. Finally we can become aware that the established order is but one of a number of possible ways of constructing our world and so become aware of the conditions of our existence in an empowering way, with a commitment to finding new, less oppressive, more just ways of structuring our existence.

Nurses, like other people in all aspects of living, do not think through in great detail their every action. This automatic thinking/action has been likened to an autopilot routine (Tripp 1987) in which we follow set patterns that govern and direct our actions. It may be that such routines have been well thought out, and may legitimately maintain an ongoing place in our practice worlds. It may be equally true that such routines may be counter productive to our interests, supporting and perpetuating a static social reality which, were we to truly examine it, we may not wish to perpetuate.

While the substance of our reflections may lie in the broadest level of our practice worlds, it may equally lie in the day to day practices and shared understandings that may have become taken for granted, just an accepted part of our practice worlds. It is, however, in theorizing in and through the concerns of everyday practice that we may begin to address the broadest scope of our nursing worlds.

JOURNALLING: ONE WAY OF REFLECTING

A journal, such as Maree uses, is a tool for engaging oneself both personally and professionally in a dialogue with nursing. Wherever we go, we take our histories with us. Every time we enter a clinical situation, we enter as the person we currently are, constantly becoming, but at any frozen moment of time the product of all that has shaped us. Street (1990) however, cites Lather (1985) who suggests that 'we are both shaped by and shapers of our world'. We are not only the product of all that has shaped us, we have contributed ourselves to what we have become. Holly (1987) notes that as adults we are able to 'look at our own looking' and analyze who we are and how we came to be that person, [that nurse]. We have the ability to be researchers of ourselves, of our own practice and engage in dialogue with ourselves about our understandings and choices.

Lather argues for a process by which practitioners can research their own practice, empowering themselves to alter their understandings and actions and the whole practice situation. In arguing for the development of 'different' research designs, Lather requests designs that:

> allow us to reflect on how our value commitments insert themselves into our empirical work. Our own frameworks of understanding need to be critically examined as we look for the tensions and contradictions they might entail...the search is for theory which grows out of context embedded in data, not in a way that reflects a priori theory, but in a way that keeps it from distorting the logic of evidence. Theory is too often used to protect us from the awesome complexity of the world (Street 1990).

The awesome complexity of nursing lies in the nature of practice. Street argues that it is imperative that nursing spend time over the difficult task of exploring practice; life in the swampy lowlands. She writes:

> It is...time to lay aside preconceived expectations and unexamined habits— time to reject mythical thinking and easy solutions to well known questions. It is time for nurses to put their role as a nurse, their nursing actions, and the clinical setting in which they practice, under close scrutiny. It is time to examine every- thing—and not just to examine; it is time to reflect on all these things and on the process of reflection itself (Street 1990).

The reflective process begins with the capturing of experience as it is lived— a gold-mine of raw data, which is recorded so that it can be analyzed. It requires writing in great detail about what happened, when, where, who was involved, how the situation unfolded.

Recording events can be done in any number of ways; often lined exercise books are adequate. A useful idea is to write on one side of the page only, allowing the blank side to be used for jottings as you reread and raise thoughts and begin to discover themes. It is helpful to date all entries and later jottings, so as you continue to reread, you identify the stages of the journey of discovery that you are undergoing. There are no rules, no right or wrong ways of journalling. Sometimes it is useful to write detailed descriptions of the days events, sometimes it is enough to write about single situations that had impact.

Journal, 16 May 1989

I've decided to focus my writing today on Robyn. I still don't feel that we are giving her the care we should. I'm struggling with just what it is that doesn't feel right. Every time I think about her I feel so desperately sad. Part of it has got to be that her kids are the same age as mine. Imagine Nikki at the tender age of 13 without a mum. I can't stand to think about all those awful adolescent years without me. Chris might be 18, but he's not as grown up as he likes to think he is. I know that he needs me too. Robyn's husband seems really capable, but will he have the sensitivity that his kids will need from him. Jason and Simone love their mum, but when I watch them all at visiting time they seem to be withdrawing. They sit back a bit from the bed now, and they don't talk as much as they used to.

Geoffrey is that reserved type of man. It is hard to get any sense of how he is feeling. I guess I'm not sure how any of them are feeling.

At least I know now that Mr Jones did tell Robyn about the biopsy report. Perhaps now we can be open with each other but I'm really finding it difficult to know how to approach this change in the family dynamic. For example, I walked in there this afternoon and found Geoffrey standing at the end of the bed, leaning on the wall and Jason and Simone watching the T.V. Robyn was just resting with her eyes closed. They all know the prognosis, but nobody is talking about it. When I am with her, she talks about it all the time, and cries a lot. What will it do to this family if they don't talk about it?

Holly (1987) writes that a personal professional journal is not just a diary of events; it includes full description of situations with all players, impressions, thoughts, motives, and feelings. It provides data that can be analyzed to permit a dialogue between the objective fact world and subjective interpretations, with the potential for surfacing the differences between them.

CHALLENGES TO JOURNALLING

Few people setting out on a journey of critical self-reflection find the journey painless. It is not easy to set aside time to write comprehensive accounts about each clinical day. Cost effectiveness and worker efficiency-driven schedules tend to reinforce a view of reflective processes as time wasting or not worthwhile. Nursing is seen as having been historically steeped in tasks and routines and the 'quick fix' solutions to known problems. Reflection is not a process that has been or is valued in such an environment. Nurses attempting to journal often make comments about not having time, hating the nature of the reflective writing style, not wanting to write about work after a whole day of doing work (Taylor 1990). These are all obstacles to be overcome and as such make the valuing of the process the first real challenge to nurses embarking on the journey of reflection on practice.

The second challenge is to remove the censor. The writing needs to be honest and detailed if it is to provide accurate and adequate data with which to work. This also is not easy. Comments from nurses include not being able to be honest in case they are not able to handle what they find and fear of wrecking the illusion that keeps them sane. Taylor (1990) writes that the actual experience of writing is not always what you think it will be. In her experience, registered nurses journalling about themselves and their practice often find the process quite painful. Examining practice to analyze where habits have come from, for example, often dredges up images from the past with 'vistas of long suppressed ogres, spectres of personal and professional ghosts, which would have been easier left unexhumed'. Taylor goes on to acknowledge the courage that it takes to continue the journey in the face of painful memories. It takes courage to shake the soothing nature of everyday life (Smyth 1987) and to grasp the opportunities for liberating ourselves and our practice.

The third challenge is to examine the writing critically, reading it, re-reading it. In doing this it is possible to begin to locate ideas, reactions, themes, and new questions. This can be quite anxiety provoking. We are exposing ourselves to scrutiny, even though it may only be our own. If we have written honestly, our dialogue with ourselves is authentic, not softened by any social niceties.

Journal, 17 May 1989

What is it about visiting times that makes families act like strangers? When I think back, I can remember lots of examples where visitors seem to spend visiting time watching everyone else in the ward, patients seem to feel that they have to 'entertain' their visitors and end up exhausted.

Robyn isn't talking, there are no other distractions really in a single room. Maybe that's why they are all so quiet, or concentrate on the T.V. So why isn't she talking? Why do I think they have to talk right now, in this strange place?

What I'd really like would be to sit down and talk through my concerns about this family, with Mr Jones. So why don't I? Am I any different from Robyn not talking to her family? I guess the rest of the staff need to talk about their concerns too. How can we support each other while we support Robyn and her family? Communication is so hard sometimes. It is one thing to know how important it is, but quite another to make it work in a place like this.

It is not easy to scrutinize our writing without justifying and rationalizing our actions, and resorting to feelings of guilt, blame, or victimization. Nurses comment that they often end up feeling that everything seems to come back to them, they are the cause of all their woes, or that they use the journal to just 'bitch' (Taylor 1990). It takes some skill to read with interest, suspending judgement. Holly (1987) quotes an unknown source when she writes that if we wish to learn from our writing, we must learn to listen 'with a quiet heart'.

PROBLEMATIZING PRACTICE

Reflection-*in*-action is reflecting on situations as they unfold in our day. This gives insights that guide immediate action. Reflection-*on*-action is that which occurs later, looking back over the events of the day, in an endeavour to make sense of why we chose the action we did. Writing about our experiences allows us the opportunity to capture the moment in order to explore it by means of reflection on action. Street (1991) reminds us that later analysis allows us to revisit our past experiences with new dimensions to our understandings and changed perspectives; often when we write, the writing is charged with the emotion of the moment, and one view of the situation dominates. Distancing allows us to see themes and patterns that we may not have been aware of; as we start to examine what it is that we know and how we came to know it, we can uncover what our personal theories of practice really are.

Journal, 19 May 1989

I can't believe it. Yesterday I called a meeting of staff to talk about Robyn, and how we were all feeling about her and her situation. I always believed that I am open, easy to talk to, approachable, all the things that a good charge nurse ought to be. They had all this stored up stuff. I feel stunned that they find me hard to approach. How can I have moved so far away from them?

It was a day full of total contradictions. I cornered Mr Jones, I felt super tense, but summoned up the courage and told him I wanted to talk to him about Robyn. I expected him to be his usual 'bolshie' self. But to my surprise, he was very helpful. We sat in the office over a cup of coffee, (his idea), and I told him all of the concerns that I feel about her. All this time I've built up an image of him as distant and brusque. Funny, he wasn't at all insensitive. I was stunned when he offered to come to a staff meeting so we could all share our concerns.

I'm starting to feel that there is a message here that I have missed. Am I the common denominator in these events? I see myself as approachable, and Mr Jones as unapproachable, wrong on both counts! Tomorrow I must have a talk to Fiona about this and see what she thinks.

Often we do not realize that we have these theories, or if we do we seldom articulate them, but they do direct our practice behaviour. Occasionally we may find examples where our 'espoused theories' are inconsistent with our 'theories in use', in that what we say we believe, has no bearing on what we actually do in practice.

Consider a dreamer, deeply asleep and dreaming about being the hero in an adventure. When we sleep, we may dream about ourselves in a situation, but we are also aware that we are watching ourselves in the dream, we are both the actor in the dream and the observer of the actor. In the same sense we need to stand back and observe ourselves in practice, to be both the observer and the observed. It is when we act as researchers of our own practice that we come to see why we act in certain ways, and what has guided the action; we begin to see that there may be other ways of understanding and acting in and on our world.

A personal professional journal is a tool which allows us to create distance, to stand back and problematize our practice, turning normal routines upside down and surfacing the real beliefs and values that guide our actions. The process of problematization in the context of critical reflection, as Tripp (1987) notes, is the process by which we treat '...as potentially suspect those things which are usually taken for granted as routine, and remarkably normal'. Often our professional lives become full of actions and reactions that are routine or habitual. We don't think to challenge our notions of what has become normal for us. Problematizing practice is learning to ask ourselves difficult questions. We are trying to turn the focus from 'quick fix' solutions to problems, toward theoretical interests (Tripp 1987). Altering the question, may well lead to different answers and different options for acting.

Street (1991) writes that the process of critical reflection can be rather like unravelling a skein of wool, in which each thread needs to be traced to its source in order to be unravelled. Sometimes we find that we cannot unravel a section because the thread is so intertwined we need to work out the relationship between each of the threads before we can start. This is a helpful metaphor. We are tracing the threads and examining relationships between them as we unravel our own personal and professional histories—how we came to be who we are, practising as we do.

Journal, 27 May 1989

I've had several chats with Fiona. I haven't written for a few days now. This whole experience has been quite painful.

Fiona was very frank but kind. She asked me questions which brought me to some cold hard truths. She got me to consider that I might be a great charge nurse, but that maybe people find me unapproachable at times because I am so busy being efficient. Do they see me as the super nurse? I certainly try really hard to have the ward run smoothly and for people to have confidence in me, perhaps this sets up a barrier that stops them seeing me...Maree?

That made me think about that paradox I located in my journal on the 19th May. Mr Jones turned out to be different from the way I had believed he was. There was me turning out to be different to what I believed of myself. Now I am starting to see that people don't always project what they intend or even what they really are. We could all be so busy acting professionally that we never really see each other.

Thinking about all of this made me go back and read over my recent journal entries. A theme that hits me is communication. One of the things I have learned is that people move in their communications at their own rate, you can't force it along. When I read back over the entry for May 16, I realise now that that is where they were at the time. When I spoke to Robyn before she went home, I discovered the family have done lots of talking, but have planned that the real talking will happen when they are at home, in their own environment and all together. I really think that we as nurses often impose our values on our patients. I am so familiar in this environment, it's a semi home for me, but it must seem such a hostile place for people who are transient and vulnerable in this setting.

The analytical process examines personal, nursing and situational specific issues, and considers them in the light of the historical, social, and political factors that have shaped them. Going back over what was written some time ago is to return to that time and view it with new eyes. Time allows an issue focus rather than an emotion focus (Cox 1990). Time, as Holly (1987) writes, provides us with 'perspective and momentum and enables deeper levels of insight to take place'.

The answers that we locate in response to our new questions, driven by theoretical analysis, become the basis for new action. This action is likely to be radically transformed in relation to the action that would have occurred without reflection. Engaging in discourse with our journal has the power to transform our consciousness both in relation to self-understandings and in terms of situating nursing within the social, political, and cultural contexts in which nursing occurs.

CONSTRUCTING OUR OWN REALITY

Sometimes in our journalling discourse, we uncover just how hard we have been working to keep things the way they are. We learn how we have come to adopt certain patterns of behaviour that support the status quo. We find that we have come to accept our world without examination without challenge. We may not even recognize our world as constraining. In this respect we are really participating in our own oppression; constructing our own reality. Reflection provides a way by which we can identify and critically examine our practice world in order to locate within it hidden elements of power and domination that we have not recognized or not challenged, and that fail to serve the interests that we would wish to acknowledge as legitimate.

Reflection assists us to identify how we are both shaped and shapers of our understandings. Reflection has the power to surface the 'false consciousness' that masks the numerous possibilities for transformative action within our practice. Old understandings lose their power. We can view ourselves as reclaiming the power to alter the conditions of our own worlds that we allowed to be imposed upon us. Hickson (1988) writes 'we are in control of our destiny if only we can recognise that we are able to act, not just react'. We can only do this, however, if we are able to see how we have been shaped by currently pervasive views of the world.

COLLABORATIVE DISCOURSE

It is often difficult for those who choose to follow the paths of critical self-reflection. Challenging our self-understandings, understandings of ourselves in practice, understandings of practice itself, and understandings of our practice worlds in general can be experienced in quite contradictory ways. On the one hand exposing ourselves and our worlds to critical scrutiny may be an exciting, liberating experience. It may also however be highly disturbing as we are faced with the tensions and contradictions which may disturb in fundamental ways our self-understandings and understandings of our worlds.

Freire (1972) alludes to this danger in acknowledging the possibility of making 'real oppression more oppressive by adding to it the *realization* of oppression [emphasis added]'. We may come to see that our understandings and activities may have been shaped in ways that serve the interests of others to our own detriment, or the detriment of those in whose interests we believed we were acting.

Reflection in isolation is difficult to sustain for a variety of reasons. There are difficulties in:

- surfacing and transcending what may be our own distorted self-understandings
- asking ourselves difficult, often self-exposing questions
- facing the difficult answers to such questions; and, perhaps most particularly
- keeping our vision directed towards new possibilities for understanding and action.

Praxis can be seen as the link between reflection and action. Freire (1972) defines praxis as 'reflection and action upon the world in order to transform it'. It is facilitated by the notion of shared (collaborative) critical discourse. Such discourse involves an engagement with others in the processes of critical self-reflection. Collaborative discourse of this nature has possibilities that isolated reflection is unlikely to achieve. Shared reflections are often far more productive and potentially liberating than isolated introspection.

Collaborative discourse may occur in a variety of circumstances with groups or individuals with whom we share common circumstances and/or common concerns. This may take the form of a 'critical friendship'—a trusting mutually supportive relationship in which critical reflection can occur. It may take the form of a collaborative group with a similar, mutually supportive critical intent. In both group and dyadic settings what is possible is a mutual relationship in which searching, perhaps difficult, questions may be asked and support given. Such support may be particularly helpful if directed towards facilitating a shift away from 'personal blaming' strategies (directed towards self or towards others) or 'system-blaming' strategies. Such strategies effectively externalize or internalize problems in a way that simply serves to reify and/or maintain existing circumstances and understandings.

EXPLORING ALTERNATIVE POSSIBILITIES: PRAXIS

In this chapter we have been working with reflection as a form of practice. Encouraging reflection on the world of practice enables possibilities for changing that reality. This is the notion of praxis. Freire's (1972) definition of praxis as 'the reflection and action of [people] upon their world in order to transform it' makes a clear link between the ways in which we understand ourselves and our worlds and the ways in which we act. All our actions are informed by what we know and believe of ourselves and our worlds. It is through reflection that we may act to transform our worlds; it is action which sustains and transforms our reflection.

It is this transformative element of action/reflection so clearly encapsulated in the above definition that is important to nurses in practice. All the insights we can gain through introspection will serve little purpose unless we are able to truly change our understandings and actions in ways that continue our search for a just and liberating existence. The value of reflection lies in its potential to transform our actions and hence our worlds, given that there is a balance between reflection and action. In relation to this point, Freire notes that words deprived of action and reflection become verbalism, and action overemphasized to the detriment of reflection becomes activism. Critical reflection therefore is not simply introspection in a 'navel-gazing' sense. Inherent in it is a commitment to transformation. This transformation is invested with a moral commitment to justice.

Carr & Kemmis (1986) capture this sense of committed, interested reflection as they note that praxis '...remakes the conditions of informed action and constantly reviews action and the knowledge which informs it. Praxis is always guided by a moral disposition to act truly and justly...' In this sense it is clear that praxis entails thought and action (theory and practice) in a dialectical relationship. Neither one is pre-eminent. The ideas which guide our actions cannot be separated from the actions themselves except perhaps artificially for the purposes of analysis. As our ideas are subject to change so too are our potential actions; the only fixed element is the moral element—the disposition to act with integrity.

We have a vision then of critical reflection as a means by which people may begin to engage in praxis, that is to move 'from being pessimistic, passive victims in an oppressive situation, to being optimistic, active recreators of victimless situations in which it is easier to love and to pursue self affirmation as responsible persons' (Alschuler 1986). There has been a tendency in nursing, as in other aspects of life, to perceive our present social circumstances as natural, immutable and essentially unchallengeable. Perceiving our worlds in such ways masks the numerous possibilities for transformative action within nursing.

Many of the constraints we experience are self-imposed to the extent that we are trapped by our own understandings. When we believe we cannot act, or act out of habit and routine, we do not search for alternative possibilities. As we come to reflect critically we may come to see that what we imagine are 'real' external constraints may well be exposed as self-limitations imposed by our own thinking. As we come to expose our worlds and ourselves to critical scrutiny we may become aware of

...the contradictory conditions of action which are distorted or hidden by everyday understandings. We may also become aware of our own potential in acknowledging that all men and women are potentially active agents in the construction of their social world and their personal lives: that they can be the subjects, rather than the objects, of socio-historical processes. The central aim of our critical reflections then must be a self conscious practice which liberates [us] from ideologically frozen conceptions of the actual and the possible (Comstock 1982).

By reflecting in a committed way we may come to see that many of our deepest beliefs about our nursing worlds may be contradicted in the ways that we think and act; and we may discover that it is not through external forces unrelated to ourselves that we are prevented from meeting our ideals but through the ways that we perceive ourselves, our actions, and our worlds. As we come to expose these self-imposed limitations then the focus of our reflection shifts towards new action, towards the ways in which we might begin to reconstruct and act differently within our worlds.

Taking on the notion of critical reflection is to embrace the possibility of transforming our consciousness, and liberating our practice. To begin to engage in such critical reflections takes courage and a willingness to step into the uncomfortable world of the as yet unknown. Smyth (1987) expresses this tension as he writes 'most of us, unless we feel uncomfortable, shaken, or forced to look at ourselves and our circumstances, are unlikely to change. It is far easier to accept our current conditions and adopt the line of least resistance'. Nevertheless, while it may take courage to expose ourselves and our worlds to critical scrutiny, the possible rewards are enormous. If critical reflection exposes forces that dominate and constrain nursing from realizing its potential, then it exposes new ways of knowing and new ways of acting within that world.

Nurses through their reflections can come to develop a new language that is directed towards exposing the potentials and exploring the possibilities of nurses and nursing. This language is one of new beginnings in which we ask ourselves: 'What if...', 'How would it be if...', 'What do we need to do to...' It is an optimistic language of possibilities in which we dare imagine how things could be different, and plan for how our dreams can become tangible (Street 1991).

The chapter began with Maree's journal entry. Maree was musing about her sore feet, 'Bloody Mr Jones', and Robyn. She was wondering about why Mr Jones intimidated her so much and whether or not Robyn was receiving enough nursing attention in her single room. Maree had invested herself in reflecting on her day to day nursing practice in a journal. In so doing, Maree was representing the experiences of her professional world in a visual form, through which subsequent analysis and change could be possible.

The connection between professional and disciplinary knowledge is embodied in the nurse who works with people in everyday nursing contexts. Professional nursing knowledge energizes people to 'do' people-work. Arising out of practice as theory, and returning again to it as right action, professional knowledge informs nurses about their work. Conversely, the knowledge of the discipline of nursing has typically been generated by nurses who work away from clinical nursing contexts, or it has been imposed on practitioners by nurses who have visited practice worlds for the span of their respective research projects.

At first glance, therefore, there would appear to be a dichotomous situation existing between professional and disciplinary knowledge in nursing, which might appear to be irreconcilable. This chapter has attempted to show that nurses working in clinical settings, who are reflecting on their worlds and committing themselves to action based on their new understandings, are indeed theorizers of their own practice. The knowledge nurses generate in and through their own practice contributes to the discipline of nursing, because practice lies at the heart of nursing and it is by illuminating and articulating this dynamic core that the nature of nursing can be made explicit.

There is no clear endpoint to our reflection; there is no ultimate ideal state of being that we can hope to reach. All we can hope for in our reflections is the surfacing new possibilities for ourselves as nurses and as people, finding new ways to express some of our possibilities, and beginning what can only ever be an ongoing search for freedom and justice.

REFERENCES

Alschuler A S 1986 Creating a world where it is easier to love: counselling applications of Paolo Freire's theory. Journal of Counselling and Development 64: 492-496

Beckstrand J 1978 The need for a practice theory as indicated by the knowledge used in the conduct of practice. In: Nicoll L H (ed) 1986 Perspectives on nursing theory, Scott Foresman, Glenview

Benner P 1983 Uncovering the knowledge embedded in clinical practice. Image: Journal of Nursing Scholarship 15(3):36-41

Benner P 1984 From novice to expert: excellence and power in clinical nursing practice. Addison-Wesley, Menlo Park

Carper B A 1978 Fundamental patterns of knowing in nursing. Advances in Nursing Science 1:13-23

Carr W, Kemmis S 1986 Becoming critical: knowing through action research. Deakin University Press, Geelong

Chinn P L Jacobs M K 1983 The emergence of nursing theory. C V Mosby, St Louis

Christman N J, Johnson, J E 1981 The importance of research in nursing. In: Williamson Y M (ed) Research methodology and its application to nursing. Wiley, New York

Comstock D E 1982 A method for critical research. In: Bredo E, Feinberg W (eds) Knowledge and values in social and educational research. Temple University Press, Philadelphia

Cox H 1990 Exploring clinical practice; a journey of critical reflection. Paper presented at the Embodiment, Empowerment, Emancipation Conference, Melbourne

Donaldson S, Crowley D M 1978 The discipline of nursing. Nursing Outlook (February) 113-120

Freire P 1972 Pedagogy of the oppressed. Penguin Books, Harmondsworth

Gortner S R 1983 Knowledge in a practice discipline: philosophy and pragmatics. Keynote Address American Academy of Nursing Meeting, Minneapolis

Hickson P 1988 Knowledge for practice. Paper presented at the Norman Peryer Forum, Christchurch

Hickson P 1990 The promise of critical theory. Paper presented at the Embodiment, Empowerment, Emancipation Conference, Melbourne

Holly M L 1987 Keeping a personal professional journal. Deakin University Press, Geelong

Moccia P (ed) 1986 Theory development and nursing practice: a synopsis of a study of the theory-practice dialetic. New approaches to theory development. National League for Nursing, New York

Pearson A 1988 Nursing: from whence to where. Professorial Lecture, Deakin University, Geelong

Schön D 1983 The reflective practitioner: how professionals think in action. Basic Books, New York

Schön D 1987 Educating the reflective practitioner. Jossey-Bass, San Francisco

Smith M C 1984 Research methodology: epistemologic considerations. Image: Journal of Nursing Scholarship xvii(2):42-46

Smyth J 1986 The reflective practitioner in nurse education. In: Conference Proceedings of the Second National Nursing Education Seminar: Visions into Practice. South Australian College of Advanced Education, Adelaide

Smyth W J 1987 A rationale for teacher's critical pedagogy: a handbook. Deakin University Press, Geelong

Street A 1990 Nursing practice; high hard ground, messy swamps and the pathways in between. Deakin University Press, Geelong

Street A 1991 From image to action: reflection in nursing practice. Deakin University Press, Geelong

Taylor B 1990 Journalling: towards critically self-reflective practice. In: Study guide, searches for meaning in nursing 2: cultural meanings and practices in nursing. Deakin University Press, Geelong

Tilden V P, Tilden S 1985 The participant philosophy in nursing science. Image: Journal of Nursing Scholarship 17(3): 88-90

Tripp D 1987 Theorising practice: the teacher's professional journal. Deakin University Press, Geelong

Visinstainer M A 1986 The nature of knowledge and theory in nursing. Image: Journal of Nursing Scholarship 18(2):32-38

19. Implications of the critical paradigm

Sue Crane

PREAMBLE

Within this chapter, a look at the phenomena of power relationships and empowerment in nursing will be explored through a literature search and reading in the areas of nursing education, nursing practice, educational theories, social theories, and feminist theories. As a result of this exploration, ways of viewing educational processes which enable professional nurse practitioners to empower themselves will be described, and the author will suggest that if nursing as a whole is to break loose from some of the cultural constraints within which it is embedded, then working within the critical paradigm may help in this process of emancipation.

The implications of this way of viewing the world for nursing practitioners—many of them participating in formal educational programs in nursing (including undergraduates)—will be explored by looking at how it changes the concept of power relationships between nurse practitioners themselves and other nurses within their environment, i.e. practitioners, educators, researchers and managers.

The present work of the author within the critical paradigm, in the development of undergraduate diploma courses, will be used as an exemplar. As the implications, she argues, for nursing are related to adopting a view of relationships with others in a caring, sharing, collaborative way, which can be liberating for those involved, this chapter is written in a traditionally academic way in the main, but it also shows appreciation for the authors as individuals by using their full names.

Within this same theme the author will also use the first person, henceforth, when sharing knowledge with the reader regarding her concurrent search for understanding and practice as a nurse practitioner, (all nurses, being students, educators, practitioners, researchers or administrators, will be viewed equally as being nurse practitioners).

I recognise that the thoughts of Maxine Greene (1978,1988), a contemporary American philosopher and educator, are predominantly being shared within this chapter, as I regard them as being very useful for nurses engaged in a search for meaning within the critical paradigm. Her exploration of meaning has developed more broadly than that described so far by other educators, such as Wilfred Carr and Steven Kemmis (1986), and John Smyth (1987).

INTRODUCTION

This chapter explores the notions of power relationships and empowerment in nursing, which are phenomena constructed and legitimated within the prevailing paradigm of the culture within which they are situated. The exploration will consider the environment within which nursing and nursing education presently seems to occur, by viewing the predominant paradigm of the western world through the eyes of Maxine Greene and several contemporary artists. The question of whether this all-encompassing paradigm is ethically and morally conducive to nursing and nursing education will be posed, and the search will continue with a look at what it means to work within other paradigms. If nurses choose to work within a paradigm, other than the predominating, then how might they view and attain power and empowerment for themselves while they are still situated within a culture where reality is still shaped by that predominant paradigm? This issue will be explored by looking at the way a few nurses are beginning to do this in nursing education.

HERE AND NOW—THE PREDOMINANT PARADIGM

Maxine Greene paints a sad picture of the socio-politico-cultural realities of the United States of America today, viewing the constraints placed upon educators who try to empower their students to reach out for liberation. She looks broadly at the historical trends in this so called free country which has caused a shift in ideals so that the predominant paradigm values economic competitiveness, technology, and power. Thus individuals who are measured as being unproductive within this type of environment are left to the wayside. In fact individuals are encouraged to be self-supporting in an increasingly uncaring world—maybe the tensions this must cause for people necessitates the need for so many psychotherapists to be used. Talk of personal freedom refers to self-dependence and self-determination; it has little to do with connectedness or being together in community (Greene 1988).

A current dilemma for some teachers relates to their attempts to maintain freedom themselves through the curricula they choose for their students, but being constrained by national educational exams, and therefore only catering for those students who will survive the inculcation of this system; receiving funding provided only for the chosen research topics; and having to support students who have heightened stress levels related to social circumstances (Greene 1988). Maxine Greene also highlights the uneasiness voiced by officials of society about the directions that everyday life is taking, with their concerns directed more and more to education, as though it is the area at fault, the victim (1988).

Are the concerns voiced by Maxine Greene applicable to Australian society, or westernised society in general? Quite clearly they are, as the values of technical control and having power predominate over respect for the environment and the individuals within it. For example, some politicians speak to the Green issues only when it is profitable for them to do so, and then, when in a position of power to create change, resume their silence. Power in this context is viewed as property which only some people own, and exert over others. Some familiar examples of this kind of power are: power of hierarchy, of command, force, secrets, and xenophobia; of opposites and division; of accummulation; of expediency and use; and of causality, results and prescription (Wheeler & Chinn 1989).

Artistic impressions

Maxine Greene (1988) enriches the above arguments with the work of twentieth century artists who have been receptive to this shift away from a society that cares, (for example T.S.Eliot 1958; and Virginia Woolf 1976). Virginia Woolf (1976), metaphorically describes living today as being 'embedded in a kind of nondescript cotton wool' in contrast to living 'consciously', the 'cotton wool' representing the safety of habits and routines—automation, rather than speaking out for individuality and innovation.

Contemporary musicians throughout the world relay similar messages to their audiences, in the hope that those with power will begin to reflect seriously on the long term effects their decisions will predictably have on our environment. For example, Bruce Cockburn recently based a tour of Australia around his chart hit song 'If A Tree Falls' which likens the removal of the rainforest remaining on our planet to 'lobotomy' (1988). Even though there is some evidence to show that the maintenance of such a resource is imperative for our own survival, Cockburn points out that the central value of felling trees from the rainforests (such as in Sarawak and the Amazon), is to generate wealth: wealth which, for some, including those having the power of making the decisions, overrides the problems treelogging will cause the wider community. Power in this context, i.e. 'Power-over', may also mean making decisions and taking actions, which you don't necessarily agree with.

Well known Australian singer/songwriters such as John Williamson and Judy Small (1985) have released similar songs voicing their concerns for the environment and the lack of caring within society—but does anybody in power hear?

In his song 'Cootamundra Wattle' John Williamson (1986) advocates that we should not bother to buy and read newspapers anymore. His reasoning relates to the fact that the type of news that sells papers is of the worst type rather than relaying acts of kindness or caring. From the perspective of a country person within the song he also describes the activities within the metropolitan areas of Australia as likened to 'hell', and advises his spouse to admire the beauty of the world surrounding them, rather than worrying for those people in the cities.

Does anybody here care?

Maxine Greene (1988) argues that even though people today are increasingly concerned about issues such as 'sickness, pollution, crime, disorder, and nuclear war', most go on 'living and partly living' (T. S. Eliot 1958) anyway. This is well illustrated in Jackson Browne's song 'The Pretender', which describes the 'ordinary man' on the street—although aware of the forces of consumerism on him, he will continue to play the game, to be a 'happy idiot' (Browne 1976). If people in positions of power do stop and think, Maxine Greene suggests that they will try to solve problems, such as 'homelessness, AIDS epidemic, teenage pregnancy, drug addiction, suicide' with technological answers rather than by caring (1988).

If people choose not to conform, as the 'happy idiot' does in 'The Pretender' (Brown 1976), then they are commonly viewed as deviants. Maggie, in Stephen Crane's novel *Maggie: A Girl of the Streets* written in 1892, experiences loneliness within the world and rejection by others. She is a victim of her culture and penny-less. She becomes a whore, but attracts no men.

At the feet of the tall buildings appears the deathly black hue of the river. Some hidden factory sent up a yellow glare, that lit for a moment the waters lapping oilily against the timbers. The varied sounds of life, made joyous by distance and seemingly unapproachableness, came faintly and died away to a silence (Stephen Crane).

Maggie cannot perceive any alternative but to drown herself.

There is a danger is using the concept of deviance, especially in education, as traditionally the people described as deviant are viewed as 'inferior' as well as 'different' (Apple 1982b).

Michael Apple explains that:

One might say here that deviance is 'earned' by the deviant, since the overt and hidden curriculum, the social relations of the classroom, and the categories by which educators organise, educate, and give meaning to the activities found in schools are perceived as being basically neutral. This claim of neutrality is, of course, less accurate than this proposition would have us believe (1982).

This gives rise again to the issue that those teachers who would disagree with the system, the way of doing things, will find difficulty in thinking and doing in a different way—there are many obstacles to change but often difficult to describe, many causes of oppression both for them and their students. Maxine Greene (1988) describes how the inherent obstacles in schools can be compared to the symbols and the images of a Nazi concentration camp for the Jewish people in World War II, and in doing so highlights that it is more comfortable for teachers not to see them. As illustrated by the life of 'Maggie', it is easier not to be a deviant.

Nurses, as well as educators, can be viewed as being exposed to tensions within their practice, stemming from the devaluing of thoughtfulness and care—the very essence of nursing. As Patricia Moccia writes,

...every day, from moment to moment, nurses witness a society characterised by alienation and dehumanisation, as they become involved in the lives of the patients who come to their institutions and agencies seeking care, compassion, and help. Every day, nurses struggle to help a growing number of people whose lives are increasingly fragmented, constricted, and impoverished as a result of public and social policies (1988).

It would be very easy for nurses to be swayed within their practice to encompass more of the technological aspects of their role, allowing these to engulf the caring aspects so much so that none will remain. This is seemingly already exhibited by the way nurse practitioners are attracted to work settings such as intensive care units rather than to elderly care settings, where commonly the 'caring' role is given to lay care assistants or enrolled nurses. Can we predict from this that the future nurse will be valued as a 'technician' rather than a 'carer'?

Referring back to Maxine Greene's point that officials (or people having 'power-over'), in voicing their concerns about the 'disorder within' and the 'disorders of' of society, direct the blame towards education, we might then ask: can education become the new saviour of society? If so how might this be approached? How can a different message even begin to be espoused and survive within the prevailing, all-encompassing paradigm? The difficulty associated with a change in direction in society, with respect to how people think and act, can be illustrated by the metaphor used by Louis Macneice (1960) in the poem 'Christmas Shopping'. Macneice describes how messages from God try to penetrate the predominating commercialisation of Christmas that he sees in London, and can be envisaged as being like the light of a lighthouse on the coast attempting to penetrate the fog in order to get its message across.

Community spirit?

Even though many people having positions of power do voice their concerns about the problems in society as illustrated previously, Maxine Greene argues that 'there is no serious talk of reconstituting a civic order, a community' (1988). One approach to viewing the way our culture has evolved and is now sustained is from a feminist stance. In this way reality for us can be seen to be dominated by a 'man's' way of knowing and doing. It could be argued therefore that if communities were structured using a 'women's' or 'feminist' process then 'peace' would be the intent or product as well as being the process by which it is achieved (Wheeler & Chinn 1989).

Charlene Wheeler and Peggy Chinn (1989) created an acronym for P.E.A.C.E. to describe what it was for them and what it was not:

Praxis
Empowerment
Awareness
Consensus
Evolvement

The acronym reflects a different way of viewing power relationships, power, within this feminist theory, being more a 'power-of-presence' rather than 'power-over' (Rowan 1984). As each component of the acronym is described you may like to reflect on what constitutes a normal day for you and whether you actually consciously engage in any of these processes.

Praxis is thoughtful reflection and action that occurs in synchrony, in the direction of transforming the world...
Empowerment is growth of personal strength, power and ability to enact one's own will and love for Self in the context of love for others...
Awareness is an active, growing knowledge of Self and others and the world in which we live...
Consensus is an active commitment to group solidarity and group integrity...
Evolvement is a commitment to growth, where change and transformation are conscious and deliberate.
(Wheeler & Chinn 1989)

Many prominent authors have expressed concern that the components of the acronym above do not generally appear within our 'free' culture, (Arendt 1958, Dewey 1927), and yet to be 'free' necessitates the engagement in these same activities (Foucault 1984, Freire 1970, 1972, 1988, Greene 1988, Habermas 1971, 1974, Schön 1983, 1987).

John Dewey, a recognised educational theorist in the States, argued for an 'articulate public' (1927) to be encouraged, i.e. being engaged in significant dialogue surrounding what should be public concerns, and as Hannah Arendt puts it 'to think what we are doing' (1958). There is very little evidence to suggest that this advice was taken either in education or society as a whole; otherwise why would we be surrounded by Virginia Woolf's 'nondescript cotton wool' (1976) or Louis Macneice's 'fog that wads our welfare' (1960)?

NURSING/NURSING EDUCATION—THE STATUS QUO

Annette Street (1991), an Australian educator involved in action research with nurses, wonders why nursing and nursing education today have developed in the way they have. She asks: 'Given that the aim of the theorist was to explain, predict and organise knowledge about nursing practice, how did the practice discipline of nursing develop along a theoretical road which has created a dichotomy between nursing theory and the reality of clinical practice?' (Street 1988). Is she correct?

Australia is undergoing a change in nursing education, whereby all pre-registration education will be totally transferred to the tertiary sector by 1992. Until now the majority of nursing curricula have been based on Tylerian technical behaviourism (Bevis 1988, Donley 1989, Perry & Moss 1989). Many nurses argue that such an approach seems to achieve very little in the preparation of the clinical practitioner (Bevis 1989, Donley 1989, Perry & Moss 1989, NLN 1988, 1989). Judith Perry and Cheryle Moss, nurses involved in nursing education in New Zealand and Australia respectively, agree with Annette Street's view of a dichotomy between theory and practice and argue that present nursing curricula are at fault as they '...are limited in their account of the relationship between theory and practice as they focus attention on the ideal rather than the real. Theory is seen as a basis for practice rather than in a dialectical relationship with practice...' (Perry & Moss 1989).

Many nurses have written about the perceived theory–practice gap in nursing, and in Australia, Deakin University (1988) and Sandra Speedy (1989) have brought this phenomenon to the fore. This gap, Sandra Speedy argues, will only begin to reduce as nurses engage in education and therefore 'see the relevance of nursing theory' and begin to locate or ground their theory in practice (1989). Surely this approach will again only perpetuate the acceptance of the 'given' within the predominating positivist paradigm, as it is the 'ideal', as decided by nursing educators, which is given value. Nursing educators may then be viewed as having 'power-over' interactions with students and nursing practitioners and be perceived as the intellectuals of nursing.

Another concern is the focus within many nursing curricula on the sciences, which flows into the way teaching content is based on the reduction of the body into systems. Technical skill acquisition also predominates within many of the activities of these educational programs. As a result, the unique ways of knowing or phenomena embedded within nursing practice related more to the arts, such as intuition (Rew & Barrow 1987) and nursing ethics (Fry 1989), are ignored. Maxine Greene argues that this is common in today's culture, where explorations in the domains of the arts are seldom allowed to disrupt or defamiliarize what is taken for granted as 'natural' and 'normal' (1988).

A dichotomy arises for undergraduate nurses: that of theory (Grand theory) and practice espoused by their educators within schools of nursing, compared with the theory (local theories) and practice they know to be used within the world of clinical practitioners. Thus oppression occurs for undergraduates as they are unable to direct their learning in a way that would become more relevant to them in the practice world.

It has been suggested by educators that a second dichotomy also arises from the Tylerian approach in the preparation of professional practitioners, that 'theorising is reserved for those having the right intellectual and academic credentials' (Carr 1982), whilst practice is 'a second class activity for those too stupid to think at a theoretical level' (Sprinthall & Sprinthall 1980). It can be argued that this dichotomy occurs in nursing, as in other practice disciplines, where the clinical practitioner, as an individual, and clinical practitioners as a group are subject to oppression as a result of their being in an environment shaped by hegemony and patriarchy; within their profession (due to bureaucracy and tradition), externally within their health care culture (Nightingale 1980, Chinn 1985, Speedy 1987) and within the attitudes held by the wider community (Clay 1987).

Disillusioned by the system, some of the better nursing practitioners are leaving it causing shortages in the richness they brought into nursing. The same can be seen to be occurring within the teaching profession (Greene 1988). Those who remain in the absence of support may elect to be silent, and by withdrawing into themselves perpetuate the automatisation of society and thereby 'no longer inhabit a resisting world' (Greene 1988). It is more usual for us, as nurses, to maintain a low profile in order to reduce the demands placed upon us, rather than to risk being labelled as deviants for not conforming with the expected (Apple 1982b, Crane 1960). Those who have 'power-over' interactions with us give out the orders and most of us will be socialised into receiving them—as Ira Shor says, 'there is little dialogue and many commands' (1980). Silence, it is suggested, has developed as a woman's way of knowing resulting from the oppression women experience within a man's world (Belenky et al 1986). Those nurses who do leave the system are perhaps angry that their caring ways are devalued. Nothing seems to have changed in this respect since Florence Nightingale's era. She described the plight of Victorian women prior to her work in the Crimean War in an essay only recently published, and asked 'Why have women passion, intellect, moral activity—these three—and a place in society where no one of these can be exercised?' (1980).

'A major contribution of feminist thinking in relation to nursing' Peggy Chinn and Charlene Wheeler write, 'is the basic tenet of feminist theory—that women are oppressed. Since nursing has traditionally been a woman's occupation, it is essential to understand the oppression of women to gain insight into some of the most persistent problems in nursing' (1985).

EMPOWERMENT FOR NURSES?

How can nursing move beyond these problems—to empower those identified within the profession as being oppressed, so that they can begin to think and take action for freedom—for nursing praxis ('informed, committed action', Carr & Kemmis 1986) rather than nursing practice, which becomes habitual? How can nursing education assist in this process and support the practitioner?

Maxine Greene's focal interest she says is in human freedom, i.e. 'the capacity to surpass the given and look at things as if they could be otherwise' (1988). This process may be assisted, as already illustrated, by viewing the world through the work of visual and literary artists. She points out that to exercise one's power of choice takes place within context: 'choice and action both occur within and by means of ongoing transactions and with objective conditions and with other human beings. They occur as well within the matrix of a culture, its prejudgments, and its symbol systems' (Greene 1988) i.e. with all the constraints and prejudices embound within it. Therefore plans for change and action must be grounded in reality, 'in an awareness of the world lived in common with others, a world which can be to some extent transformed' (Greene 1988).

The implications for nursing would be that the clinical setting and the practitioners in it become the focus of descriptive research to reveal the local theories embedded within their actions, which could then be relayed to undergraduates by their educators. Patricia Benner's work (1984) formed a milestone within nursing research in this respect, however as the researcher, she attempted to interpret the ways of knowing embedded within practice *for* the practitioner. There is a danger here as Wilfred Carr and Stephen Kemmis (1986) point out—that 'only the practitioner has access to the understandings and commitments which inform action in praxis, [and] only the practitioner can study praxis'. John Heron (1981) agrees, arguing that no researcher can predict outcomes or describe truths for any human research subject, as to do so would neglect the notion of intelligent agency. People, individually and as members of groups, generate new ideas and insights for themselves all the time, and the intention of their actions is based upon ways of knowing developed over time within the culture they shape, which is externally shaped also (Heron 1981). Therefore the ways of knowing (or local theories) embedded within nursing practice within a variety of settings are not readily accessible to another person by them merely observing nurses (John Heron 1981). The implications here for nursing research are that nurses only explore their own practice, so that they are collectively 'co-researchers' and 'co-subjects' within their culture, 'participating fully in the action and experience to be researched' (Heron 1981).

Donald Schön (1983) advocates the need for practitioners 'to learn to read their own lived worlds', engaging in a process of 'reflection-in-action' and so explore the knowledge base they are working from. Henry Giroux and Peter McLaren (1986) also argue that a shift in the conceptualisation of practitioners (referring to teachers) is desirable. Here they 'extend the traditional view of the intellectual as someone who is able to analyze various interests and contradictions within society to someone capable of articulating emancipatory possibilities and working towards their realization' (Giroux & McLaren 1986). Nursing practitioners could establish themselves as 'transformative intellectuals' (Giroux & McLaren 1986) by viewing themselves, and being viewed by others, in this way.

This perspective is in keeping with the 'critical' paradigm, and within nursing we could envisage researchers becoming 'co-subjects' and encouraging practitioners to become 'co-researchers', and so collectively they could explore their own culture and themselves, with critical theory and action research as methodology and method respectively. In this way we may begin to realise how our common understandings have been shaped as a result of consciously or unconsciously conforming to domination and begin to move forward beyond the given, consciously rejecting 'power-over' types of power (Carr & Kemmis 1986, Kemmis & McTaggart 1988, Chinn 1989).

Therefore this collective awareness raising would be for the purpose of change, arising from and for our actions (nursing praxis) and for empowerment—similarly P.E.A.C.E., a process and product as described by Charlene Wheeler and Peggy Chinn (1989). In this way we can begin to address the tensions, the constraints and the puzzles arising from praxis collectively, by surfacing them, engaging in critique, reconstructing and moving on beyond our historically static ways of knowing, allowing multiple ways of knowing to become legitimate.

This chapter I hope does not appear to be ideological—for we as nurses surely have to acknowledge that the first step towards creating a community, which values the essence of caring and peace, is to start where we are—'the here and now'. We also need to acknowledge that if we as nurses chose to view power relationships in a different way than the 'predominating', and seek our own and collective empowerment, then we need to learn how to surpass the obstacles to change that we will continuously encounter. Peggy Chinn (1990) and Judy Small (1985) suggest that we could envisage these obstacles as walls which presently serve to segregate us, not only as nurses but also as women, affecting the power relationships between ourselves and others within our area of work, between ourselves and other nurses, ourselves and other women. Such walls could, for example, explain the recent need for some of us to focus our discussion on the 'theory/practice gap' in nursing (Speedy 1989, Deakin University 1988). Peggy and Judy also describe that in contrast there are windows within us, 'through which we can begin to envision a different way of being' (Chinn 1990). As nurses by verbally sharing our visions in a collective way we could begin to know how similar the experiences and issues arising from them within nursing are, begin to accept the differences between us as contributing to the richness of our community, and begin to experience as well as continuing to seek peace (Chinn 1990; Small & Humphries 1985). In this way dialogue may occur between all practitioners (previously labelled clinical practitioners, educators, students, administrators and researchers) providing forums for groups of people (all learners) to come together within their cultural matrix and find 'openings' for freedom (Greene 1988), to find windows for P.E.A.C.E. (Wheeler & Chinn 1989).

There is general agreement in that 'the search for some kind of critical understanding is an important concomitant of the search for freedom' (Greene 1988), within the philosophies of neo-Marxists: Jürgen Habermas (1971, 1974, 1979), Paulo Freire (1970, 1972, 1988), Henri Giroux (1979, 1981, 1984, 1985), Antonio Gramsci (1971), Michael Polanyi (1964), Donald Schön (1983, 1987), Michel Foucault (1984), John Dewey (954) Merleau-Ponty (1962/1967), Michael Apple (1979, 1982a, 1982b), and Maxine Greene (1979, 1988). Neo-Marxists focus on critical consciousness, using self-reflection to expose how the socio-politico-historical aspects of culture impact on thought and therefore action, thought which can be self-modified. 'Thought', wrote Michel Foucault, 'is freedom in relation to what one does, the motion by which one detaches oneself from it, establishes it as an object, and reflects upon it as a problem' (1984).

Therefore there is a continuous double dialectical relationship established between thought and action (theory and practice) and individual and society (nurse versus nursing culture), (Carr & Kemmis 1986). Wilfred Carr and Stephen Kemmis conceptualise that self-reflective communities could progress forward in a 'self-reflective spiral of action research', constantly 'relating retrospective understanding to prospective action' (1986). Therefore empowerment (a liberating power) of individuals and/or groups may be gained through raising awareness of self and identifying the internal and external constraints to liberation. Freedom may then be gained by them seeking out pathways, or opening spaces, within the existing structure.

John Dewey (1934) also looks at the concept of thought; 'mind' he argues could be thought of as a verb, i.e. to denote 'all the ways in which we deal consciously and expressly with the situations in which we find ourselves'. He argues for the need for 'all sorts of persons to learn to read their own lived worlds', thus generating critical conciousness. Paulo Freire worked with Brazilian peasants, helping them to develop both literacy of the written word and 'critical literacy' collectively in order to promote social changes for democracy (Freire 1970, 1972, Freire & Macedo 1987). Within the critical paradigm, groups of people who view themselves as oppressed may actively generate change, but '...the great humanistic and historical task of the oppressed [is] : to liberate themselves and their oppressors as well' (Freire 1972). Paulo Freire's notion of change is a process of transformative action, through problematization, to concientization leading to praxis (1970).

Jürgen Habermas also proposes that change can occur through the development of what he terms 'emancipatory knowledge' which can be generated from reflection and give power to the oppressed in any political struggle (1971, 1974, 1979, Held 1980, Carr & Kemmis 1986). He contends that there are at least three types of knowing or 'interests' embedded in human activity: technical, practical and emancipatory, which are associated with the empirical, the hermeneutic and the critical sciences respectively (Habermas 1971). All three 'interests' can be viewed as inherent in the development of knowledge required for nursing praxis: technical nursing knowledge being scientific and procedural; practical nursing knowledge being used to provide holistic, empathic care; and emancipatory nursing knowledge arising through critical reflection to provide creative and liberating aspects of care (Deakin University School of Nursing 1988, Perry & Moss 1989). Though, as previously described, many nursing curricula continue to focus mainly on the technical interest, the only knowledge perceived to be valid within the 'predominant' paradigm.

Empowerment for nurses engaged in education?

If we choose to operate within the critical paradigm in formal nursing education curricula, then what does it all mean? How will this approach be beneficial and is it presently used anywhere internationally?

Within the last section of this chapter we explored the possibility of nurses forming critical self-reflective collectives for the purpose of awareness raising, or bringing into their consciousness, those repressive aspects of their culture in order to review them and move forward. We could envisage the same collective processes being developed within educational settings in order for the participants of formal nursing programs to seek out their collective learning needs and explore different ways of learning. The learning needs of a group of participants would be generated by their individual engagement in clinical praxis—again relating their '*retrospective* understandings to *prospective* action' (Carr & Kemmis 1986). The participants may be graduate nurses who are able to reflect on their wealth of experiences as practitioners. Undergraduate nurses do not necessarily have experiences within nursing practice, but, by joining with other participants and engaging in reflective and collective processes, they can explore the 'here and now' for themselves with regard to their notions of nursing. Their own knowledge of nursing may have been developed for example, by reading books about nursing during their childhood, by watching hospital based soap operas on the television, or listening to the stories of their aunt who was a nurse way back in the 1930s. By engaging in such processes they are able to direct their own learning needs, that they view as being relevant at the time, in contrast to the educator, as an 'expert', but removed from the realities of clinical practice, deciding what it is they should learn and when. Liberation is therefore of the kind as defined above by Paulo Freire (1970), and understandings related to praxis will be explored within the realms of the three human 'interests' as described by Jürgen Habermas (1971).

Em Bevis (1988) describes the role of nursing educators then becoming one of 'metastrategists', as they 'provide the climate, the structure, and the dialogue to promote praxis'. They design processes which allow nurses (including undergraduates) to reflect on the mysteries they find embedded in their own praxis or observed praxis/practice, from multiple standpoints, so that eventually patterns are seen, awareness is gained, and future praxis developed. By learning collectively: 'multiple interpretations constitute multiple realities; "the common" itself becomes multiplex and endlessly challenging, as each person reaches out...toward what might be, should be, is not yet' (Greene 1988).

Maxine Greene conceptualises freedom as 'an opening of spaces as well as perspectives, with everything depending on the actions we undertake in the course of our quest, the praxis we learn to devise' (1988). This enhances the developed view of the role of nurse educators within the critical paradigm i.e. to create 'openings' in order for nurses to empower themselves, 'to engage in some sort of praxis, engaged enough to name the obstacles in the way of their shared becoming' (Greene 1988).

The implications for educators who choose to work within the critical paradigm are that they will need to engage in reflective processes themselves, focusing on how they interact with their students. Are those interactions presently authoritative or collaborative? Are students 'silenced' within learning sessions due to the educator speaking to them for the whole duration of those sessions? Are students valued as people with rich knowledge bases as gained through previous life experiences (Bevis 1988); 'subjects of decisions' rather than 'objects' (Freire 1970)? Are the labels 'student' and 'teacher' avoided so that the educator is viewed by all as a learner as well?

Learning in nursing could become a collaborative, shared, and participatory ongoing experience which may, by its very nature, remove the horizontal and hierachial oppression which occurs within the profession both in and between practice and in educational settings. Learning in nursing could become a continuous preoccupation for all nurses, rather than an occupation for only a few (who choose to specialise in that area) and learning would not be dichotomised from praxis (adapted from Freire 1972). Power within relationships of this context can be described as power: of the whole; of unity, integration, collectivity and distribution; of nurturing, intuition, and sharing; of process; of consciousness; and also of diversity, of letting go, and responsibility (Wheeler & Chinn 1989). Thus the purpose of nurse educators, researchers and managers would be to support the nurse clinician, so that all are equal nurse 'practitioners' engaged in praxis, and directing the future of nursing. It could be assumed that this nurturing and focus on caring for others within the profession would also be transmitted to those people for whom nurses engage in care.

GENERATING ALTERNATIVES

Nursing academics in the United States of America (U.S.A.) have during the past few years advocated a need for a curriculum revolution in nursing in the form of a paradigm shift, from the positivist to the critical. This is evident from themes of national nursing education conferences (N.L.N. 1988, 1989), a recent Post-Doctoral Conference on 'Critical and Feminist Theories and Nursing Inquiry' (Clemson University,1989) and publications (Bevis & Watson 1989, N.L.N. 1988, 1989, 1990, Thompson 1987, MacPherson 1983). Rosemary Donley (1989) reflected that: 'Everyone [who attended the national nursing education conference in 1987] was inspired by a powerful mandate to create fundamental changes in the way we educate nurses—a mandate that called for a transformation of nursing curricula from a training model to a schema that would educate caring, critically thinking health professionals', as she spoke at the national nursing conference in 1988. In the same paper she urged her colleagues to move 'from concept to implementation' (Donley 1989) and used for the change the analogy described by Donald Schön (1983), being from the 'high hard ground' to the 'messy swamps'.

This same analogy was used by Annette Street (1991), indicating that the transition will be a difficult one for educators to face as it entails moving from 'the safe ground of a clear-cut, objective, and highly refined training model to the ambiguous notion of health as human caring [which] lacks the road map and cognitive surety of making simple, true and false choices' (Donley 1989). Rosemary Donley (1989) also asserts that once the journey is commenced then it will never end, which we begin to realize when we view praxis as the process and the product within a framework of critical or feminist theory.

Peggy Chinn is a nurse educator in the U.S.A. working within a feminist frame of reference for formal nursing education programs. She views the concept of feminist praxis as seeking 'personal empowerment and exercise of personal power in the world that leads to growth, transformation, unity, justice, and peace' (Chinn 1989). In the past she has participated with graduate nurses within doctoral programs where the feminist processes, as described within her book jointly written with Charlene Wheeler, are explored and developed (Chinn 1989, Wheeler & Chinn 1989). By engaging in these processes the hierarchal nature of course objectives, course design (for example lectures), and evaluation (as in examinations and gradings) is removed. This approach requires a dramatic shift, as for example it influences the way educators view their purpose, the way they interact with participants, the language they use, how students are able to achieve excellence within their programs, and the resources they use (Bevis 1989, Bevis & Watson 1989, Chinn 1989, Weiler 1988). The participants may also experience difficulties in accepting a change of role compared to their previous experiences as students. Thus there is a need for all nurses engaged in these radical processes to support each other, and the following authors can assist in their collective understanding of the reactions they may experience.

Em Bevis and Jean Watson (1988) in the second chapter of their recent publication describe a 'learner maturity continuum' along which learners engaged in processes within the critical paradigm will need support in differing ways from their educators. As the learners increasingly take control over what and how they learn, the educator role needs to adapt to cater for this shift, i. e. from low learner / high educator to high learner / low educator structure (Bevis & Watson1989). Alfred Alschuler (1986), refering to Paulo Freire's critical theory, describes how people will pass through three stages as they become more exacting as a result of becoming more aware of the dialectics in their culture. The stages are a magical conforming stage; a naive reforming stage; and a critical transforming stage where 'it is easier to love and to pursue self-affirmation as responsible persons'.

Although there are now several nurse academics in the U.S.A. espousing the need to work within the critical paradigm their work has not been by an exemplar in actual nursing education or praxis. Instead a critique of the American Nurses' Association's 'Social Policy Statement' (Allen 1987); a look at the implications for research methodology (Stevens 1989, Hedin 1986); and an explication of how 'critical scholarship' can 'reweave' reality for nursing (Thompson 1987), are found. Therefore we find there is a general lack of clarity, where in some cases the critical paradigm is viewed as a traditional type of critique process (i.e. negative), which does not encourage others to really consider this paradigm as a way of re-viewing their world.

There are many American and Australian nurses who consider that there is only a choice of two paradigms in order to access nursing knowledge, i.e. the logical positivist, and the interpretive (Dzurec 1989, Leonard 1989), the former being quantitative research and the latter qualitative. This is evidenced within the majority of nursing research texts (e.g. Chenitz & Swanson 1986, Sarter 1988) and therefore these nurses are either unaware of or choose to disregard the emancipatory critical paradigm as a valuable way of exploring the knowledge base of nursing.

There are currently only a few schools of nursing internationally who are endeavouring to incorporate learning processes in keeping with the critical paradigm into their educational programs (e.g. Massey University and Auckland Institute of Technology in New Zealand, Deakin University and The Flinders University of South Australia). The Diploma of Nursing curriculum document of Deakin University (1988) provides one exemplar of a nursing curriculum developed with a critical theory stance, drawing on the philosophies of Jürgen Habermas (1971), Paulo Freire (1970, 1972) and Donald Schön (1983, 1987). The work of Deakin's Faculty of Education, describing the use of critical theory and action research in the development of the professional schoolteacher for praxis (Carr 1980, 1982, Carr & Kemmis 1986, Holly 1984, Smyth 1987) was instrumental in the establishment of the School of Nursing (Geelong Campus). Judith Perry and Cheryle Moss (1989) describe more fully the reason for the School's philosophical stance. The engagement in reflection-in-action, facilitated by keeping a personal-professional journal, by all practitioners of the Deakin School of Nursing at Geelong (i.e. staff and nurses enrolled in formal programs) is one of the many learning processes (Holly 1984, Smyth 1986). This enables these nurses to develop their praxis collectively (as debate of issues arising from journal entries is part of this process) and this is research in itself, in and for nursing, in comparison to research in the positivist and interpretive paradigms, which would be research on and about nursing (adapted from Carr & Kemmis 1986).

As illustrated by the present situation in the United States, it is one thing to espouse a philosophy but another to actually use it to direct all aspects of an educational nursing program. All practitioners connected with Deakin University School of Nursing are experiencing continuous personal and collective learning, related to a shift in paradigm. As a result the units of study which some of them develop reflect where they are 'at' in their own thinking. My own work, within this school, involving the constant development of pre-registration nursing units in 'Nursing Elderly People', for second year nurses, and 'The Discipline of Nursing', an initial unit for first year nurses, may serve as exemplars which I am as willing to share with you as I am to explore yours. The conference paper I delivered at 'The First

International Self-Care Deficit Nursing Conference' (Crane 1989) details the learning processes engaged in by all participating practitioners involved in the elderly care unit and the roles they developed as learners, in a joint search for meaning whilst engaging in praxis within elderly care settings.

Exemplars of nursing research conducted within the critical paradigm are also few in number (Hickson 1988, Perry 1985, Street 1990). Pat Hickson (1988) recently completed a Masters thesis which explored the 'practice worlds of four nurses' with a critical approach. Annette Street (an educator) is presently directing nursing action research studies within the Royal Children's Hospital in Melbourne (1990). If we as nurses are going to direct our future pathway towards a discipline, then we could surely benefit from being able as practitioners to describe the unique ways of knowing embedded within our practice, ways of knowing which value more than solely the technical.

CONCLUSION

This chapter has attempted to explicate the phenomena of power relationships and empowerment in nursing and nursing education by viewing the socio-politico-cultural reality within which nursing is embedded. It was argued that the predominating paradigm of society values power, being 'power-over' in nature, and technology/technological knowledge. Within this paradigm knowledge is 'asocial' and static, as there are accepted modes of thought which are never questioned or challenged and so no alternatives are ever explored. Messages from the arts relating to the lack of care and the lack of community spirit within society are deliberately ignored as these modes of thought are not perceived to be valuable, or legitimate. What is more these messages are dangerous for those having power as they bring into question the morality of 'power-over' interactions occurring between people. How people impose internal constraints on themselves, as well as being subject to the external, due to their compliance with the 'given' and their silence, was discussed. To speak out, though, is frowned upon and people risk being labelled as a rebel or a deviant.

The status quo within nursing and nursing education was viewed as having been shaped by, and also perpetuating, this mode of thought and action. It was implied that the use of 'power-over' within the profession transmits itself into the ways in which nurses view their interactions with patients and students respectively. A gap was perceived to exist between theory and practice, between the ideal and the real, between the educator and the practitioner, so that nursing students become exposed to the tensions this creates. Being encouraged to be assertive, autonomous and accountable for their actions, a true patient advocate, some practitioners and nursing students try such an approach within their praxis, only to continuously hit what seems to be a 'brick wall'—the external modes of thought are too static to allow any small changes. It becomes easier to assume silence and not to think, thus taking refuge from the ambiguities of the outside world.

It was proposed that the perceived lack of care and community spirit within society was ethically and morally opposing the essence of nursing, and therefore alternative ways of knowing were advocated, especially by working within the critical paradigm. The way that some critical theorists, educational theorists and feminists reject the use of knowledge and power as described above was explored. Instead knowledge was viewed as arising from a combination of many ways of knowing as it is constantly developed within a particular social context. Individuals and groups may become conscious of this knowledge as they engage in self-reflection, and begin to realise how their understandings have been shaped by internal and external constraints, as a result of consciously or unconsciously conforming to domination.

Within the critical paradigm power-of-presence relationships and empowerment for nursing practitioners were described. The need for all nurses as practitioners to engage in self-reflection as co-researchers was highlighted. In this way we could collectively explore our ways of knowing embedded within our praxis, consciously identify those walls between us, accept our differences and move forward towards what we envisage for ourselves and our patients within a peaceful and free world. In this way dialogue will be encouraged between all practitioners (previously labelled educators, clinical practitioners, students, administrators and researchers), as co-learners within their cultural matrix. Within this paradigm the focus is on nursing praxis, as both a process and product, and therefore there is no concept of any gaps between theory and practice, the 'real' and the 'ideal', as they are one and the same within praxis. There is never a 'right' way or an 'only' way developed, no domination, and therefore the tensions or dialectic relations addressed within praxis will never be finally resolved. Therefore if nursing practitioners begin to strive for freedom within the predominant paradigm, they should also realise that it will be a never ending journey. The resistance and the obstacles to change will always be there and so they will have to face the anguish and frustrations related to being accountable for their praxis.

The implications of the critical paradigm for nursing education were described, and how the roles of the educators and the students change as they become learners together seeking their collective empowerment. Examples of how a few nurses are using alternative learning and research processes within the critical paradigm were described, although this approach is advocated by many in nursing.

Finally it can be seen that the future pathway that nursing will take, towards disciplinary status or not, is within our hands—all nursing practitioners are responsible for the actions or non-actions they take within the presently dominating paradigm of society. The critical paradigm has been presented as an alternative way of viewing ourselves and our culture which may allow us to empower ourselves individually, and collectively, in and for nursing praxis.

So do we remain silent, allowing for the 'power-over' relationships in nursing to persist? The Australian singer-songwriter Judy Small tells us:

...we are foolish people who do nothing
Because we know how little one person can do
Yes we are foolish people who do nothing
Because we know how little one can do

('One Voice in the Crowd', Judy Small 1985)

or do we join together in 'power-of-presence' relationships in a common search for liberation for nursing using reflective processes?

Do you think of me as enemy and could you call me friend
Or will we let our differences destroy us in the end?
The wall that stands between us could be a window too
When I look into the mirror I see you

('Walls and Windows', Judy Small & Pat Humphries 1985)

Passages from 'One Voice in the Crowd', words and music by Judy Small, and 'Walls and Windows', words and music by Judy Small and Pat Humphries, reproduced with permission. From the album One Voice in the Crowd, available from Crafty Maid Records, PO Box 304, Fairfield, Victoria 3078. Copyright © Larrikin Music Publishing Pty. Ltd.

REFERENCES

Alschuler A S 1986 Creating a world where it is easier to love: counselling applications of Paulo Freire's theory. Journal Of Counselling and Development 64:492-496
Allen D G 1987 The social policy statement: a reappraisal. Advances in Nursing Science 10 (1):39-77
Apple M 1979 Ideology and curriculum. Routledge & Kegan Paul, London
Apple M 1982a Education and power. Ark Paperbacks, Boston
Apple M 1982b Cultural and economic reproduction in education. Routledge & Kegan Paul, London
Arendt H 1958 The human condition. University of Chicago Press, Chicago
Belenky M F, Clinchy B M, Goldberger N R, Tarule J M 1986 Women's ways of knowing, the development of self, voice, and mind. Basic Books, New York
Benner P 1984 From novice to expert: excellence and power in clinical nursing practice. Addison-Wesley, Menlo Park
Bevis E O 1988 New directions for a new age. In: National League for Nursing. Curriculum revolution: mandate for change. N.L.N., New York
Bevis E O, Watson J 1989 A new direction for curriculum development for professional nursing: a paradigm shift from training to education. N.L.N., New York
Browne J 1976 The Pretender. In: The pretender (album) Elecktra/Asylum/Nonesuch Records, Los Angeles
Carr W 1980 The gap between theory and practice. Journal of Further and Higher Education 4(1):0-69
Carr W 1982 Treating the symptoms, neglecting the cause: diagnosing the problem of theory and practice. Journal of Further and Higher Education 6(2):19-29
Carr W, Kemmis S 1986 Becoming critical: knowing through action research. Deakin University Press, Victoria
Chenitz W C, Swanson J M 1986 From practice to grounded theory—qualitative research in nursing. Addison-Wesley, Menlo Park

Chinn P L, Wheeler C E 1985 Feminism and nursing, can nursing afford to remain aloof from the women's movement? Nursing Outlook 33(2):74-77

Chinn P L 1985 Nursing patterns of knowing and feminist thought. Nursing and Health Care (February): 71-75

Chinn P L 1989 Feminist pedagogy in nursing education In: Curriculum revolution: reconceptualizing nursing education. N.L.N., New York

Chinn P L 1990 Feminism and nursing: what has it to offer? In: A dialogue with six international scholars of nursing, conference papers. Deakin University Faculty of Nursing, Geelong

Clay T 1987 Nurses, power and politics. Heinemann Books, London

Clemson University 1989 Critical and feminist theories and nursing inquiry. In: The eleventh annual Clemson University post-doctoral conference proceedings (November 10-12). Clemson University, Clemson

Cockburn B 1988 If a tree falls. In: Big Circumstance (album). Liberation Records, New York

Crane S (1871-1900) 1960 Maggie: a girl of the streets. Fawcett World Library, New York

Crane Sue 1989 The development of a diploma course unit in nursing elderly people using the Self-Care Deficit Nursing Theory, and reflection-in-action. In: The first international Self-Care Deficit nursing conference proceedings (abstract only). University of Missouri-Columbia, Columbia

Deakin University School Of Nursing 1988 Diploma of Nursing curriculum document. Deakin University Press, Geelong

Donley Sr. R 1989 Curriculum revolution: heeding the voices of change. In: Curriculum revolution: reconceptualizing nursing education. N.L.N., New York

Dewey J 1927 The public and its problems. Republished 1954 Swallow Press, Athens, Ohio

Dewey J 1934 Art as experience. Minton, Balch & Co, New York: 268

Dzurec L C 1989 The necessity for and evolution of multiple paradigms for nursing research: a poststructural perspective. Advances in Nursing Science 11(4):69-77

Eliot T S 1958 The complete poems and plays 1909-1950. Harcourt Brace, New York

Foucault M 1984 The Foucault reader. Rabinow P (ed) Pantheon Books, New York

Freire P 1970 Cultural action for freedom. Center for the Study of Social Change, Cambridge, Massachusetts

Freire P 1972 Pedagogy of the oppressed. Ramos M B (trans) Pelican Books, London

Freire P, Macedo D 1987 Literacy: reading the word and the world. Routledge & Kegan Paul, London

Freire P 1988 The politics of education. Culture, power and liberation. Bergin & Carvey, Massachusetts

Fry S T 1989 Toward a theory of nursing ethics. Advances in Nursing Science 11(4):9-22

Giroux H 1981 Critical theory and educational practice. Deakin University Press, Geelong

Giroux H 1979 Schooling and the culture of positivism; notes on the death of history. Educational Theory 29(4):263-284

Giroux H 1984 Marxism and schooling: the limits of radical discourse. Educational Theory 34(2):113-135

Giroux H 1985 Introduction. In: Freire P The politics of education. Macedo D (trans). Macmillan, London

Giroux H, McLaren P 1986 Teacher education and the politics of engagement: the case for democratic schooling. Harvard Educational Review 56(3):213-238

Gramsci A (1891-1937) 1971 Selections from the prison notebooks of Antonio Gramsci. Hoare Q, Smith G N (eds and trans) International Publications, New York

Greene M 1978 Landscapes of learning. Teachers College Press Columbia University, New York

Greene M 1988 The dialectic of freedom. Teachers College Press Columbia University, New York

Habermas J 1971 Knowledge and human interests. Shapiro J (trans) Heinemann, London

Habermas J 1974 Theory and practice. Veirtel J (trans) Heinemann, London

Habermas J 1979 Communication and the evolution of society. McCarthy T (trans) Beacon Press, Boston

Hedin B 1986 Nursing, education and emancipation: applying the critical theoretical approach to nursing research. In: Chinn P L (ed) Nursing research methodology. Aspen Publishers, Rockville pp 133-145

Held D 1980 Introduction to critical theory: Horkheimer to Habermas. University of California Press, Berkeley

Heron J 1981Philosophical basis for a new paradigm. In: Reason P, Rowan J (eds) Human inquiry. John Wiley and Sons, Chichester

Hickson P 1988 Knowledge and action in nursing: a critical approach to the practice worlds of four nurses (thesis). Massey University, Palmerston North

Holly M L 1984 Keeping a personal–professional journal. Deakin University Press, Victoria

Kemmis S 1985 Action research and the politics of reflection. In: Boud D, Keogh R, Walker D (eds) Reflection: turning experience into learning. Kogan Page, London, pp 139-163

Kemmis S, McTaggart R 1988 The action research planner. Deakin University Press, Geelong

Leonard V W 1989 A Heideggarian phenomenologic perspective on the concept of the person. Advances in Nursing Science 11(4):40-55

Macneice L 1960 Christmas Shopping. In: Hewett S (selector) This day and age, an anthology of modern poetry in English. Edward Arnold, London

MacPherson K I 1983 Feminist methods: a new paradigm for nursing research. Advances in Nursing Science 5(2):17-25

Merleau-Ponty M 1962/1967 Phenomenology of perception. Humanities Press, New York

Moccia P 1988 Curriculum revolution: an agenda for change. In: Curriculum revolution: mandate for change. N.L.N., New York, pp 53-64

National League for Nursing 1988 Curriculum revolution: mandate for change. N.L.N., New York

National League for Nursing 1989 Curriculum revolution: reconceptualizing nursing education. N.L.N., New York

National League for Nursing 1990 Curriculum revolution: redefining the student–teacher realtionship. N.L.N., New York

Nightingale F (1820-1910) 1980 Cassandra. The Feminist Press, New York

Perry J 1985 Theory and practice in the induction of five graduate nurses : a reflexive critique (thesis). Massey University, Palmerston North

Perry J, Moss C 1989 Generating alternatives in nursing: turning curriculum into a living process. The Australian Journal of Advanced Nursing 6 (2):35-40

Polanyi M 1964 The logic of tacit inference. In: Greene M (ed) 1969 Knowing and being. University of Chicago Press, Chicago

Rew L, Barrow E M 1987 Intuition: a neglected hallmark of nursing knowledge. Advances in Nursing Science 10(1):49-62

Rowan G 1984 Looking for a new model of power. Women of Power, Spring

Sarter B (ed) 1988 Paths to knowledge: innovative research methods for nursing. N.L.N., New York

Schön D 1983 The reflective practitioner: how professionals think in action. Basic Books, New York

Schön D 1987 Educating the reflective practitioner. Jossey-Bass, San Francisco

Shor I 1980 Critical teaching and everyday life. University of Chicago Press, Chicago

Small J 1985 One voice in the crowd. In: One Voice In The Crowd. (album). Crafty Maid Music, Sydney

Small J, Humphries P 1985 Walls and windows. In: One Voice In The Crowd (album). Crafty Maid Music, Sydney

Smyth W J 1986 Reflection-in-action. Deakin University Press, Victoria

Smyth W J 1987 A rationale for teachers, critical pedagogy: a handbook. Deakin University Press, Geelong

Speedy S 1987 Feminism and the professionalization of nursing. The Australian Journal of Advanced Nursing 4(2):20-28

Speedy S 1989 Theory–practice debate: setting the scene. The Australian Journal of Advanced Nursing 6(3):12-20

Sprinthall N, Sprinthall L 1980 Adult development and leadership training for mainstream education. In: Corrigan D, Howey K (eds) Special education in transition: concepts to guide the education of experienced teachers. The Council for Exceptional Children, Reston, Virginia

Stevens P E 1989 A critical social reconceptualization of environment in nursing: implications for methodology. Advances in Nursing Science 11(4):56-48

Street A 1991 Nursing practice: high, hard ground, messy swamps and the pathways in between. Deakin University Press, Geelong

Street A 1990 Myths in action. In: The fourth national nursing education conference proceedings, Myth mystery and metaphor. Melbourne

Thompson J L 1987 Critical scholarship: the critique of domination in nursing. Advances in Nursing Science 10(1):27-38

Weiler K 1988 Women teaching for change, gender, class and power. Bergin & Carvey, Massachusetts

Wheeler C E, Chinn P L 1989 Peace and power, a handbook of feminist process, 2nd edn. National League for Nursing, New York

Williamson J 1986 Cootamundra Wattle. In: Mallee Boy (album). Emusic, Sydney

Woolf V (1882-1941) 1976 Moments of Being. Harcourt Brace Jovanovich, New York

20. The construction of nursing: ideology, discourse, and representation

Sheryl Delacour

INTRODUCTION

Nursing has been constructed by powerful discourses including those of medicine and gender, in which our society's dominant ideologies are enshrined. From the level of connotation, socio-cultural myths are produced from female stereotypes which circulate in common currency as part of 'common sense' notions—those which 'go without saying'—operating to foreclose a space for alternative representations and meanings. These constitute the primary fodder for representations of nurses and nursing in the mass media. The centrality of mass media in shaping and reinforcing dominant patriarchal values, attitudes, and ways of perceiving is undeniable. Moreover, media imitate other media whose cultural products are plundered, reproduced, repeated, and recycled.

In this way, even stereotypes regarded as dubious may, after a measure of exposure, become internalized and naturalized; they are thereby metamorphosed into categories of the normal, the real, and the healthy and desirable. Further, the concentration of media ownership works against the possibility of a multiplicity of discourses on nursing. The codified essences of archetypal myths, put to work in representations which project nursing as the quintessential occupation for women, structure public perceptions of nurses and nursing, including patients, key policy-making figures, and our colleagues in other health care professions. Certainly, these coalescing forces operate dynamically within individual nurses' psyches as well as permeating professional subjectivity, ensuring that, at least in part, we continue to replicate these dominant, ideological paradigms in our own professional roles and relationships.

Nursing has been 'spoken' by others until recently and the current representations appear to have been dipped in formaldehyde at the beginning of the 20th century. The gap between professional nursing discourses, changes in nurse education, nursing roles, and the dominant cultural construction is enormous. Certainly it is important that we analyze the processes through which dysfunctional images and discourses are maintained. Moreover, it is useful to regard reading media as a politically situated and critical activity for the nursing profession. This kind of reading position promotes the view that media may be approached as texts to be deconstructed. These practices will assist in clarifying the systematic mapping of nursing, based on gender difference, and energize our efforts to ameliorate the effects of nursing representations and the discourses which cross these.

It is alarming that a significant proportion of people generally derive the bulk of their knowledge and perceptions about nurses, nursing, medical and health issues from the mass media. These notions are gleaned, in particular, from commercial television and radio, tabloid newspapers, women's magazines, and romance fiction. It is imperative, therefore, that we analyze these familiar images and representations and their derivation, so that we map more effectively their dynamics, implications for women, and counterproductive perceptions which they structure. Further, we need to explore the unwelcome effects on the development of the discipline. Some of the latter include a diminished sense of personal worth and effectiveness, and a lack of positive professional regard for colleagues (leading to the well-documented 'horizontal violence'). It is difficult, also, to gain widespread public acceptance of the need for higher degrees in nursing. These attitudes, in turn, make inroads into an affirmative sense of the profession's value, role expansion, collegiality, and our ability to orchestrate cohesive political action and commitment to policy development and implementation. In addition, we need to confront the plethora of personal and professional developmental issues and conflicts lying psychodynamically at the interface between professional image and professional identity. Initially, this analysis teases out the role of ideology, discourse, and hegemony, as well as historical influences on nursing. The common images and representations, disseminated through the mass media, are explored in terms of film, television, and romance fiction. Some tools for analyzing these media are discussed. Representations of nursing and nurses derived from reports on nurse education and nursing historiography are explored. This analysis does not include the construction of psychiatric nursing.

IDEOLOGY, DISCOURSE, AND HEGEMONY

Ideology includes not only consciously held values and beliefs, but myths, images, representations, and ways of perceiving. Dominant discourses are shaped by ideology. People are socially constructed by the powerful discourses of dominant institutions, for example, medicine, education, and religion; and potent discourses are prescriptive and can colonize parts of the social domain and spread into areas beyond their own. Kress (1985) elaborates: 'If the domination of a particular area by a discourse is successful it provides an integrated and plausible account...which allows no room for thought; the social will have been turned into the natural. At this stage it is impossible to conceive of alternative modes of thought or else alternative modes of thought will seem bizarre, outlandish, unnatural'. If our profession is more conscious of these features, we will become more rigorous in, for example, our analysis of knowledge and practices which work against an appropriate theorizing of nursing around women's health and our approaches to intervention. Discourses collapse contradictions and suppress differences, and domains of social life become subjected to homogenizing influences. Certain features are highlighted in discourse and privileged, and the choices are always heavily ideological. Baudrillard (1981) reflects on the closure of discourse and its general homogenizing tendencies: '...this logical mirage that is the effectiveness of ideology. It is the abstract coherence, suturing all contradictions and divisions, that gives ideology its power of fascination'.

Foucault (1972) asserts that our subjectivity and identity are linked and brought into play by discursive strategies and representational practices. His analysis foregrounds the crucial role of discourse and its capacity to produce and sustain hegemonic power, through which all categories of the normal (natural) as well as the abnormal (unnatural) are exposed as social constructs. Dominant discourses are hegemonic, and it follows that particular views have prominence. Hegemonic texts contain features which operate to privilege certain views over others which are silenced or marginalized. It is possible to examine the processes through which this occurs and to reveal the strategies through which conflict is glossed over or naturalized so that the text appears seamless and natural.

Discourses of knowledge are not neutral. Medical discourse is a discourse of power and authority; it is hegemonic. It is helpful to recognize the centrality of hegemony, that is, the existence of constellations of beliefs which operate to legitimate existing power relations. Nursing ideology and discourse have been heavily influenced by the normalizing disciplines of medicine, religion, the military, pedagogy, psychology, science, and technology. Medical dominance in the health care field has facilitated wide acceptance of medical views on gender, health, illness, and the proper role for nursing in the health care industry. It is useful, then, at this point to recall Lukes' (1974) supple and penetrating exposition of the power of hegemony:

> Is it not the supreme and most insidious exercise of power to prevent
> people, to whatever degree, from having grievances by shaping their perceptions,
> cognitions and preferences in such a way that they accept their role in the existing
> order of things, either because they can see or imagine no alternative to it or
> because they see it as natural and unchangeable, or because they value it as
> divinely ordained and beneficial?

It is apparent that nurses have grasped this essential insight and are now working positively to develop their own discourses for their discipline. The above insight contributes explanatory power around the socially constructed set of values: qualities and characteristics found commonly in nurses at least until the late 1970s. Studies in personal inventories into role orientation and self-images of nurses were highly revealing on this point—these reflected, in replicated studies, the desire to be needed by patients and an equally strong desire to serve doctors. Satiric images frequently contain the kernel of truth from which we may tend to flee into the refuge of overblown rhetoric and the manic defence of grandiose professional images.

HISTORICAL INFLUENCES ON NURSING'S CONSTRUCTION

Australia, as a British colony, incorporated many of the features of Britain. There are three archetypal paternalistic systems which were formative for Australian nursing—the institutions of medicine, religion, and the military. Early Australian schools of nursing, established along the lines of the Nightingale school, were permeated by predominant notions of female roles from late Victorian England, socially appropriate at that time and centring around women as subservient helpers whose raison d'etre was to serve the needs of men and, in so doing, derive vicarious satisfaction and self-esteem. Nightingale, a product of class and gender relations during that period, modelled the characteristics of the ideal nurse on 'ladies' of her own class, elaborating the nurse's role along the lines of the striking sexist division of labour of that time. The assertion here is not meant in a judgemental sense; strategies adopted during that historical moment may well have been functional for that period. Kingston's (1975) model of the Victorian family is analogous to the structure of hospital hierarchy—matron as a superior model of 19th century housewife; doctors as frequently absent husbands and rulers of the hospital household; and the probationers and trainees as the daughters doing the unpleasant chores. Certainly until quite recently this model had a discordant resonance for nursing in general hospital settings.

There is a long history, furthermore, of medical discourse around women's mental health. These discourses circulated freely during the 19th century and were still evident, albeit in a more minor key way, in obstetric and gynaecological texts into the 1970s. Ideologies of gender and 'proper' roles for women are inextricably bound up within this discourse, with motherhood and mothering roles. Indeed, the latter was regarded as a culmination of psychosocial development and a condition necessary for full mental health.

It is hardly revealing, then, that characteristics, needs, qualities, and roles assigned and ascribed as those befitting women, decisively informed medical discourse on nursing and the construction of congruent representations of the nurse. Doctors were deified, and remnants of this status and cultural authority were still reasonably prominent into the 1970s. These self-serving myths, in terms of the symbiotic fit between nursing and medicine, operating within their ideological scaffold, were reified as fact.

In analyzing the potency of the construction of nursing as the fulfillment, in the workplace, of the natural role for women it may be useful to reflect on the binary system of oppositional thought which characterizes patriarchal societies. Derrida (1967) and Cixous (1980), in their seminal critiques of binary logic in western philosophical thought, contend that meaning is produced precisely through binary oppositions, for example, masculine/

feminine. This system is markedly evaluative and constricting closures are inherent, multiples cannot be accommodated, that is, it is not possible to think 'this' and 'that', without the norm (male) which is positively valued, and the deviant (female). The implicit privileging of the male position is codified. Through the working of discursive alignment male myths become human myths, and it is not possible to 'think' woman for her subjectivity is denied. Many feminist writers have suggested recently that woman (and we may impose 'nurse' here) operate as a metaphor for the undefined, for western philosophy is unable to deal with the feminine. In developing an alternative nursing discourse on female psychosexual development, with its practice implications, we may use the insights of the above critiques to inform our developing discourses.

Some other binary oppositions cited by Cixous (1980) are relevant for the construction of women and nurses, and shed understanding on the construction of the nurse-doctor relationship as one of symbiosis. These are: Activity/Passivity, Culture/Nature, Head/Emotions, Intelligible/Sensitive and Logos/Pathos. Moi (1985) contends that 'Each opposition can be analyzed as a hierarchy where the "feminine" side is always seen as the negative, powerless instance. The fundamental "couple" male and female, is the central determining structure'. A plethora of studies indicate the significant point that the qualities and characteristics attributed to mentally healthy males, when applied to females are regarded as indicators of mental ill health (Chesler 1972). The hidden positive/negative evaluation can be traced as the underlying paradigm. The dynamics circulating around these unconsciously determined perceptions and valuations are almost palpable in lending support, and produce their effects on the subordination of nurses, as well as in controlling and delimiting their sphere of practice.

MASS MEDIA

It has been argued above that people learn important ideological lessons about social life and nursing from the mass media. These messages are contained within a time warp whereby contemporary radical reworkings in our construction of nursing and its partial realization in new educational and practice dimensions are notable for their absence from the mass media's input into the public domain. Tuchman et al (1978) posit that: 'The societal need for continuity and transmission of dominant values may be particularly acute in times of rapid change...'. The reflection hypothesis explores the notion that mass media reflect dominant societal values and the corporate characteristics of commercial media induce program planners and managers to design programs which appeal to the largest audiences, offering programs consonant with widely held values and perceptions. Moreover, it has been acknowledged that audiences generally do not welcome change. Dominant ideologies form a vast reservoir of ideas for program development and these are incorporated into symbolic representations of society, rather than literal ones. Further, content and representation are prescribed by the popular generic codes which dictate form and structure. Examples here are the genres of romance fiction represented within nurse-doctor pulp paperbacks, film melodrama, and 'soaps', a hybrid form of which, 'The Young Doctors', is an example from television. It is clear, also, that symbols are subject to slower evolvement than material conditions—that is, 'culture lag'.

Women and nursing are symbolically annihilated by the mass media as Tuchman et al (1978) observe: 'Newspapers' very emphasis upon establishment institutions and those with institutionalized power ... most information in the general sections concerns people in power and newspapers justify this emphasis by stressing that such people work in or head societal institutions that regulate social intercourse'. This partly explains the absence of nursing discourse and perspectives on bioethical issues, in which nurses are as involved as doctors whose views are prominent in articles dealing with these matters. Johnstone's (1989) research confirms this impression. Nursing's construction in the electronic media's soapy melodramas trivializes, stereotypes, and sexualizes the nurse. The dynamics of cultural management revolving around representation of nurses include discrediting by caricature in cartoons, potent examples of which reached a new height during the 1986 Victorian nurses' strike; or through picking up on threatening or provocative features and distorting these to mobilize conventional sentiment against nurses. Media personnel frequently regard women—and therefore nurses—as a special category, relegated to a position requiring only token attention, for their cultural products are, in the main, designed and positioned to attract buyers to their advertisements.

Women's magazines frequently carry triumph over tragedy stories which relate to bioethical concerns and medical technologies. Expressed in 'cozy you' private language, with generous interpolations from medical experts, these issues appear in vacuo—detached from their related societal ramifications. Biographical and personalized, this genre has no place for nursing perspectives.

TOOLS FOR DECONSTRUCTING DISCOURSE AND MEDIA

Implicit in the methodology of Barthes's (1973) studies in popular culture was an undermining of the bedrock distinctions between cultural objects and the qualities and values supposedly inherent within them. His elegant and engaging analyses of the ideological role of cultural products unequivocally reject the manner in which mass media represent social constructions—the outcome of historical and political struggles—as simply 'natural' or common sense. He indicated that myth represses dialectically forged reality. The seamless, plausible, authentic flow is manufactured for audiences. Media criticism generally is positioned and structured within very constricted paradigms—these are set by the dominant media.

Myths which construct nursing in the public arena are ideological impositions, and it is important that we adopt critical reading/viewing positions if only as a means of partially inoculating ourselves against their noxious effects. As metaphors are ways of decorating according to individual ideological positions, for example, 'termination of pregnancy' or 'killing an unborn child', we do well to heed Barthes (1973) : 'Metaphors are the language of our mythologies and our mythologies to a large extent construct us, construct notions of reality and are part of the ideological and political structure of reality'. We become used to these and no longer think of them as metaphoric; we become unable to think critically about them: the names given to them are right. If we are to re-fashion the representation of nursing we must grapple with the power of mass media to impose cultural assumptions and reflect the dominant living ideology of our society, and tease out the implications of our naturalized metaphors for the evaluative power embedded within them. A range of methods may be used to assist us to unmask and hence subvert the reinforcement of negative constructions of nursing.

General questions

These may be brought to bear on any medium or discourse, including our own: Who has speaking rights? Who says what? Which position? On behalf of whom? Who is silenced? What are the assumptions? What is privileged in the text? What is ignored, glossed over or marginalized? Who is the target audience and how is the reading/viewing position constructed to promote a 'preferred' reading? Which genre and its codes and effects? What type of publication/program and resultant status of discourses? How are power and knowledge articulated? How are gender, sexuality, roles and relationship, race, class, deviance and normality constructed? Which rhetorical devices? Which linguistic features?

Electronic media

It is possible to analyze the textual system by studying the film grammar—that is, its cinematic language system. The following elements of film form may be teased out: the mise-en-scene comprising lighting, sets, costume, setting, behaviour of figures, props, and use of space. How does the mise-en-scene contribute motifs viewed in the film? What relationship and psychosocial effects are established and underscored by framing, composition and territory? How are point of view, emotions, identification, distance, and interiority expressed through camera angles, different kinds of shots—for example extreme close-ups, reaction shots, two shots? How does the sound track support or add counterpoint, irony and the like to the visuals? What ideological positions are marked off by editing devices?

Film genre effects

Many cinematic techniques are used to simulate 'actuality' and they provide 'guarantees of truth'. These are relevant especially for decoding documentaries and TV news report genres and derive from *cinema vérité*: direct gaze, voice-over, 'on the spot' eyewitness, focus shifts, hand-held camera work, indepth focus, apparent haphazard mobile framing and monochromatic images. Generating their own simulations of reality, these techniques are frequently used within an investigative structure. They seduce the viewer into believing that the representations and discourses replicate reality per se along with quintessential truths. The authority of the discourses are, then, underscored by these elements of film form.

Nursing content analysis

Kalisch & Kalisch (1983) were involved in pioneering work on content analysis of images of nurses and nursing. Their checklist for monitoring the media comprises 11 sections containing key questions we may use to develop the major features of media depictions. The categories are as follows: prominence in plot, demographics, personality traits, primary values, sex objects, career orientation, role of the nurse, professional competence, education, administration, and overall assessment. These tools are a helpful way into analyzing media and it is suggested that nurses become familiar with them. Deeper analyses will be undertaken more easily after a series of this kind of exercise.

PULP ROMANCE FICTION GENRE

A dozen novels from the Mills and Boon subgenre of doctor-nurse romances were examined and this fruitful sample reflects the contradiction of women's status and roles. All texts share a sense of the insufficiency of female selfhood, beyond that required for narrative development of the quest and the uncomfortable happy endings intended to make whole the heroine who is constituted, at the outset, as 'women as incomplete'. These features are not peculiar to the subgenre but form part of the generic code generally, for all genres are influenced by 'commonsense' understandings. It is possible that pop Freudian notions, extrapolated from psychiatric discourse and part of readily accessible common 'knowledge', reflect the highly contested aspect of Freudian theory around 'penis envy'. Lacan's (1977) re-reading of Freud develops this theme along the lines of the phallus as the major signifier and related concepts exploring 'women as lack'.

   Fiedler (1988) suggests that 'In the popular mind the deep psyche of the mass audience...nurse, equals woman'. At a profounder, mythological level, woman equals nurse. Etymologically, the root of nurse is *'nutrire'*, to nourish. At the level of connotation—from which spring myths generally—

powerful metaphors for women and nurses are evoked. These include nourishing mother and its ecclesiastical overtones. Further, the connotative level is compounded and confused by an ambivalently regarded sexuality. It is understandable then, that this subgenre sells well, and new titles, along with reissues of best sellers are available each month. Nursing is a serviceable theme, for many readers can identify with aspects of the caring nurse role as an added extra to the satisfactions derived from the familiar romantic quest in which the battle of the sexes is central. The essential ingredients in this formulaic genre dictate the features which are to be included in each version of the form. In this way the publisher and editor, in highly specific ways, control aspects of the author's 'creation'. As there is a guaranteed market, this approach is not risky, it is cheap, and authors comply with a rather rigid formula.

It would be a fiendishly difficult task, indeed, for us to attempt to subvert this subgenre! Try, as an exercise in sheer futility, to rewrite one of these romances using non-sexist language and discourse. Radway (1984) alerts '...each romance is, in fact, a mythic account of how women must achieve fulfilment in a patriarchal society'. In my view this rather grim prognostication, whilst not lacking in a degree of plausibility, explores only one aspect of the possible reader response. Perhaps closer to the point is Snitow's (1983) observation: 'The ambiguity of the books indicates a central truth: romance is a primary category of the female imagination'. It needs to be noted here that this salient concern of women is not addressed adequately by feminist theory.

Audience identification is increased by the denatured quality of these texts in which most heroines have familiar service jobs (a marketing strategy) such as teaching, nannying, and nursing. The subgenre analyzed fails to capture nurses' changing conditions and roles. It is suggested to authors that these fantasies mirror the appeal and pleasure experienced by children's initial exposure to fairytales (Snitow 1983). Nevertheless, we are able to engage in an ideological interrogation of these texts.

The nurse-doctor subgenre enshrines and celebrates major discourses, including those of family, medicine, science, and gender. Patients are classified by conditions, become disease entities to be managed and represent a mass of impersonal problems generally. Noun phrase examples are 'a cardiac arrest' and 'Thursday clinics'.

Doctor/male

The heroes are very much in the same mould as a 1960s television prototype, the famous Hippocratic heart throb, Ben Casey. A male 'writ large', he embodies feral magnetism and is arrogant, impatient, patronizing, enigmatic and supremely self-assured. Kinetic and proxemic elements support his command of space, and these are indices of status, power, and dominance. Many linguistic structures combine to express coercion and denote purpose; he acts and others react. Mere looks from these powerful figures are capable of ending discussion.

Physical descriptions of these stock male doctors revolve generally around their sheer physicality, attractiveness: he is stalwart, has broad shoulders, possesses a deep authoritarian voice and has dark hair, and there appears to be a magnetic aura about his eyes—with these he invades and controls space and others, and his glance is capable of awakening a constant state of sexual excitation in the heroine.

The power differential between nurse and doctor is crystallized in the doctor's manner of relating—a parent-child typology is used. Linguistically, he makes many declarative statements and is liberal with coercive imperatives and threatening and judgmental interrogatives. These are often buttressed by coercive expressions of possessive modality and also index power—'we', the royal plural. Modal auxillaries strongly reflect a parental ego state—obligation, necessity, authority, giving orders, expressing expectations, and prescribing standards are typical examples.

Nurse/female

The complementary role of the woman/nurse, the subservient partner, is established fully in the opening pages of each text. A salient feature is the relentlessly self-effacing behaviour of the young woman, bolstered by her reactive style of hesitant interaction, and expressions of anxiety of which we read a great deal at the level of bodily manifestations. Many of the common images of nurses—as nonentity, follower, handmaiden, bimbo, sex-symbol and girl-next-door may be observed in the texts.

The relatively weaker, less rational construction of the nurse heroine is conveyed by many processes which over determine the image. She has fewer speaking rights than the doctor despite her positioning as an average example of female subjectivity, from whose point of view, ostensibly, the story is told. Whilst the main character, frequently she is introduced to the reader after the doctors and patients. Her modes of feeling, valuing, perceiving, preoccupations, dependence, limited options, and fretful ambivalences maintain characteristics ascribed to women and nurses. She 'mentally decides', conveying an interesting and redundant term which indicates, possibly, that thinking is either new, hard work, or a hazardous task. Non verbal expressions are congruent with the common affective state of agitation and consternation: embarrassment, blush, adjust hairclip, insides lurching. And all the while, fetching, attractive and desirable—no mean feat.

It is highly revealing that the nurse's first real (and trivial) action is frequently described in a lengthy passage, for example, that of 'adjusting a white hair clip' which is 'holding the frilly cap on her honey blonde curls'. She could hardly be a real Nightingale nurse without the cap. In the reader's first introduction to the heroine, a male, often a patient, is acting upon her: he is the agent and she the affected, as he perhaps 'slips his arm around her trim waist'. Her figure commands a great deal of attention and reference to it is via a prenominal position, thus coding its emphasis: 'the trim waist of young Sister Briony'. Despite the attention of male patients, the nurse is depersonalized and this feature is embedded in the linguistic structures: 'They're a great bunch of nurses' as the patient directs his attention to a representative of that group.

Impersonality and the power relations of hospital hierarchies are reproduced. Possessive pronouns are used liberally to denote nurses as dutiful daughters. Moreover male patients get to use possessives in terms of women/ nurses. Doctors are referred to variously as 'doctor', 'doc', 'the registrar'. Other categories of nursing staff receive uncharacteristically punctilious attention to their places within the hierarchy, for example 'Senior Sister McCullagh', 'Student Nurse Newman', 'the girl', 'the junior'. It is not an infrequent occurrence for the doctors to address the heroine with an impersonal 'you'—'you carry on'.

Myth of holy marriage between nursing and medicine

Ashley (1976) contended that 'the relationship between nursing and medicine is based on the myth of holy marriage between nursing and medicine'. A precarious relationship indeed and mirrored by the construction of heterosexual love and relationships in these texts. At the conclusion to the novels, the status of the hero will console the heroine for her own lack of status and self-esteem. Mirrored here is what has been conceptualized as the 'the narcissistic fit between nursing and medicine' (Muff 1982).

TV NURSE/DOCTOR MELODRAMA AND SOAPS

A detailed analysis of these is not essential for they construct similar representations of nursing, and are sustained by the same ideologies situated within the interstices of the formative discourses as those in nurse/doctor romance fiction. These images match substantially those described by Muff (1982) and Kalisch & Kalisch (1982a, b). United States culture has colonized much of the western world because of the ubiquity of the cultural products of their film and television industries. The range of representations—nurse as nurturant mother, angel of mercy, handmaiden, sex symbol, battleaxe, and token torturer—ride in tandem with those exposed by Muff (1982).

'A Country Practice' is a well meaning attempt to portray nurses in more positive ways, albeit '...still unwittingly reinforcing dominant ideology' (Crisp 1987). 'Over the top' stereotypes are avoided and this realization may be attributed partly to the significant proportion of women involved in all major aspects of the production side. On the other hand, whilst muted, some seductively reasonable (and therefore 'palatable') stereotypes emerge, including the sympathetic portrait of an older nurse as a motherly figure who supports and sustains. Moreover nurses' work commands a more credible representation: a recent episode contained a segment of a younger sister competently performing an emergency tracheostomy. 'The Young Doctors', juxtaposed against the above, reinforces nurses' infantalization in the TV hospital soaps in terms of the trivial activities in which they are involved. The central concerns and driving focus are on romantic relationships, commonly between nurses and doctors. The officious matron is drawn from the battleaxe image.

'Let the Blood Run Free', a 1990 program, is in the genre of satirical comedy and its subgenre category is that of health care. This deliciously frivolous program is not without its seductive attractions, not the least of which are distilled gems of truth which are outrageously overblown. Moments of recognition for nurses are thick on the ground. This program sends up its genre, form, and discourses. Matron Dorothy is an overdetermined site for the projection of multiple fears of the powerful mother figure and nurse as battleaxe and token torturer. Some gems from the second episode include the recap at the beginning of the program which begins, 'In last week's power struggling episode'; and 'matron's reign of terror' is intoned like a magic incantation as matron, resplendent in war medals, a nun's black veil and a sheik's headdress stretches out her arm in a classic, catatonic Hitler pose. In this way references to other terrors are invested in the materiality of the Matron, and it may be argued, thereby expresses the degree of emotion she triggers. The nurses, thus far, are labile, dizzy dames with lots of hair, cleavages, mini level uniforms and the de rigeur caps and aprons. Matron is far more interesting and she metamorphoses into other nursing personas in the blink of a quick dissolve or fade to black. The Ministering Angel's grey uniform is wickedly played off against that of nurse as torturer, when matron delivers a vigorous kick to the Chief Executive Officer's stomach.

This sequence elegantly expresses the psychodynamic splitting process which is a central ego defence operating in many of the conflicting attributions to the nurse as both nurturant and dangerous. This process is due to the failure to assimilate and synthesize less than perfect significant care givers in childhood; whole subjects are not internalized, and each end of the ambivalence or polarity—good and bad—is idealized and disparaged. Transference invokes intense affects and revives the infant/parent relationship. The feelings which belong to the key childhood players are, as in the above matron segment, evoked by superficial similarities—a powerful, ambivalently held mother figure.

RECENT RESEARCH ON PUBLIC PERCEPTION OF NURSES

Lumby &Zetler (1990) alert us to the disquieting lack of change in public perception of nurses, despite their tertiary education and extended roles. They note that 'The media soon reassures us, however, that most of these changes remain hidden or are of no interest to the public'. Their investigation into the 'nature of stereotyping of occupation role information' illuminated that the enduring stereotype, as identified in the United States study they replicated, was 'feminine, nurturant, follower, altruistic...nurses fell into the helping dimension as opposed to the achievement dimension and were on the middle range of intelligence levels just below a repair person, a therapist, a librarian and a business executive'. There are important implications here in regard to positioning and marketing nursing and the enduring stereotypes invite research into the current reasons for attraction to nursing.

NURSING HISTORIOGRAPHY

Many histories of nursing reveal, though they do not reflect critically about, the subjugation of nurses to psychological, emotional, and bodily disciplines. Beyond the first half of this century histories of nursing are replete with rigorous protocols for behaviour and dress on and off duty, and discipline books record a range of petty misdemeanours. Socially constructed qualities of the good nurse are naturalized in the discourses as attributions to nature. Nursing is constructed as a 'calling' requiring the womanly virtues of trustworthiness, neatness, sobriety, quietness, honesty, endurance, obedience, devotion, and unselfishness (Trembath & Hellier 1987, Brodsky 1968, Game & Pringle 1983). Other important features point to the instillation of perfectionistic practices and authoritarian perceptions. Doctors, wary of nurses who 'may not know their place', teach and direct nurses, and ensure that they are not given texts with scientific knowledge. It is noted with interest that these concerns still feature in newspaper articles, letters to the editor pages in newspapers and TV pronouncements by doctors.

Nurses work for love—not money, is a clear ideological construction throughout many histories of nursing. This clever ploy to ensure cheap labour dovetailed for many nurses who perceived a dichotomy between 'professionalism' and 'industrialism'. Brodsky's (1968) history refers to the 'inspired calling'. His chapter headings add a gloss and mobilize prominent nursing metaphors and symbols, for example, 'Rich is the Heritage', 'Miss Nightingale suggests' and 'A new Lamp Shines'. The title is considered unnecessary on the cover: instead three gold embossed lamps suffice. The tone of the text, written by a male doctor, is set by the quote chosen to feature on the page following the table of contents.

Delivered as a speech, on the occasion of a nurses' graduation in 1897, in the author's view it is apparently still relevant in 1968: 'There is no higher mission in life than nursing God's poor. In so doing a woman may not reach the ideals of her soul; she may fall short of the ideals of her head, but she will go far to satiate the longings of her heart from which no woman can escape'! As Brodsky displays no concerns around his right to 'speak nursing history' it is likely that he regarded it as a branch of medical history—not an uncommon overvalued idea—and therefore one on which he could pronounce with authority. This overdeveloped sense of entitlement accords with his assessment of the above quote as an apt one.

Serving God's poor certainly did not yield material rewards for the nurse—for example, the nurses' quarters at the Royal Melbourne Hospital as late as 1910 were known as 'Ratland'. In 1897, Hansard records a parliamentary debate centred around nurses' conditions at the Coast Hospital (Prince Henry). There is an eerie similarity. At that time nurses worked 77 hours per week with one day off per month. Male workers at the same hospital, enjoying the advantage of unions and the vote, worked 8 hours per day. The argument which swayed the debate was put forward by a doctor and his case rested on the view: 'The mother tends her child 10 hours a day, why should not the Sister of Mercy, also?'.

A trenchant gem (Tracy 1908) provides an interesting counterpoint to the above ideologies. She stated:

Clamouring to want to be placed on waiting lists for nursing and to be ministering angels despite 18 hour days, made it possible for employers to impose sweating conditions ... the idealistic convention of nursing life is a pretty phantasy built upon a shelf-full of sixpenny editions and a pile of coloured pictures...and candid truth is better kindness than canting rhapsody!

For the most part until the 1980s, nursing historiography shared many of the features of Whig history, that of the great man in history or in these cases, women, and all come out faultless. Mythologies of history generally are structured on uncritical ideas of progress and triumph. Analogously, 19th century Darwinian notions and crude, linear understandings of psychosexual development are relevant. Further, they tend to be history 'from above'. Feminist historians are rewriting history/herstory, the 'history from below', and exploring how women felt, from an interior perspective. Too frequently histories of nursing have been told from the points of view of doctors, matrons, and administrators. The nature of the discourse is exterior and this is a denial of the feminine and its interiority. It is a masculine discourse which talks about the externals of the social world. These approaches are heavily imbricated in a patriarchal ideology, structuring a domain which functions to keep nurses in submission to medical dominance and reinforcement of the medical model.

It is encouraging that recent seminal work (Curry 1989) maps the rise of medical hegemony in New South Wales psychiatry. This investigation unearthed a medical conspiracy to depose the first administrator (a nurse) at Tarban Creek—now Gladesville Hospital. The evidence of doctors was central and the point of view of administrator Digby was silenced within the dominant institution of the juridical. The positioning of dominant discourse structured the result: a doctor became the administrator. This change effected the adoption of similar models.

NURSES SPEAK THEIR OWN STORIES

Following closely on the decision to transfer nurse education to the tertiary sector, nurses are constructing their own discourses in the fields of research, education, clinical practice, and administration. Caring, nurses as change agents, health promotion, nursing theories and diagnoses are examples of frequent topics of conference papers. Critical theory and other methodological and disciplinary tools are advanced to inform our analysis of nursing.

Nursing texts embody many of the significant features of medical and scientific discourses and have a marked tendency towards classification. Indeed, this may not be avoidable. On the other hand, it is helpful to be aware of the effects of our discourses for these are depersonalizing: the impersonal health care system is reproduced in the texts' linguistic structures. Our discourses are embedded in these classificatory systems. Patients are named after the disorder or symptoms and in the course of this naming, the disorder becomes focal. The patient recedes and is removed to the blurred margins of perception.

Patients' behaviours are presented in linguistic terms which make them appear separated from them, for example, 'non compliant medication taker' (Hodge & Kress 1988). Their behaviours are presented as individual objective entitites which are then reattached to the patient as a disease or symptom. As a consequence, the patient ceases to be regarded as an active, responsible participant in events. Therefore, causation and agency centre around the nurse. A certain kind of displacement operates to reclassify people into nursing categories, so that the term/category, for example, 'non-compliant patient' becomes the name of, and stands in for, the person. Many managerial metaphors are used in this kind of discourse and the individual becomes lost. Once established, the linguistic forms, when in common currency in nursing classification, valuation, and metaphor, as Kress (1985) indicates, 'seem to exert power autonomously'. We need to be vigilant, then, with regard to a careful development of nursing diagnoses which will feature within our developing discipline. Our discourse is now replete with rhetoric around 'holistic care' and 'client centred nursing'. We need to ensure that we adopt a critical approach to our discourse to uncover the possible homogenizing and alienating effects.

NURSING DOCUMENTARIES

'Handmaidens and Battleaxes' (Gillespie 1989) and 'Running Out of Patience' (Everill & Brown 1988) herald a refreshingly critical and empowering approach to the construction of nursing and the legitimate politicized nurse's role in which the cognitive dissonance associated with industrial activity has dissipated. 'Running Out of Patience' was rejected, on the grounds of unacceptable production values, by the Australian Broadcasting Corporation and Special Broadcasting Service. Certainly, due to the circumstances surrounding the filming, the colour at times lacks range and balance and some of the focus pulls needed cleaning up, but as Special Broadcasting Service frequently show experimental films and have a policy of providing air space to independent film-makers, this rejection is most unfortunate. The film is cleverly edited to highlight changed attitudes and values, and contains stills, archival footage, news reports, scenes from the 1986 Victorian nurses' 50-day strike, and interviews with young and older nurses from all levels of nursing. Presented are multiple comments on the strike, reflections on nursing history and socialization, and the powerful feelings surrounding the strike. It is clear that nurses are no longer to be conned and cajoled by the invidiously attractive, vicarious rewards of confusing slavish adherence to the system with catering to patients' needs; and holding, without guilt, expectations for themselves and their profession—like other self regarding groups. These relatively recent convictions are reinforced in the documentary by cutting to archival footage which was constructed propaganda. It served to reinforce the nurse-mother nexus. This heavily ideological footage used heavy-handed symbolism. Its expression in film grammar, connoting of deification of woman as nurse, was pure, demure, and saintly.

NURSE EDUCATION: REPORTS AND VIEWS

The history of the transfer of nurse education in New South Wales from hospital-based settings to the tertiary sector has been well documented (Duffield 1986, Russell 1989). As indicated previously, the public perception of nurses and their roles equates closely with the role and status of women generally within a patriarchal society. The inherent assumptions and values which structure these perceptions were translated and enshrined also in many of the nurse education reports from the 1940s through to their traces in the 1970s. The theory of the 'born nurse', 'nursing as calling' and 'role for women par excellence', makes it all too easy to devalue nursing's complexity, to focus overly on desirable female qualities and to put forward 'bandaid', cosmetic changes in nurse education. If nursing is an inherently female occupation and nurses are born then they require little education. We would do well to remember that work that is valued in our society is heavily ideologically loaded and biased towards upper middle-class males.

The earliest report on nurse education (Kelly 1943) was prepared by a twenty-eight person committee, of whom eleven were doctors. Many others were nurse administrators. This composition was reflected also in many of the other 'expert' inquiries into nurse education, and nurse educators generally were not represented on the committees until the late 1970s. As Russell (1989) notes: 'All produced reports containing many often conflicting recommendations'. Awareness of committee composition is crucial to understanding many of the inbuilt biases and prejudices in the reports. Arguments tended to be based not on educational considerations, but rather service needs, for hospitals were heavily dependent on a large student workforce to keep down costs. It was difficult for doctors and administrators to challenge the foundations of a system of which they were integral parts.

Representations of nurses and nursing which imbue the Kelly report (1943) reflect clearly a role which is an extension into the workplace of the nurturing female role in the home. It is noted with interest here, that probationers' pay is to be regarded as an allowance rather than a wage. The merged nurse-mother role was still evident in reports in the 1960s, and the Bailey Report (1963) declares: 'It must be remembered that we have not at any time...set out to educate nurses—we have concentrated on giving a technical training in support of physical medicine'. The Saint report (1971) reflects a nebulous understanding of nurses' roles and emphasizes qualities such as warmth and sympathy, derived from public perceptions of the ideal woman. The reports from 1943 to 1978 are recommended as a rich primary source of ideology and discourse around the ambivalence with which nursing is regarded generally.

The medical profession has been at the forefront of opposition to the transfer of nurse education to tertiary settings. As Duffield (1986) observes wryly: 'They were concerned that the control of nursing education would be removed from their hand and placed in the domain of educationalists, or worse, nurses themselves'. During the protracted struggle in the late 1970s surrounding the appropriate education for nurses, much press was given to the views of doctors, and prominent members of that profession continued to appropriate speaking rights on behalf of nursing. Legge (1977) stated: 'No surgeon on earth would start an operation assisted by college sisters' in an article entitled 'Academic Nursing Just Won't Work'. Madison (1977), Dean of Medicine at Newcastle, asserted: 'I fear that it [nurse education] could come to be associated with a gradual loss of credibility and relevance and increasing apprehension from the population whom it is our task to serve'.

The public perception of nursing's status is mirrored in the views of editors of print media well into the 1980s. Spence (1989) was granted two full pages to attack changes in nursing education and practice in his article 'Tender Loving Academics'. The editor of that paper printed one small letter of reply from a nurse and refused to accept an article I had written as a response. Certainly neither the editor, nor Spence, nor the Royal Australasian College of Surgeons, from whose report (1987) Spence drew his recommendations, recognized the inappropriateness of one profession setting out recommendations for the education of another profession. These are compelling examples of the pressing need to change public perceptions of nursing.

The subservient, handmaiden nursing role which inspires much medical opinion is not incongruent with that shared by the public. In addition, the following comment, overheard in the mid 1980s, on the occasion of nurse educators and administrators graduating at a college of advanced education in which graduates from other disciplines were participating, speaks for itself: 'Oh, they're giving diplomas to nurses now -they'll be giving them to the garbos next'. In a recent sympathetic article (Stynes 1990), the traces of medical hegemony are evident in the title of the article 'Medical Professionals at Last'.

CONCLUSION

Historically, nurses have been cloistered, disciplined, and shaped by a medically dominated authoritarian hierarchy. This has been, in large measure, internalized by nurses. Their individual psyches have been subjected to structuring by powerful ideologies centring around medicine, family, and gender. Nursing has been spoken by others. Projected fears around women and their ascribed characteristics have assisted the cultural production of dysfunctional myths and stereotypes of nurses and nursing. The devaluing of nurses, and women, has been a consequence. We need to examine the processes which make the following unconsciously induced association so automatic—and enshrine it in the print media. In an article entitled 'East Sydney Residents Want Brothels Licensed', Totaro (1983) outlines recommendations from a State Government report, which includes 'It says that younger prostitutes could be trained to move to other areas of work and that this re-education could be effected by implementing rules currently applying to nurses'. For those interested in a damning example of a fusion of both roles and images, the personal column of *The Glebe* (Anon 1990) has this to offer: 'Attractive nurse gives erotic examinations at her home'.

It is time to attempt to close the gap between media, medical, and nursing representations of nurses and their roles. It is imperative that we develop a coherent national nursing policy and strategic plans to ameliorate the current constructions in the public domain which work against and subvert our claims for autonomy and accountability to our own profession. The discipline of nursing will not advance unless there is radical revision in the public perception of nurses and nursing. Further, the current images make it difficult for patients to enter a trust relationship with us, and it is also difficult to mobilize support for independent practice roles, including those centred around the nurse as primary therapist or caregiver. The task is a difficult one, and some of the constraints have been highlighted in this chapter.

The Kalisch team (1983) provide many helpful strategies and suggest avenues through which we may begin to make incursions. They indicate that negative public images and perceptions may foster attraction to nursing for ill conceived reasons. (This in turn impacts on retention rates in the profession.) They also claim that policy makers' decisions and perceptions of other health professionals are informed by negative public images.

An important first step in changing public perceptions would involve data collection. As part of national policy, our professional organizations could set up and coordinate state and regional centres for systematic mass media monitoring.

State committees would be well placed to devise standardized material for media analyses and guidelines including protocols. Subsequent to media monitoring, we need to implement a multi-dimensional strategic plan to comment on media portrayals and to reconstruct public perceptions and images. The avenues include: 'letter to the editor' columns; writing articles for women's magazines in an easily readable style; using networks to lobby broadcasters; offering scriptwriters the free consultation service of specialist nursing groups; developing relationships with print journalists who specialize in health issues; gaining airtime on talkshows and in alternative broadcasting services; providing media information kits on nursing, including specialist policy documents, to relevant media personnel.

This chapter has been structured by my deliberate choices of discursive alignment. Examples of my partial deconstructions of dominant discourses and representations, along with selections of analytical tools, suggest ways of revealing ideologies from a critical reading position. As Speedy (1987) has observed: 'If the opportunity for an alliance between nursing and feminism is rejected, nursing may spend its future fighting the same battles it has for decades, and nothing could be more wasteful!'. Moreover, the rejection of this alliance serves to undermine attempts to work towards the establishment of the discipline. It is imperative that the prerequisite radical revision of public perceptions of nurses and nursing be foregrounded urgently as agenda for national nursing policy directions.

REFERENCES

Anon 1990 Advertisement in personal column. The Glebe, 15 March, Sydney
Ashley J 1976 Hospitals, paternalism and the role of the nurse. Teachers College Press, New York
Bailey D 1963 Survey on nurse education in Western Australia for the Nurses Registration Board, Perth
Barthes R 1973 Mythologies. Granada, London
Baudrillard J 1981 For a critique of the political economy of the sign. Telos Press, St Louis
Brodsky I 1968 Sydney's nurse crusaders. Old Sydney Free Press, Sydney
Chesler P 1972 Women and madness. Doubleday, New York, p 67-68
Cixous H 1980 Where is she. La jeune nee. In: Marks E, de Courtivron I (eds) New French Feminisms. Harvester, Brighton, p 90-91
Crisp J 1987 No message, no sex, just good fun: dealing with gender representation in popular films. Hecate 13 (1): 76
Curry G 1989 The select committee on the lunatic asylum Tarban Creek, 1846: The medicalization of mental nursing in New South Wales. MA dissertation, unpublished
Derrida J 1967 L'Ecriture et la differance. Seuil, Paris
Duffield C 1986 Nursing in Australia comes of age! International Journal of Nursing Studies 23(4): 282
Everill S, Brown C 1988 Running out of patience. Australian Film Institute, ACT
Fiedler L 1988 Images of the nurse in fiction and popular culture. In: Jones A (ed) Images of nurses. Perspectives from history, art, and literature. University of Pennsylvania Press, Philadelphia, p 101
Foucault M 1972 The archaeology of knowledge. Tavistock, London

Game A, Pringle R 1983 Gender at work. Allen & Unwin, Sydney
Gillespie R 1989 Handmaidens and battleaxes. The real story of nursing. Silver Films Production, Australian Film Institute, ACT
Hodge R, Kress G 1988 Social semiotics. Polity Press, Cambridge
Johnstone M 1989 Bioethics. An Australian nursing perspective. Harcourt Brace Jovanovich, Melbourne
Kalisch B, Kalisch P 1983 Improving the image of nursing. American Journal of Nursing 83 (January): 48-52
Kalisch P, Kalisch B 1982a Nurses on primetime television. American Journal of Nursing 82 (February): 264-270
Kalisch P, Kalisch B 1982b The image of the nurse in novels. American Journal of Nursing 82 (August): 1220-1224
Kelly C (Chairperson) 1943 First Report for Committee for reorganization of the nursing profession. Government Printer, Sydney
Kingston B 1975 My wife, my daughter and poor Mary Ann. Women and work in Australia. Nelson, Melbourne
Kress G 1985 Linguistic processes in sociocultural practice. Deakin University Press, Geelong, p 61
Lacan J 1977 Ecrits. A selection. Tabistock, London
Legge D 1977 Letter on nursing education. The Age, 5 December
Lukes S 1974 Power. A radical view. Macmillan, London p 24
Lumby J, Zetler J 1990 Images of nursing—1980 or 1990? Paper presented to Royal Australian College of Nursing, Australia Conference, Sydney
Madisson D 1977 Letter on nursing. Newcastle Morning Herald, 28 May:
Moi T 1985 Sexual/textual politics. Routledge, London p 104
Muff J (ed) 1982 Socialization, sexism, and stereotyping: women's issues in nursing. C V Mosby, St Louis, p 300-306
Radway J 1984 Reading the romance. Women, patriarchy and popular culture. University of North Carolina Press, Chapel Hill, p 17
Royal Australasian College of Surgeons 1987 Submission to inquiry on professional issues in nursing. Melbourne
Russell R L 1989 Nursing education: a time for change 1960-1980. Australian Journal of Advanced Nursing 5(4):36
Saint E 1971 (Chairperson) Report of the Committee of Inquiry into Nursing, 'Nursing in Queensland'. Royal Australian Nursing Federation, Brisbane
Snitow A (ed) 1983 Desire. The politics of sexuality. Virago, London, p 264, 274
Speedy S 1987 Feminism and the professionalization of nursing. Australian Journal of Advanced Nursing 4(2):27
Spence D 1989 Tender loving academics. The Independent Monthly (September):40-41
Stynes J 1990 Medical professionals at last. Financial Review, 25 September:42
Totaro P 1983 East Sydney residents want brothels licensed. Sydney Morning Herald, 15 February:5
Tracy B 1908 Ministering Angels. The Lone Hand, Sydney
Trembath R, Hellier D 1987 All care and responsibility: a history of nursing in Victoria 1850-1934. Florence Nightingale Committee, Melbourne
Tuchman G, Daniels A, Benét J (eds) 1978 Hearth and home. Images of women in the mass media. Oxford University Press, New York, p 3, 28

FURTHER READING

Baudrillard J 1983 Simulations. Semiotexte, New York
Birckhauser-Oëri S 1988 The mother. Archetypal image in fairy tales. Inner City Books, Toronto
Bolinger D 1980 Language. The loaded weapon. Longman, London
Bonney B, Wilson H 1983 Australia's commercial media. Macmillan, Melbourne
Coward R 1983 Patriarchal precedents. Sexuality and social relations. Routledge & Kegan Paul, London
Culler J 1983 On deconstruction. Theory and criticism after structuralism. Routledge &

Kegan Paul, London

Davies C (ed) 1981 Rewriting nursing history. Croom Helm, London

Eco U 1981 The role of the reader. Explorations in the semiotics of texts. Hutchinson, London

Eisenstein H 1984 Contemporary feminist thought. Unwin Paperbacks, Sydney

Foucault M 1973 Madness and civilization. A history of insanity in the age of reason. Vintage Books, New York

Foucault M 1976 The birth of the clinic. An archaeology of medical perception. Tavistock Publications, London

Foucault M 1979 Discipline and punish. The birth of the prison. Vintage, New York

Foucault M 1980 Power/Knowledge. Selected interviews and other writings 1972-1977. The Harvester Press, Sussex

Foucault M 1980 The history of sexuality. Volume 1: An introduction. Vintage Press, New York

Kress G, Hodge R 1981 Language as ideology. Routledge, London

Maggs C 1987 (ed) Nursing history: the state of the art. Croom Helm, Kent

Miller J 1978 Toward a new psychology of women. Penguin Books, Middlesex

Modleski T 1984 Loving with a vengance. Mass-produced fantasies for women. Methuen, London

Rich A 1979 On lies, secrets and silence. Selected prose 1966-1978. Norton, New York

Sontag S 1977 Illness as metaphor. Penguin Books, Middlesex

Vance C 1984 (ed) Pleasure and danger. Exploring female sexuality. Routledge & Kegan Paul, London

21. Theory: where are we going and what have we missed along the way?

Colin Holmes

'Would you tell me, please, which way I ought to go from here?'
'That depends a good deal on where you want to get to', said the Cat.
'I don't much care where—' said Alice.
'Then it doesn't matter which way you go', said the Cat.

(*Alice's Adventures in Wonderland*, 'The Pig and the Pepper', Lewis Carroll)

INTRODUCTION

I wish to argue that nursing theorists have failed to address a number of fundamental issues, and to suggest a few areas of scholarship which may serve as a springboard for more comprehensive theorization. Among other things, nurse theorists fail to provide substantial accounts of the relationship between theory and practice; to explicate a notion of nursing as political action; and to substantiate adequately descriptions of nursing as scientific or aesthetic activity. It is imperative that nurses explore the possibilities for a consciously designed future for nursing, and I have supplied extensive references so that readers may find their own starting points. In view of the extensive literature around nursing ethics, I have omitted discussion of related notions of nursing as an ethical activity. In conclusion, however, I have ventured some brief speculations concerning the directions which nursing theory may eventually take.

THE THEORY–PRACTICE RELATIONSHIP

Theory has traditionally been viewed as being developed through deductive or inductive processes, that is arguing from the abstract to the specific or vice versa. Whilst the inductive approach regards practice as a research resource from which to infer theory, the deductive approach utilizes abstract ideas to construct theory, which is then tested through research. These processes thus imply, if not entail, certain constraints on the theory-practice relationship. Deductive methods suggest that theory stands in a superior position to practice, and that unlike theories in the natural sciences, which have traditionally been representational (even accounting for unpredictability, uncertainty, and sudden discontinuities), nursing theories have a normative role, attempting to influence practice in ways which, for example, will lead to better nursing care. Ironically, whilst it seeks to provide ideals and inform the aspirations of practitioners, a major problem with this theory-down approach is that practice actually comes to be regarded as having little inherent value in the construction of theory, except as a testing ground. Indeed, the biggest challenge for deductivists may be to avoid the charge of elitism, by convincing practitioners that their own experiences and insights are inherently valuable. That much nursing theory is regarded as irrelevant and obscure is testimony to a failure to acknowledge the importance of, and to communicate effectively with, the ordinary practitioner, and to develop theories that are adequate to everyday practice needs.

Sandra Speedy (1989) feels that the main problem with over valuing theory is actually that 'we may search for ever for one theory to explain every nursing situation and then adhere to it'. This seems contradictory. How can we adhere to a single theory, if we are searching forever for that theory? If we will never find it, how can we adhere to it? In any case, there does not appear to be anything inherently wrong with undertaking such a quest, even if it is interminable, since it could be viewed as a search for excellence and may serve valuable purposes. Furthermore, placing theory before practice does not actually entail a search for a single, all-encompassing theory as she suggests, nor does it imply that a stage would be reached in which the development of theory would come to an end. Such a conclusion would only be thinkable in the context of an outmoded positivist epistemology which incorporated a simplistic representational theory of truth, taken to refer to a single, static reality. As soon as one casts off the shackles of Platonic absolutism, however, and admits that reality is constructed, socially or otherwise, deductivism is liberated and becomes pregnant with multiple possibilities.

Benner & Wrubel (1989) describe practice and theory as being 'in dialogue', and are concerned that if theory is separated from, and valued above practice, it will be imposed on practice. In fact this appears to have been exactly what has happened over the last decade or so, and one ironic consequence has been the devaluing of theory by practitioners. Benner & Wrubel's account identifies abstract theory as referring to 'an imagined ideal of nursing', and then disparages this by emotively juxtaposing it with 'actual expert nursing as it is practised today'. But here's the rub! Firstly, much nursing 'as it is practised today' is probably not expert in the way that Benner uses that term, and is not an appropriate basis from which to draw inferences about good practice—which must surely be the kind of practice on which nursing theory ought to be predicated. It may be countered that Benner & Wrubel specifically induce theory from *expert practice*, but this only raises another problem—how are we to recognize expert practice? What parameters should we employ? How will we know that the nursing is the best possible under the circumstances? Any answers to these questions must draw on concepts of health, nursing, person, and so on, in other words on nursing theory, and we are back to where we started!

Finally, how can we improve nursing practice unless we have something greater than practice to draw on—something that transcends practice, to guide us forward? Practice-derived theory actually appears to be logically incapable of providing a way forward, because it has no foundation on which to construct ideals for practice other than practice itself. At the very least, it exhibits an inflated estimation of practice which blinds it to the need for progress, and an insularity which prevents it from providing the vision which will inspire practitioners. Just as theorists working from abstract principles or metatheories must be wary of making theory so abstruse that it becomes incomprehensible to practitioners, theorists working from an explication of practice must be careful not to become a party to the mystification of practice, by which it assumes unjustifiably esoteric significance. If Benner's (1984) rehabilitation of practice is the major reason for the increasing popularity of her work, theory is clearly being employed for its rhetorical and political value. It cannot be denied that theories are implicit in practice, as indeed they are in the way in which we conduct ourselves in the world at large and in the way we make sense of that world. That is, after all, what a theory is supposed to help us do. This much is clear from the work of social psychologists, especially those working in cognitive psychology, and in particular attribution theory (Hewson 1983), which seeks to uncover such phenomena as 'lay epistemologies' (Kruglanski 1980, Kruglanski & Jaffe 1983), 'implicit personality theories' (Furnham 1989), implicit ethical theories (Lerner 1970, Semin & Manstead 1983), and theories of causality (Jaspars 1983). These are characterized by the whole gamut of internal psychodynamic and cognitive strategies to which humans are prone, contributing to a whole panorama of misconceptions and misinterpretations, which in turn lead to prejudice, racism, sexism, ageism, homophobia, unreasonableness, and so forth. Just as we would not wish these to serve as guides for social policy or practice, so we should not want implicit theories of nursing alone to underpin the philosophy of nursing and its practice.

NURSING AS SCIENCE

The majority of nurse academics have regarded 'nursing theory' as a stepping-stone to the growth of nursing as a science, and some have acknowledged that this was in turn a means of establishing professional autonomy. In other words, it served unashamedly political purposes. American authors in particular consistently assumed, however, particularly during the 1970s, that a purpose of nursing theory was to establish nursing as a science, as many of the important papers reproduced in Nicoll (1986) testify, including those by Abdellah, Chinn & Jacobs, Fawcett, Gortner, Hardy, Jacox, Dorothy Johnson, Leininger, Peplau, and Silva & Rothbart (Carper's monumental paper stands as a glorious exception). Although it is difficult to distinguish strategic from rational discourse here, it is clear from their addended comments that many of the authors continue to take this view, and some, Parse for example, even prefer the phrase 'nursing science' to nursing theory, and 'nurse scientist' to nurse theorist.

Now all this talk of science and scientists might not be a matter for concern if these writers subscribed to a view of science which acknowledged that natural, social, and human sciences have much in common that transcends outmoded positivistic philosophy. Some nurse theorists and practitioners have rejected such a philosophy and preferred to go down the track suggested by Jean Watson (1985a, 1985b) of anti-positivist humanistic, holistic, person-oriented philosophies, but in doing so many have simply repeated criticisms of positivism which were elaborated at the turn of the century by neo-Kantian German social philosophers (notably Windelband, Rickert, and Dilthey). They have thus addressed a long-discarded scientism which sees all true knowledge to derive from science alone. We may say that this approach has been conceived as mechanistic, analytic, objective, static, and reactive, and is often contrasted with nursing's aspirations, which are increasingly holistic, subjective, dynamic, and interactive (Holmes 1990). However, metatheories of science are being developed which are not simply antipositivist (see summaries in Stockman 1983), but which actually attempt to place these approaches within a single unified metatheory (see Outhwaite 1987, for a review).

These metatheories would allow the word 'science' to be used legitimately of positivistic and alternative approaches without infidelity to a coherent articulation of underlying philosophy. Those who have worked in this direction include the critical school, notably Jürgen Habermas (beginning with Habermas 1968), Anthony Giddens (1979, 1982), and the neorealists such as Mary Hesse (1980) and Roy Bhaskar (1978, 1979, 1986). Mary Hesse, for example, views the tenets of early Habermasian post positivism as part of the new scientific orthodoxy. If this new rapprochement was acknowledged by the nurse theorists and their commentators when they use the word 'science', our concern would be unfounded and our attention would shift to the integrity of their metatheoretical position. Unfortunately, I do not generally find this to be the case. Time and time again, nursing theory is submitted to analysis of the most blatantly positivist kind (Hardy 1974, Menke 1983, Winkler, Fitzpatrick & Whall 1983).

Consider a recent example. Barbara Sarter (1990) disappointingly reiterates the old arguments in favour of nursing science and rigorous scientific investigation, even listing the goals of science to include not only description, explanation, and prediction but also control. This is rather surprising in view of her recent championship of an exciting holistic nursing theory based on the philosophy of 'evolutionary idealism' (Sarter 1987). According to this philosophy, which echoes the theories of Martha Rogers and Margaret Newman, the fundamental substance of the universe is consciousness, and like the post-Hegelian antirationalism of Bergson and Teilhard de Chardin, it sees that consciousness as being in a process of constant evolution. One of its strengths, as Sarter sees it, is that this conceptualization actually encompasses the whole range of human experience, including mystical and moral, as well as scientific, in a way that is not possible within a materialist, positivist philosophy. It certainly seems odd that she feels impelled to refer to it as providing a metaphysical foundation for holistic nursing science, and to characterize that science in such conventional terms. It seems nonsensical to construct theories in one paradigm, and then evaluate them using criteria drawn from another.

Perhaps some comfort could be drawn from the frequent appeals of nurse theorists to Thomas Kuhn's (1962) antipositivistic work on scientific revolutions and the notion of paradigms. His thesis has been profitably used by many leading nurse academics, including Susan Gortner (1983), Margaret Newman (1990), and Hildegard Peplau (1987), and by Munhall & Oiler (1986) in their influential research textbook. Now, although Kuhn's work suggested that the development of scientific knowledge is necessarily both non-rational and non-cumulative, it is also clear that his arguments drew exclusively on the history of the natural sciences, and none of these authors has ever attempted to justify its translation into the field of nursing. This is either a serious oversight, or they see nursing as paradigmatically a natural science. The insights of Kuhn's work are based on his examination of forms of scientific enquiry with a very long history, which have been applied specifically to the physical world, in an attempt to explain the continuities and discontinuities which characterize it. The objects and purposes of such an enterprise, and the social and intellectual contexts in which they occurred, were quite different to those of present-day nursing. In any case, Kuhn had 'second thoughts' (1977) and modified his views in ways which have generally not been accounted for by nurse theorists (Fry 1990). Furthermore, his arguments have been strongly criticized by a number of philosophers of science (Laudan 1977, Shapere 1981), and have been admitted as problematic in relation to the social sciences, to the extent that Holland (1990) refers to a 'paradigm plague' which demands curative and preventive measures. It is fair to claim that the dominating position in the philosophy of science assumed by Kuhn's views, as they appeared in 1962, has largely been usurped by those of Laudan (1977) and his respondents, and one of the points Laudan makes is that the notion of rationality being employed by Kuhn's supporters is too narrow and equates too directly with outmoded logical positivism.

Nursing theory is beset by a problem not encountered with such force in the natural sciences, and that is the conflict between generalism and specificity. A comprehensive theory of nursing should provide generalized characterizations which apply to nursing in all its forms, and lately it is the characterization of 'care and caring' which has taken 'pole position' in the race to substantiate a unique and overriding professional characteristic. However, whether it is abstracted from principles or derived from practice, if nursing theory is to have relevance for practitioners it must be applicable, and in order to be applicable it must have insights and consequences which are specific enough to guide practice in particular cases. In the natural sciences the problem of specificity rarely arose in the past because theories were predicated on the assumption of a stable and consistent universe, in some sense pre-existing and waiting to be ever-more precisely represented in theory. Even the discontinuities, inconsistencies, and randomness, which have been discovered in such areas as particle physics and astrophysics, are 'accounted for' in the associated theories, drawing, for example, on probability theory and computer modelling. As Laudan (1977) points out, the evaluative criterion for scientific theory has traditionally been, and largely remains, the extent to which it may be considered true, rather than in terms of its usefulness. In nursing, such a 'natural science' approach would be misguided for several reasons.

Firstly, nursing theory which simply mirrored reality, or conversely, was a purely hypothetical abstraction, would be quite valueless unless it had implications for practice. Unlike positivistic scientific theories, nursing theories could be seen as having an inherently prescriptive role, in which theoretical statements have implications for the conduct of nursing as well as vice versa. This means that they are engaged in a dialectical relationship with complex social processes, as well as with individual social actors. Nursing theories are therefore required to address issues arising at both the macro- and micro-level simultaneously and interactively. Herein lies at least one major problem. Because they are either too general to apply in a given case, or too specific to have any transferability, nursing theories which seek to inform practice appear, from a traditional positivist perspective, to be caught in a no-win situation.

Furthermore, because nursing addresses such a complex network of human phenomena, simplistic notions of discoverable truth might reasonably be thought out of the question. It is heartening to admit that many nurse researchers have already left such disputes far behind, albeit unresolved, and are drawing on a mixture of introspective, reflective, ethnographic, grounded-theory, phenomenological, hermeneutic, critical, and feminist methods. Some have even begun to adopt post structuralist methodologies (Dzurec 1989, Dickson 1990, Hazelton 1990, for example), drawing on the work of Foucault and others. Even allowing for the inevitable delay in absorbing new philosophies, it seems that whilst nurses display great creativity in the construction of their nursing theory, they generally fail to capitalize on the insights developed by epistemologists, and philosophers of science which increasingly inform nursing research.

NURSING AS POLITICAL ACTION

In a recent search of two major international computerized data facilities, which incorporate all nursing and sociological literature published during the last 15 years, inputting the word 'nursing' resulted in thousands of references. The word 'Marxism' similarly yielded a few thousand references. The two words together, however, yielded not a single one in either facility! This is remarkable in itself, and would not occur in any other arena of social or intellectual endeavour. Given nursing's history of oppression and exploitation, the recent interest in 'the politics of nursing', and an increasingly political agenda, this lacuna is truly amazing. Jo Ann Ashley (1978), a true nursing visionary, made an impassioned plea for politico-historical study in nursing. She wrote: '...studying and understanding the past gives one the courage to create and respond to what is new without fear of losing one's identity with the whole of humanity'. The purpose and value of historical research, she maintained, is 'to help people to creatively overcome the binding chains of the past'—in other words it is political. The complete failure to acknowledge nursing's socio-historical embeddedness, and to articulate any political position, never mind construct any specific political program, must be considered major weaknesses in contemporary nursing theory. Substantive theoretical analysis cannot be isolated from historical and contextual critique, and nursing desperately needs the kind of critical-historical analyses which will enable its theories to be viewed in their wider sociopolitical and intellectual contexts. These must be recognized and their significance appraised if we aspire to 'create and respond to what is new' as Ashley (1978) suggested.

It has long since been established that the notion of politically neutral theory is logically as well as practically impossible, even if that theory falls clearly within the framework of natural science (see Keat 1981, Popkewitz 1984, and consider the political significance of androcentric scientific discourse described by feminist scholars). That the theorist is a participant in the reality which she/he seeks to explain, has consequences not only for positivism but also for the notion of scientific objectivity, and Weber's arguments against the possibility of value-free science have been repeatedly elaborated and extended (Keat & Urry 1975).

In fact, the very language in which theories are framed has political significance (Burton & Carlen 1979, for example), and is considered by critical theorists and post structuralists alike to constitute a major vehicle through which dominant ideologies are transmitted, sustained and reproduced. The ideological partisanship of language has recently become especially apparent to nurses through feminist critiques (Macdonnell 1986, Weedon 1987), and is particularly significant in nursing's struggle to overcome subjugative power structures (Garmarnikow 1978, Willis 1983). The use of oppressive discourse has recently been nicely exposed in the case of Australian medical domination, by Hazelton (1990). To use the language of the marketplace reduces health care to a commodity, and implies attitudes and beliefs founded on political preferences regarded by some as incompatible with prevailing nursing values. McGivern (1988) suggests that nurses ought to learn and use such language, but see, for example, the controversial comments of Myra Levine, (1989). The language of quality assurance is particularly vulnerable to this kind of criticism because, wherever it develops, its concepts and practices inevitably constitute a reproduction of the dominant political ideology (Harris 1987, Mulkay, Ashmore & Pinch 1987, Holmes 1989, for example, on the use of 'QALYS').

The development of self-care notions in nursing and the readiness with which they have been translated into practice, and the phenomenological and humanistic philosophies of Paterson and Zderad, Watson & Benner, are products of the fierce individualism ('you-are-what-you-make-yourself') which underpins the political conservatism of the United States. According to this ideology, as former English Prime Minister Margaret Thatcher insists, there is no such thing as society...there are only individuals. Society is simply an aggregation of individuals, and any attempt to explain or understand it except in such terms amounts to reification. All notions of socially constructed knowledge, or of rationality itself as socially constructed—indeed any of the so-called 'externalist theories' which seek to establish the locus of control outside individuals—are rejected. It is partly for these reasons that the sociology of knowledge is repeatedly described as fraudulent by conservative thinkers (apparently including Laudan, 1977), and in the wake of the international resurgence of conservatism we are undoubtedly witnessing a return to internalist theories, which regard the individual as the locus of control for social behaviour.

Whilst Levine (1989) criticizes the stress placed on person-centred approaches and the responsibility of the individual vis-a-vis her/his involvement in health care decisions, and choice of particular lifestyles and values, she fails to see that these reflect concepts of the person and of social relations which are products of the ideology underlying North American capitalism. More substantially, Williams's (1989) critique of individualistic health promotion is harnessed to a summary of critiques of classical liberalism. The individualist model assumes that individuals' health status is determined primarily by their own behavioural and circumstantial choices, that individuals are responsible for their own health status and, furthermore, that individuals therefore have a responsibility to undertake self-care and adopt a healthy lifestyle (Hill & Smith 1985, Pender 1982). Williams's earlier research (1987) suggests that these beliefs are typical of many nurses. She concludes that they are at odds with the explicit commitment of the American Nurses' Association to egalitarianism, and suggests that the community may be better served through the adoption of a model based on a feminist conception of health. She calls for a redefinition of nursing practice that will 'orient nurses and nursing towards interventions at the macrosocial level to promote health' (1989). She calls us to political activism in the service of health, and to begin our preparation for this by examining our own experiences of structurally imposed constraints on personal choice.

Sara Fry (1990) claims of Laudan (1977) that 'he offers nursing a view of scientific rationality that can be properly called the philosophy of nursing science'. Bearing in mind some of the implications of Laudan's position, I wonder if this is really what nurses want? He rejects all forms of historicism (and with it Kuhn's historical interpretation), the whole sociology of knowledge enterprise, and the thesis I suggested above, namely that scientific theory is necessarily sociopolitically or ideologically coloured. The consequences of this philosophy for nursing are profound, and I believe that we would do well to devote some time considering our position.

There is resistance, particularly in the United States, to anything that smacks of Marxism, but a couple (literally) of brave nurses have ventured into that territory. One (Crowley 1989a), has analyzed the political significance of the development of 'nurse consultants' in terms of Marxist accounts of the aspirations of the petit bourgeois. The other, Jo Ann Ashley, has pointed out that nursing has long been an industry and that nurses are part of the world of industrial alienation and economic domination. She calls on nurse theorists to incorporate economic theories into their analyses, and writes '...a Marxist interpretation of our struggles and difficulties is imperative for providing new understandings of our plight in the world...such an interpretation would also shed light on the dehumanization and disintegration observable within the North American health care system, as well as the class struggles within the nursing profession and medical hierarchy' (1978). She goes on to provide a brief class analysis of the American system, and shows how closely it fits the Marxist analysis of class struggle. Whilst I am not arguing that we should all necessarily be Marxists, I am saying that the political issue is one that nursing theory cannot avoid. As Jean Watson (1990) points out, 'the personal is political'; and we may add that nursing is political, and nursing theory is political. To let it remain implicit is itself a political act, substantiating and perpetuating the status quo, and repeating all the mistakes that have sustained nursing's oppression in the past. It gives nurses the impression that nursing is apolitical, that politics is to do with governments and institutions rather than with individuals, that they have nothing to say that is politically significant, that they are politically powerless, and that they are safe to remain in a state of political naivety. But we know that need not be the case (for examples and advice, Spengler 1976, Archer & Goehner 1982, Kalisch & Kalisch 1982, Mason & Talbott 1985, Salvage 1985, White 1985, Clay 1987).

Nursing theories conceived within a metatheoretical context of 'critical theory', would embody a concept of emancipation which is relevant here, and Frankfurtian or Habermasian versions are just beginning to be evidenced in the literature. In addition to the well-known but brief paper by

Holter (1988) on critical theory and nursing, and the reply by Lorenson (1988), a number of nurse academics and clinicians have noted that critical theory may have something to offer nursing (Thompson 1983, 1985, 1987, Hickson 1988, Kendall 1989). In Australia, Deakin University School of Nursing has begun to attract attention as a testing-ground for curricula which draw on Habermasian theory, and for its explorations of critical approaches to nursing theory (witness contributions to the present volume; also Street 1988, Hickson 1990). Furthermore, a number of its undergraduate, Masters and Doctoral students, are presently utilizing forms of critical research paradigm or researching nursing's relationship with critical theory. The writings of Anneli Sarvimäki (1986, 1988a), from the University of Helsinki, have drawn on Habermas's theory of communicative interaction, and her Doctoral thesis (Sarvimäki 1988b) contains critiques of a wealth of alternative epistemological frameworks, many of which are virtually unknown to Anglo-American scholarship. Adoption of such theories constitutes an explicit politicization of nursing theory. Habermas's genealogy through the Frankfurt School is essentially neo-Marxist of course, and an unequivocal objective of his social philosophy is the end of traditional capitalist forms of society (Habermas 1985).

He wants to see an end to structures of oppression and domination, in favour of a society in which social differences cease to be important, and his notion of the 'ideal speech situation' (Habermas 1970) as the medium for emancipatory action (Broniak 1988) appeals to many nurses today for obvious reasons (i.e. Brown 1989).

It is interesting to note that, whether or not it is fair to abbreviate aspects of Habermas in this way, his own approach is one of deconstruction and reconstruction through historical analysis. Of course, historicism, in the form of historical materialism, is a central plank of the Marxist method. It represents another reason why nurses who sympathize with these approaches should undertake the writing of the critical history of their profession, through which they can draw understandings to construct theories that are politically explicit, ideologically unequivocal, and socio-economically informed.

It is regrettable that the diverse factors which have recently stimulated a reinterpretation of nursing through the eyes of feminism—a reinterpretation which involves the deconstruction and reconstruction of some of the most fundamental nursing phenomena like caring, pain, health, and illness—have not yet attracted a socio-historical contextual analysis. Feminist perspectives interlock with post modernism on one hand, with its rejection of universals, its deconstruction and reinterpretation of the familiar, and its promise of a radical new worldview; and with critical social theories on the other, with their subordination of science, their methodological flexibility and emancipatory intentions. What underlying tensions, what changes in thinking, in sociopolitical circumstances, in the philosophy of knowledge, have created the circumstances in which this can happen, and eventually impact on nursing? Miller (1988) attempted to answer some of these questions from a critical social science perspective, and confirmed that key themes which interlocked feminism with nursing included the notion of the personal as political, marginality and invisibility, and the paradoxicality of nursing goals. Other nurses generating, and caught up in, these changes will need to explore the issues by entering into a self-reflective process through which they become sensitive to the larger intellectual, social, and political forces which are shaping their thought.

NURSING AS AESTHETIC ACTIVITY

Most nurse theorists concede that nursing is both an art and a science, and some place great value on the artistic component, seeing it as the dimension which adds quality to technical proficiency. But where is the understanding of nursing as an art expressed in nursing theory? We are beset by problems when we insist that nursing is an art, and yet nurse theorists have consistently failed to draw on the vast literature which has developed since the earliest times around the subject of aesthetics and the theory of art. We need to draw on such theories and insights in order to clarify and elaborate our own aesthetic vocabulary. How else can we articulate our notion of, and questions about, nursing as an art? The accumulated insights of philosophical aesthetic traditions would surely give greater coherence and clarity to our ideas, and provide us with a foundation for entering into the discussions taking place in other disciplines concerning, for example, the nature of artistic performance, aesthetic evaluation, and the art-craft-technology nexus. It would perhaps be churlish to suggest that this is another case of interdisciplinary learning being sacrificed on the altar of professional autonomy, but it could justifiably be regarded as a case of intellectual arrogance serving only to alienate, rather than win over, colleagues in other academic disciplines.

Even though Osborne (1968) is surely right in suggesting that 'we need to clarify and elaborate our own aesthetic vocabulary...for without words in which to clothe them our ideas lack coherence and our thinking and apprehension are muddled', following Paterson & Zderad (1976) we can frame some fundamental questions, and perhaps I can list some of the more obvious ones. In what sense is nursing an art? What right have we to insist that nursing *is* an art? To what does the word *art* refer here? How important in this context is the *process* of art as compared to the *product*? What epistemological and ontological status has *aesthetic knowledge*, and is it to be identified with that derived from the apprehension of a work of art? Ought we to characterize expert nursing as a *craft*, and if we do, is that different to saying it is an art, or is craft a category of art? Where do *artistry and skill* fit into the picture? Is all therapeutic nursing a form of art, and is all artistic nursing therapeutic? What is the significance of the relationship between the notion of nursing as art, and the posited relationships between art, truth, and beauty? What is the relationship of aesthetic experience to other types of human experience? How does this perspective help us to improve the quality of nursing care? How does it articulate with the way we conceive the ultimate objectives of nursing care?

Generally, nurse theorists have not asked such questions, and if they are slow to respond to the latest philosophies of science, they are even slower to introduce an explicit aesthetic component into their work. Certainly, Carper (1978), Watson (1979, 1985a), and Benner (1984) have made concessions in this direction, but they have not attempted any prolonged or detailed theorization on nursing aesthetics. Jean Watson regards human science as subsuming aesthetics, ethics, intuition, and process discovery, and she has utilized Heidegger's philosophy of language as a basis for analyzing clients' poetic expression, but at no point does she articulate an explicitly aesthetic theoretical component. Some effort is beginning to be made (Diers 1990, O'Brien 1990, 1991, Lumby 1991), but most nurse academics simply acknowledge that nursing is a science and an art, then concentrate exclusively on the scientific component, so that whilst Nightingale's characterization is in some sense true, that sense still awaits explication in nursing theory.

Aesthetics and nursing as art

As an introduction to what aesthetics may have to offer nurses, I put before the reader a rather haphazard hors-d'ouvres made up from a miscellany of influential positions and opinions. Detailed accounts and analyses of most of these can easily be pursued in aesthetics texts such as Hospers (1969), Dickie & Sclafani (1977), or Margolis (1980). I begin with a few ideas on the nature of aesthetics, move to the issue of what constitutes art, aesthetic knowledge, and end with some views on art, craft, and artistic production. Aesthetics, the philosophical study of art, is a relatively young branch of philosophy, having developed primarily from the work of Kant, especially his Critique of Aesthetic Judgement (1790). Before this time it had been a metaphysical and epistemological enquiry concerning either sense data generally, or the relationship between beauty and truth. Even now, aesthetics continues to be preoccupied with questions concerning its own content and methods (Novitz 1990).

Concerning the terminology of aesthetics, Lipman (1973) has suggested the following distinctions:

1. The philosophy of art—inquires into the place of art in the entire panorama of human activity;
2. Aesthetics—involves enquiries into specific philosophical problems within the domain of art;
3. Meta-aesthetics—is concerned with the way in which we talk about art, and the methodological aspects of aesthetics itself.

Mead (1952) adopts a broader view of aesthetics, including the beautiful and expressive areas of experience, and this might be useful in explicating the beauty which may be discerned in artistic nursing care. Quinton's (1977) description is broader still, taking in natural objects such as scenery and bodies. According to Dickie & Sclafani (1977), whose volume brings together some of the most important statements on these issues, aestheticians concern themselves with both the theory of art and with the aesthetic response. The polarities represented in their work are referred to as 'the subjective approach' and 'the objective approach'. The subjective approach is most powerfully represented by Tolstoy (1975), who argues that the value of a work of art rests on its power to transmit emotion. Typical of the objective approach is Clive Bell's (1947) theory of significant form, in which the starting-point for all systems of aesthetic experience is a peculiar emotion. The objects that promote this emotion are called works of art. All works of art, and only works of art, have the power, through the characteristic use of significant forms, to evoke aesthetic emotion. This view points to an absolute set of characteristics manifested in objects and events that are responsible for the aesthetic emotion, and again raises the question of the relationship between art and qualities such as beauty and truth. A theory of aesthetic value pursuing such a stand would require that these qualities, if that is what they are, also possess value. Whilst for Urmson (1957) aesthetic values are unique and irreducible to other values, Beardsley (1969) has developed an instrumental theory of aesthetic value, in which, whilst not denying the value of inherent moral and aesthetic effects, the ultimate value of art appears to be its role in fostering psychological and social well-being. Similarly, for Dewey (cited in Cross 1977), art has moral functions inasmuch as it helps us to perceive the world more clearly. For Hobbs (1977), on the other hand, an aesthetic experience occurs when a person is preoccupied with an object or event as an end in itself rather than as a means to some other end, whether religious, moral, or economic.

Whilst a number of tentative criteria have been offered by aestheticians, including Morawski (1974), it has been suggested by others, such as Rosenberg (1962), that like science, art cannot be unambiguously defined. These authors adumbrate various typologies of art theory, which, although unambiguously centred on the so-called 'fine arts', may help in clarifying our ideas. Weitz (1970) insists that to ask 'what is art?' is to ask the wrong question, but distinguishes five traditional theoretical positions.

1. Formalist Theory: art is a unique combination of certain elements in their relations; anything which is art is an instance of significant form; and anything which is not art has no such form.
2. Emotionalist Theory: the requisite defining property is not the significant form but rather the communicative expression of emotion in some sensuous public medium.
3. Intuitionist Theory: art is not some physical, public object but rather a

specific creative, cognitive and spiritual act. It is really a first stage of knowledge in which certain human beings (artists) bring their images and intuitions into lyrical clarification or expression.
4. Organicist Theory: art is really a class of organic wholes consisting of distinguishable, yet inseparable, elements in causal relationships which are presented in some sensuous medium: anything that is a work of art is, in its nature, a unique complex of interrelated, interacting parts.
5. Voluntarist Theory: art is essentially three things: embodiment of wishes and desires imaginatively satisfied, language which characterizes the public medium of art, and harmony which unifies the language with layers of imaginative projections.

It might be a useful exercise to ascertain the extent to which these criteria are subsumed in our concepts of nursing. We must also consider the various social and emancipatory theories, often associated with socialist philosophy. Kavolis (1968) and Hadjinicolaou (1973), for example, consider the social function of art, pointing to its role in reinforcing existing social conditions through reflecting, and thereby confirming, their legitimacy, and in effecting change through social critique and transmission of new attitudes. For Marxism, artistic praxis is an integral part of human praxis, and the force behind artistic conceptions is political and social revolution (Arvon 1973). Nurses must also consider what ontological and epistemological status may be ascribed to the aesthetic components of nursing. Hirst (1973) asserts that the knowledge embodied in art cannot be expressed in ordinary language, but only through the medium of the work of art itself. Although this would suggest a form of aesthetic knowledge, and is reminiscent of Carper's (1978) paper which speaks of aesthetic ways of knowing, Hirst is adamant that whilst such knowledge is direct and immediate, it is not 'real' knowledge (Ross 1983). On the other hand, according to Heyfron (1983), who harnesses Sartre's (1962) phenomenological theory of the emotions, aesthetic emotion does constitute a form of real knowledge, allowing not only apprehension of, but also insight into, the nature of the world. More recently, Dorter (1990) has acted as apologist for Plato's dismissal of aesthetic knowledge as sophistry, insisting that although providing less certain and less accurate knowledge than rational procedures, he recognized art as furnishing a valid way of knowing reality. When nurses examine the epistemological status of aesthetic knowing it will surely prove necessary to consider not only the relationship between aesthetic knowing and rational processes, but also the nexus between aesthetic knowledge and intuitive knowledge, that is between art and intuition. This is particularly timely in view of the rehabilitation of that concept, particularly in connection with Bergsonian antirationalism, into epistemology (through Polanyi 1958, 1967, 1969), into psychology (i.e. through Johnson 1975, on whom Jean Watson drew from in her 1979 text), and into the nursing literature (Benner 1984, Agan 1987, Rew & Barrow 1987, Rew 1988).

Nursing conceived as a craft seems to present a less problematic entrée into the notion of nursing as art, but raises the difficult conundrum concerning the relationship between artistry and craftsmanship. The relationship between art, craft, and technology is an area of study which nurse theorists must begin to explore. Art theorists tend to adopt one of the following positions:

- that art subsumes craft, that craft subsumes art, or that they are extremes of a continuum;
- that art and craft are closely related but separate activities;
- that there is an overlapping, or dialectical relationship between art and craft.

In contrast to art, craft has been thought to emphasize predetermined ends, skill, materials, function, and popular appeal, whilst Schwartz (1970) views the distinction as largely cultural, rather than implicit in artifacts. He argues that it may be more productive to regard craft as the collective processes by which objects are produced, and art as the design formulation, attendant overtones and images produced by these objects. Some theorists have attempted to distinguish art from craft on the grounds of function, and in considering the role of 'usefulness' in the arts Dewey, for example, attempted to describe the qualities by which a 'useful' object was liberated and became an aesthetic object. In an attempt to clarify the issues through the delineation of crafts pursued for different ends, Williams (1978) has categorized craft ideologies as follows:

1. Critical Productive: use of craft as a means of self-expression
2. Social Vocational: the individual production of quality crafts as a vocation
3. Vocational Industrial: long production runs of saleable items for economic security
4. Social Avocational: crafts as a hobby or leisure pursuit
5. Therapeutic: as a contribution to a person's well-being.

Nurse theorists approaching the notion of nursing as a craft might find these distinctions useful.

Descriptions of skill in nursing have followed protocols developed primarily in technical contexts. Over the years we have championed models formulated by a succession of educationalists—Gagné, Bloom, Bruner, the Knowlesian androgogues, and more recently the reflective practitioner approach of Schön (Powell 1989), and emancipatory learning of Freire. Now the Dreyfus 'novice to expert' model (reiterated in Dreyfus & Dreyfus 1986), adopted by Benner (1984), is also making an impact, perhaps because of its thesis that expert practice is non-rational. It would be interesting to explore ways in which these characterizations could articulate with aesthetic theories, such as those of Walter Pater (1897), which posit excellence, wherever it occurs, as a source of aesthetic value. Benner's scheme was initially developed from a study of the coping skills of pilots faced with emergency situations, and then supported by drawing on the characteristics of chess players and other skilled performers.

Because of their radically different processes and objectives, conceptions of the development of nursing artistry, however, may require alternative formulations. Drawing on studies of art education, Clark & Zimmerman (1978), for example, propose a continuum between the naive and the sophisticated artist/practitioner, whilst Gilliatt (1980) provides an overview of approaches which have been proposed for the development and enhancement of aesthetic sensitivity. In approaching both art and craft, we must also consider questions concerning what comprises artistic activity. Cross (1977), for example, asserts that in art the process is more important than the product, whilst in craft the reverse might be the case. The clear lesson here is that in defining nursing as art or craft, nurses must enter the debate concerning the relationship between product and process, form and content. Mattil (1971) believes it is important to distinguish between procedures and techniques. Procedures are the various activities that can be explained within the general framework of the project, whilst techniques are the highly individualized use of the materials involved. He adds that one can teach procedures and this may help the student to develop his or her own technique, whereas aesthetic judgement can develop only when the student has the freedom to make choices in his or her work. This looks quite promising as a basis for exploring the nursing process as an art form.

Finally, one of the most obvious ways in which nursing can be viewed as an art form is in terms of performance. Whilst a number of established accounts of dramatic performance have effectively pursued the old part-truth that 'all the world's a stage', at the macro-level the 'dramaturgical' social interaction theory of Erving Goffman (1959, 1963, 1969a, 1969b, 1971, 1974) is perhaps the only one with which nurses may be familiar. At the micro-level, Birdwhistell (1970) has also provided interesting accounts of momentary responses and fragmentary elements of behaviour that make up 'kinemes', or social performances. I would like to draw attention, however, to the literature which is emerging from a developing confluence of aesthetic, anthropological, and theatrical scholarship on the subject. Significant contributions include Armstrong (1981), Burns (1972), Schechner (1985, 1988), and Turner (1974, 1982, 1986). The recent collection edited by Schechner & Appel (1990) contains a wealth of material exploring the relationships between social dramas, rituals, and theatre, and the papers by Myerhoff on their role in the transformation of consciousness, Blau on the essence of performance itself, and especially Schechner on levels and magnitudes of performance, are particularly promising springboards from which to begin exploring the notion of nursing as aesthetic performance.

THE FUTURE OF NURSING THEORIES

What then of the future for nursing theory? I am forewarned of the dangers in attempting to answer such questions by a recent plan for the development of nursing knowledge (Stevenson 1990), which seems to run counter to all my expectations! Whereas I would predict a radically new and revitalized theorization in nursing, Stevenson suggests that we pursue a conventional path along familiar lines. With trepidation, therefore, I would like to suggest briefly that there are grounds for expecting quite different, far-reaching developments. First, referring back to the competing demands of specificity and generality, those theories that claim to be single, unifying 'grand theories', like that of Rogers, seem to be regarded by practitioners as suitable for guiding practice in some settings but not in others. Nurses prefer the discriminating eclecticism which has long been necessary in the context of contradictory and competing perspectives, and they actually employ a mixture of theories aimed at meeting the very specific requirements of their particular clinical setting. It is reasonable to expect that these tensions will lead to the development of a range of theories with applicability at specific levels of analysis. Grand all-explaining, all-encompassing theories of the kind advocated by Rogers, will continue to be developed alongside small scale ones which have direct implications for very specific practice settings. If I read her aright, this is the view of Meleis (1985), and the recent literature (e.g. Marriner-Tomey 1989) does suggest that it is the trend.

Second, consistent with the progressive pattern of theory development presented by Meleis, although nursing theories will continue to draw eclectically and critically on the work of other disciplines, the move to pluralism will surely be accompanied by an increasing theoretical independence. Although we are just starting out in some aspects of nursing theory, this trend is already underway in the context of research, with the continuing development of alternative research paradigms (Chinn 1986, Keddy et al 1987, Hedin & Duffy 1988, Morse 1989). Third, whilst nursing theory will become increasingly independent, there are many intellectual insights and traditions that have not been tapped—I've already alluded to political, economic, and aesthetic theories—and it is to be hoped that these will enter more obviously into nursing theory. A theory in which characterizations of nursing as an art truly counterbalance those of nursing as a science has been gestating for a long time, and surely the birth pangs cannot be far away. It is now 12 years since the appearance of Carper's famous article on fundamental ways of knowing in nursing, and it is sometimes forgotten that she posited aesthetic knowing as the highest form, in the sense that it was concerned with the balancing and integration of the other forms, and with acting in relation to projected outcomes. We should, therefore, look forward to the day when we have a 'theory of nursing aesthetics' to balance all those 'theories of nursing science'!

There are good reasons to expect critical theory, especially the Habermasian variety, to assume greater importance for nursing theory. Apart from the promise of a coherent philosophy which subsumes a number of irritatingly persistent disputes about the nature of science, it incorporates a notion of emancipation which has obvious appeal to nursing (Hedin 1986), and there are strong links with feminism (particularly the debates over language, science, and morality, Habermas 1990). It also clarifies the theory-practice relationship (Habermas 1974) through a notion of praxis developed in the context of critical pedagogy (Freire 1972, Misgeld 1975, Shor 1980, Freire & Shor 1987), which is already familiar to educationalists (Carr & Kemmis 1986, Bell & Schniewind 1987, Grundy 1987, Schön 1987, Smyth 1987, Moore 1988), and is figuring increasingly in nursing curricula (Brown 1989). Other contemporary notions of praxis may also prove useful. The humanistic Marxism of the Yugoslavian theorists, Markovic and Stojanovic, is founded on a strongly normative notion of praxis. They ground their views in a theory of the good, namely that human beings can and should be beings of praxis, or 'theoretico-practical persons'. This version of praxis represents a standard for individual excellence and an axiological principle for social critique of present formations and possible futures (Crocker 1973), and may prove an attractive alternative to the non-normative concept offered by other critical theorists, providing a nexus with the ethical components of nursing practice. Furthermore, as part of its program of ideologiekritik, critical theory has a longstanding role in the critique of culture, and through the pioneering work of Benjamin and Adorno, has built up an extensive aesthetic theory (Edgar 1990 for an introduction). It will be interesting to see whether nursing's engagement with critical theory finds this a useful resource.

Undercutting many of these debates are the new feminist epistemologies (Harding & Hintikka 1983, Bleier 1984, 1986, Belenky et.al. 1986, Harding 1986, 1987, Gergen 1988, Hare-Mustin & Marecek 1988, Crawford 1989), which reject most, or all, of the assumptions underlying the greater part of the Western intellectual tradition, including positivism. They identify Baconian method, in which knowledge is identified with power, as instrumental in creating the mechanistic world view that facilitated the development of capitalism, which they see as substantiating male dominated society (Merchant 1980). Some point to the centrality of sexual metaphors ('a penetrating analysis' for example) in articulating conceptions of knowledge, which in turn constrain the questions that may be asked about nature, self, and society (Keller 1983).

Harding (1986) attempts to synthesize a range of feminist positions, and identifies three different positions:

1. Feminist empiricism—which puts androcentrism down to 'bad science' and seeks correction through increased rigour vis-a-vis gender factors
2. Feminist standpoint—which seeks to replace androcentrism with a feminist alternative

3. Feminist post modernism—which seeks to reject all claims that there are universals which circumscribe and characterise reason, science, language, and existence.

Feminist theories' emancipatory intentions, their potential for radical personal revitalization, and their revaluing of women and their experiences, have an obvious relevance and appeal to nursing. Feminist critique has an explicitly political function (Benhabib & Cornell 1987), and as Jansen (1990) says, for radical feminists science is also a way of practising politics by other means. In light of the strong and wide-ranging influence of feminist ideologies in nursing (Ashley 1980, Benner 1984, Chinn & Wheeler 1985, Speedy 1987, Andrist 1988, Hedin & Duffy 1988, Miller 1988, Crowley 1989b, Hedin & Donovan 1989, Watson 1990), and the uncharacteristic rapidity with which feminist epistemologies have found a place in nursing literature (MacPherson 1983, Chinn 1986, 1988, Hagell 1989), feminism will undoubtedly have a profound and lasting impact on conceptions of nursing science.

Finally, it is unfortunately not difficult to identify some very powerful influences which may delay these developments, and will certainly contribute to the ideological standpoint of nursing theory for some time to come. First, there is the development of 'glasnost' and the associated political upheavals in Eastern Europe, which have surely damaged the credibility of the whole Marxist perspective on economic theory, political theory, and theories of history and science (Monthly Review 1990a,b, Davies 1990, Survey 1988, 1989).

Second, there is the current upsurge of international conservatism, which will lead to increased emphasis on individualism, on personal responsibility, on internal explanations and positivistic approaches to social problems. In the United States there has always been opposition to any active socialism, but this has recently become even more deeply entrenched, and more clearly manifest in social policies worldwide. Consider, for example, recent changes in labor law; increasing governmental control over higher education; the obstinate commitment to Keynesian economic policies; welfare and fiscal policies which increase the gap between rich and poor; the privatization of basic utilities and community services; the formal substantiation of health as a commodity; and the attendant changes in popular, as well as 'official' discourse which place economic considerations above the well-being of the people.

Third, there are correspondingly tighter controls exercised over educational and health care establishments by governments, which will pressure nursing in both settings to subscribe to the dominant paradigm of uncompromising individualism, ruthless conservatism, and capitalist economics. Consider, for example, the outrageous contraction of routine health care services in order to fund prestigious, high-tech ventures of marginal value to the community. What we are left with are economic stringencies in the face of increasing societal need, i.e. a system which sees health care as a commodity, and the sick left to suffer because there is no bed, or because they cannot afford one.

It is my hope that there will eventually be a backlash in academia to these developments, and that a strongly neo-socialist approach to nursing and its theorization will emerge which will provide a basis for the transformation of nursing into a politically and socially relevant discipline. Participating in the application and critique of the latest developments in epistemology and the philosophy of science will also increase the credibility of our theoretical statements. But more than this, I believe that by developing the notion of nursing as an aesthetic activity, emphasizing the unity of theory and practice, we shall contribute to the authentication of our discipline, and to a spiral of ever improving care.

REFERENCES

Agan R D 1987 Intuitive knowing as a dimension of nursing. Advances in Nursing Science 10 (1):63-70
Andrist L C 1988 A feminist framework for graduate education in women's health. Journal of Nursing Education 27 (2):66-70
Archer S E, Goehner P A 1982 Nurses: a political force. Wadsworth, Belmont
Armstrong R P 1981 The powers of presence: consciousness, myth and affecting presence. University of Pennsylvania Press, Philadelphia
Arvon H 1973 Marxist esthetics. Cornell University Press, Ithaca
Ashley J A 1978 Foundations for scholarship: historical research in nursing. Advances in Nursing Science 1 (1):25-36
Ashley J A 1980 Power in structured misogyny: implications for the politics of care. Advances in Nursing Science 2 (3):3-22
Beardsley M 1969 The instrumentalist theory of aesthetic value. In: Hospers J (ed) Introductory readings in aesthetics. Free Press, London
Belenky M F, Clinchy B M, Goldberger N R, Tarule J M 1986 Women's ways of knowing: the development of self, voice and mind. Basic Books, New York
Bell C 1947 Art. Chatto & Windus, London
Bell L, Schniewind N 1987 Reflective minds / intentional hearts: joining humanistic education and critical theory for liberating education. Journal of Education 169 (2):55-57
Benhabib S, Cornell D (eds) 1987 Feminism as critique: essays on the politics of gender in late-capitalist societies. Polity Press, Oxford
Benner P 1984 From novice to expert: excellence and power in clinical nursing practice. Addison-Wesley, Menlo Park
Benner P, Wrubel J 1989 The primacy of caring. Addison-Wesley, Menlo Park
Bhaskar R 1978 A realist theory of science, 2nd edn. Harvester Press, Brighton
Bhaskar R 1979 The possibility of naturalism. Harvester Press, Brighton
Bhaskar R 1986 Scientific realism and human emancipation. Verso, London
Birdwhistell R 1970 Kinesics and context. Penguin, Harmondsworth
Bleier R 1984 Science and gender: a critique of biology and its theories on women. Pergamon Press, New York
Broniak C 1988 What is emancipation for Habermas? Philosophy Today (Fall):195-206
Brown J 1989 Emancipation through praxis: the reflexive relationship between theory and practice. Paper presented to National Nursing Theory Conference. In: Koch T (ed) Theory and practice—an evolving relationship. School of Nursing Studies, Sturt, South Australian College of Advanced Education
Burns E 1972 Theatricality: a study of convention in the theatre and in social life. Harper Torchbooks, New York

Burton F, Carlen P 1979 Official discourse: on discourse analysis, government publications, ideology and the state. Routledge & Kegan-Paul, London

Carper B A 1978 Fundamental patterns of knowing in nursing. Advances in Nursing Science 1:13-23

Carr W, Kemmis S 1986 Becoming critical: knowing through action research, 2nd edn. Deakin University Press, Highton

Chinn P (ed) 1986 Nursing research methodology: issues and implementation. Aspen Systems, Rockville

Chinn P 1988 Nursing patterns of knowing and feminist thought. Nursing and Health Care 1:71-75

Chinn P, Wheeler CE (1985): Feminism and nursing. Nursing Outlook 33(2):74-77

Clark G, Zimmerman E 1978 A walk in the right direction: a model for visual arts education. Studies in Art Education 19(2):34-49

Clay T 1987 Nurses, power and politics. Heinemann, London

Crawford M 1989 Agreeing to differ: feminist epistemologies and women's ways of knowing. In: Crawford M, Gentry M (eds) Gender and thought: psychological perspectives. Springer Verlag, New York

Crocker D A 1973 Praxis and democratic socialism: the critical theory of Markovic and Stojanovic. Humanities Press, Atlantic Highlands

Cross J 1977 For art's sake: a strategic approach to teaching art in schools. Allen & Unwin, London

Crowley M A 1989a The entrepreneurial nurse consultant: a Marxist analysis. Journal of Advanced Nursing 14:582-586

Crowley M A 1989b Feminist pedagogy: nurturing the ethical ideal. Advances in Nursing Science 11(3):53-61

Davies R W 1990 Gorbachev's socialism in historical perspective. New Left Review 179:5-28

Dickie G, Sclafani R (eds) 1977 Aesthetics: a critical anthology. St Martin's Press, New York

Dickson G L 1990 A feminist poststructuralist analysis of the knowledge of menopause. Advances in Nursing Science 12(3):15-31

Diers D 1990 The art and craft of nursing. American Journal of Nursing January 90(1):65-66

Dorter K 1990 Conceptual truth and aesthetic truth. Journal of Aesthetics and Art Criticism 48(1):37-51

Dreyfus H L, Dreyfus S E 1986 Mind over machine: the power of human intuition and expertise in the era of the computer. Free Press, New York

Dzurec L C 1989 The necessity for and evolution of multiple paradigms for nursing research: a poststructuralist perspective. Advances in Nursing Science 11(4):69-77

Edgar A 1990 An introduction to Adorno's aesthetics. British Journal of Aesthetics 30(1):46-56

Fitzpatrick J J, Whall A L (eds) 1983 Conceptual models of nursing. Prentice-Hall, Englewood Cliffs

Freire P 1972 Pedagogy of the oppressed. Penguin, Harmondsworth

Freire P, Shor I 1987 A pedagogy for liberation: dialogues on transforming education. Macmillan, London

Fry S 1990 The development of nursing science: theoretical and philosophical issues. In: Chaska N L (ed) The nursing profession: turning points. C V Mosby, St Louis

Furnham A 1989 Lay theories: everyday understanding of problems in the social sciences. Pergamon Press, Oxford

Garmarnikow E 1978 Sexual division of labour: the case of nursing. In: Kuhn A, Wolpe A (eds) Feminism and materialism: women and modes of production. Routledge & Kegan-Paul, Oxford

Gergen M M (ed) 1988 Feminist thought and the structure of knowledge. New York University Press, New York

Giddens A 1979 Central problems of social theory. Macmillan, London

Giddens A 1982 Profiles and critiques in social theory. Macmillan, London

Gilliatt M 1980 The effects of habituation, the Feldman-Mittler methodology and studio activities on expanding art preferences in elementary students. Studies in Art Education 21(2):43-49

Goffman E 1959 The presentation of self in everyday life. Penguin, Harmondsworth
Goffman E 1963 Behaviour in public places. Free Press, New York
Goffman E 1969a Interaction ritual. Penguin, Harmondsworth
Goffman E 1969b Strategic interaction. University of Pennsylvania Press, Philadelphia
Goffman E 1971 Relations in public: microstudies in the public order. Basic Books, New York
Goffman E 1974 Frame analysis: an essay on the organization of experience. Harvard University Press, Cambridge
Gortner S 1983 The history and philosophy of nursing science and research. Advances in Nursing Science 5(2):1-8
Grundy S 1987 Curriculum: product or praxis? Falmer Press, London
Habermas J 1968 Knowledge and human interests. Heinemann, London
Habermas J 1970 On systematically distorted communication. Inquiry 13:205-218
Habermas J 1974 Theory and praxis. (Translated by Viertel J 4th edn Theorie und praxis) Heinemann, London
Habermas J 1985 Civil disobedience: litmus test for the democratic constitutional state. Berkeley Journal of Sociology 30:95-116
Habermas J 1990 Moral consciousness and communicative action. (Translated Lenhardt C, Nicholsen. S) MIT Press, Cambridge
Hadjinicolaou N 1973 Art history and class struggle. (Translated Asmal L, 1978) Pluto Press, London
Hagell E I 1989 Nursing knowledge: women's knowledge. A sociological perspective. Journal of Advanced Nursing 14:26-233
Harding S 1986 The science question in feminism. Cornell University Press, Ithaca
Harding S (ed) 1987 Feminism and methodology. Indiana University Press, Bloomington
Harding S, Hintikka M B (eds) 1983 Discovering reality—feminist perspectives on epistemology, metaphysics, and philosophy of science. Reidel, Dordrecht
Hardy M 1974 Theories: components, development, evaluation. Nursing Research 23:100-107
Hare-Mustin R, Marecek J 1988 The meaning of difference: gender theory, postmodernism, and psychology. American Psychologist 43:455-464
Harris J 1987 QALY-fying the value of life. Journal of Medical Ethics 11:142-145
Hazelton M 1990 Medical discourse on contemporary nurse education: an ideological analysis. Australian and New Zealand Journal of Sociology 26(1):107-125
Hedin B A 1986 Nursing, education, and emancipation: applying the critical theoretical approach to nursing research. In: Chinn P (ed) Nursing research methodology: issues and implementation. Aspen Systems, Rockville
Hedin B A, Donovan J 1989 A feminist perspective on nursing education. Nurse Educator 14 (4):8-13
Hedin B A, Duffy M E 1988 Researching: designing research from a feminist perspective. Proceedings of the conference 'Caring and nursing: exploration in the feminist perspectives', Denver (June 17-18): 363-374
Hesse M 1980 Revolutions and reconstructions in the philosophy of science. Harvester Press, Brighton
Hewson M (ed) 1983 Attribution theory: social and functional extensions.Blackwell, Oxford
Heyfron V 1983 The objective status of aesthetic knowing. In: Ross M (ed) The arts: a way of knowing. Pergamon Press, Oxford
Hickson P 1988 Knowledge and action in nursing: a critical approach to the practice worlds of four nurses. MA(Nursing) thesis, Massey University, Palmerston North
Hickson P 1990 The promises of critical theory. Unpublished paper presented at the conference, 'Embodiment, empowerment, emancipation: critical theory, reflectivity, and nursing practice', held in Melbourne, February 1990
Hill L, Smith N 1985 Self-care nursing: promotion of health. Prentice-Hall, Englewood Cliffs
Hirst P 1973 Literature and fine arts as a unique form of knowledge. Cambridge Journal of Education, Michaelmas
Hobbs J 1977 Is aesthetic education possible? Art Education 30(1):30-32
Holland R 1990 The paradigm plague: prevention, cure, and inoculation. Human Relations 43(1):23-48

Holmes C A 1989 Health care and the quality of life: a review. Journal of Advanced Nursing 14:833-839

Holmes C A 1990 Alternatives to natural science foundations for nursing. International Journal of Nursing Studies 27:187-198

Holter I M 1988 Critical theory: a foundation for the development of nursing theories. Scholarly Inquiry for Nursing Practice 2, 3:223-232.

Hospers J (ed) 1969 Introductory readings in aesthetics. Free Press, London

Jansen S C 1990 Is science a man? New feminist epistemologies and reconstructions of knowledge. Theory and Society 19:235-246

Jaspars J 1983 The process of causal attribution in common sense. In: Hewson M (ed) Attribution theory: social and functional extensions. Blackwell, Oxford

Johnson R E 1975 In quest for a new psychology: toward a redefinition of humanism. Human Sciences Press, New York

Kalisch B J, Kalisch P A 1982 Politics of nursing. Lippincott, Philadelphia

Kant I 1790 The critique of aesthetic judgement. (Translated Meredith J C) Oxford University Press, Oxford

Kavolis V 1968 Artistic expression: a sociological analysis. Cornell University Press, Ithaca

Keat R 1981 The politics of social theory. Blackwell, Oxford

Keat R, Urry J 1975 Social theory as science. Routledge & Kegan-Paul, London

Keddy B, Acker K, Hemeon D, et al 1987 Nurses' work world: scientific or "womanly ministering"? Resources for Feminist Research 16 (4):37-39

Keller E F 1983 Gender and science. In: Harding S, Hintikka M B (eds) Discovering reality—feminist perspectives on epistemology, metaphysics, and philosophy of science. Reidel, Dordrecht

Kendall J 1989 Child psychiatric nursing and the family: A critical theory perspective. Journal of Child Psychiatric Nursing 2(4):145-153

Kruglanski A W 1980 Lay epistemo-logic—process and contents: another look at attribution theory. Psychological Review 87:70-87

Kruglanski A W, Jaffe Y 1983 Lay epistemology: a theory for cognitive therapy. In: Abramson L Y (ed) An attributional perspective in clinical psychology. Guildford Press, New York

Kuhn T 1962 The structure of scientific revolutions. University of Chicago Press, Chicago

Kuhn T 1977 Second thoughts on paradigms. In: Suppe F (ed) The structure of scientific revolutions. University of Illinois Press, Urbana

Laudan L 1977 Progress and its problems: towards a theory of scientific growth. University of California Press, Berkeley

Lerner M J 1970 The desire for justice and reactions to victims. In: Macaulay J, Berkowitz L (eds) Altruism and helping behaviour. Academic Press, New York

Levine M 1989 The ethics of nursing rhetoric. IMAGE: Journal of Nursing Scholarship 21(1):4-6

Lipman M 1973 Introduction to chapter one. In: Lipman M (ed) Contemporary aesthetics. Allyn & Bacon, Boston

Lorenson M 1988 Response to "Critical theory: a foundation for development of nursing theories". Scholarly Inquiry in Nursing Practice 2(3):233-236

Lumby J 1991 Nursing: art or science. Deakin University Press, Geelong

Macdonell D 1986 Theories of discourse: an introduction. Blackwell, Oxford

McGivern D O 1988 Teaching nurses the language of the marketplace. Nursing and Health Care 9(3):126-130

MacPherson K I 1983 Feminist methods: a new paradigm for nursing research. Advances in Nursing Science January:17-25

Margolis J 1980 Art and philosophy: conceptual issues in aesthetics. Humanities Press, Atlantic Highlands

Marriner-Tomey A 1989 Nurse theorists and their work, 2nd edn. C V Mosby, St Louis

Mason D J, Talbott S W (eds) 1985 Political action handbook for nurses. Addison-Wesley, Menlo Park

Mattil E 1971 Meaning in crafts. Prentice-Hall, Englewood Cliffs

Mead H 1952 An introduction to aesthetics. Ronald Press, New York

Meleis A 1985 Theoretical nursing: development and progress. Lippincott, Philadelphia

Menke E 1983 Critical analysis of theory development in nursing. In: Chaska N L (ed) The nursing profession. McGraw Hill, New York

Merchant C 1980 The death of nature: women, ecology and the scientific revolution. Harper and Row, New York

Miller K L 1988 Feminist ideology in nursing: a foundational inquiry. Doctoral thesis, University of Colorado Health Sciences Center, Denver

Misgeld D 1975 Emancipation, enlightenment, and liberation: an approach toward foundational inquiry into education. Interchange 6(3):23-37

Monthly Review 1990a Perestroika and the future of socialism I and II. Editorial articles. Monthly Review 41(10):1-13, and 41(11):1-17

Monthly Review 1990b The future of socialism. Whole issue of Monthly Review 42(3)

Moore B 1988 Towards a theory of curriculum decision-making: insights from critical praxis (Jürgen Habermas). South Australian College of Advanced Education, Adelaide

Morawski S 1974 Inquiries into the fundamentals of aesthetics. MIT Press, Cambridge,

Morse J M (ed) 1989 Qualitative nursing research: a contemporary dialogue. Aspen Systems, Rockville

Mulkay M, Ashmore M, Pinch T 1987 Measuring the quality of life: a sociological invention concerning the application of economics to health care. Sociology 21(4):541-564

Munhall P L, Oiler C J 1986 Nursing research: a qualitative perspective. Appleton-Century-Crofts, Norwalk

Newman M 1990 Nursing paradigms and realities. In: Chaska N L (ed) The nursing profession: turning points. C V Mosby, St Louis

Nicoll L H (ed) 1986 Perspectives on nursing theory. Little Brown, Boston

Novitz D 1990 The integrity of aesthetics. Journal of Aesthetics and Art Criticism 48(1):9-20

O'Brien B 1990 Nursing: craft, science and art. Paper presented at the Conference 'Dreams, deliberations, and discoveries', Nursing Research in Action, 11-13th June 1990,.Royal Adelaide Hospital, Adelaide

O'Brien B 1991 Artistry in nursing. Faculty of Nursing Monograph. Deakin University Press, Geelong

Osborne H 1968 Aesthetics and art theory: an historical introduction. Longman, London

Outhwaite W 1987 New philosophies of social science: realism, hermeneutics and critical theory. Macmillan, Basingstoke

Pater W 1897 Appreciations. Macmillan, London

Paterson J G, Zderad L T 1976 Humanistic nursing. John Wiley, New York

Pender N 1982 Health Promotion in nursing practice. Appleton-Century-Crofts, Norwalk

Peplau H 1987 Nursing science: a historical perspective. In: Parse R R (ed) Nursing science: major paradigms, theories, and critiques. W B Saunders, Philadelphia

Polanyi M 1958 Personal knowledge: towards a post-critical philosophy. University of Chicago Press, Chicago

Polanyi M 1967 The tacit dimension. Routledge & Kegan Paul, London

Polanyi M 1969 Knowing and being. Routledge & Kegan Paul, London

Popkewitz T S 1984 Paradigm and ideology in educational research: the social functions of the intellectual. Falmer Press, London

Powell J H 1989 The reflective practitioner in nursing. Journal of Advanced Nursing 14:824-832

Quinton A 1977 Entry on 'aesthetics'. In: Bullock A, Stallybrass O (eds) The Fontana dictionary of modern thought. Collins/Fontana, London

Rew L 1988 Intuition in decision-making. IMAGE: Journal of Nursing Scholarship 20(3):150-154

Rew L, Barrow E M 1987 Intuition: a neglected hallmark of nursing knowledge. Advances in Nursing Science 10(1):49-62

Rosenberg H 1962 The tradition of the new. Thames and Hudson, London

Ross M (ed) 1983 The arts: a way of knowing. Pergamon Press, Oxford

Salvage J 1985 The politics of nursing. Heinemann, London

Sarter B 1987 Evolutionary idealism: a philosophical foundation for holistic nursing theory. Advances in Nursing Sciences 9(2):1-9

Sarter B 1990 Philosophical foundations of nursing theory: a discipline emerges. In: Chaska N L (ed) The nursing profession: turning points. C V Mosby, St Louis

Sartre J-P 1962 Sketch for a theory of the emotions. Methuen, London

Sarvimäki A 1986 Skapande interaktion. Forskningar No.10, Helsingfors svenska sjukvardsinstitut, Helsingfors

Sarvimäki A 1988a Nursing as a moral, practical, communicative and creative activity. Journal of Advanced Nursing 13:462-467

Sarvimäki A 1988b Knowledge in interactive disciplines. PhD thesis. School of Education, University of Helsinki, Helsinki

Schechner R 1985 Between theater and anthropology. University of Pennsylvania Press, Philadelphia

Schechner R 1988 Performance theory (second revised edition of Essays in performance theory, 1977). Routledge, London

Schechner R, Appel W (eds) 1990 By means of performance: intercultural studies of theatre and ritual. Cambridge University Press, Cambridge

Schön D 1987 Educating the reflective practitioner. Jossey-Bass, San Francisco

Schwartz F 1970 Structure and potential in art education. Ginn & Blaisdell, Waltham

Semin G, Manstead A 1983 The accountability of conduct: a social psychological analysis. Academic Press, London

Shapere D 1981 Meaning and scientific change. In: Hacking I (ed) Scientific revolutions. Oxford University Press, New York

Shor I 1980 Critical teaching and everyday life. Black Rose Books, Montreal

Smyth W 1987 A rationale for teacher's critical pedagogy: a handbook. Deakin University Press, Geelong

Speedy S 1987 Feminism and the professionalisation of nursing. Australian Journal of Advanced Nursing 4(2):20-28

Speedy S 1989 Nursing theory and practice: risks and rewards. Paper presented at the National Nursing Theory Conference, Sept.8-9. In: Koch T (ed) Theory and practice— an evolving relationship. School of Nursing Studies, Sturt, South Australian College of Advanced Education

Spengler C 1976 Womanpower and health care. Little Brown, Boston

Stevenson J S 1990 The development of nursing knowledge: accelerating the pace. In: Chaska N L (ed) The nursing profession: turning points. C V Mosby, St Louis

Stockman N 1983 Anti-positivist theories of the sciences. Reidel, Dordrecht

Street A 1988 High, hard ground, messy swamps and the pathways in between. Faculty of Nursing Monograph. Deakin University Press, Geelong

Survey 1988 Unnamed author(s). Gorbachev and glasnost. Survey: a journal of East and West studies 30(3)

Survey 1989 Unnamed author(s). Perestroika and Soviet history. Survey: a journal of East and West studies 30(4)

Thompson J 1983 Toward a critical nursing process: nursing praxis. Doctoral dissertation, University of Utah, Salt Lake City

Thompson J 1985 Practical discourse in nursing: going beyond empiricism and historicism. Advances in Nursing Science 7(4):59-71

Thompson J 1987 Critical scholarship: the critique of domination in nursing. Advances in Nursing Science 10(1):27-38

Tolstoy L 1975 What is art? and essays on art. Oxford University Press, London

Turner V W 1974 Dramas, fields, and metaphors. Cornell University Press, Ithaca

Turner V W 1982 From ritual to theatre: the human seriousness of play. Performing Arts Journal Press, New York

Turner V W 1986 The anthropology of performance. Performing Arts Journal Press, New York

Urmson J O 1957 What makes a situation aesthetic? Proceedings of the Aristotelian Society, Supplement 31:75-92

Watson J 1979 Nursing: the philosophy and science of human caring. Little Brown, Boston

Watson J 1985a Reflections on different methodologies for the future of nursing. In: Leininger M (ed) Qualitative research methods in nursing. Grune & Stratton, New York

Watson J 1985b Nursing: human science and human care: a theory of nursing. Appleton-Century-Crofts, Norwalk

Watson J 1990 The moral failure of the patriarchy. Nursing Outlook 38(2):62-66

Weedon C 1987 Feminist practice and poststructuralist theory. Blackwell, Oxford

Weitz M 1970 The role of theory in aesthetics. In: Weitz M (ed) Problems in aesthetics: an introductory book of readings. Macmillan, London

White R (ed) 1985 Political issues in nursing: past, present and future, Vol 1. Wiley, London

Williams D 1978 The practices and ideologies of craft. In: Craft Australia 4 (September): 28-35

Williams D M 1987 Nursing and health promotion: contraindications between the goals of the profession and its model of health promotion. Dissertation. College of Urban Affairs and Public Policy, University of Delaware, Newark

Williams D M 1989 Political theory and individualistic health promotion. Advances in Nursing Science 12(1):14-25

Willis E 1983 Medical dominance: the division of labour in Australian health care. Allen & Unwin, Sydney

22. Threads of an emerging discipline: praxis, reflection, rhetoric and research

Judith Lumby

We need languages that regenerate us, warm us, give birth to us, that lead us to act and not to flee (Chawaf cited by Marks & Courtivron 1981).

WHAT WE SAY AND WHAT WE DO

Do we tell our story?

Annette Street in her exploration of nursing practice (1988) tells us that clinical nurses have developed a stereotyping which goes something like this:

Nurses do not read about nursing
Nurses do not think about nursing
Nurses do not talk about nursing
Nurses do not write about nursing
Nurse administrators do not support clinical staff
Nurse academics have lost touch with practice

While we could all question these assertions, the reality for nursing is that these are perceptions of practitioners who deliver our message of caring. And they deliver important messages for those of us who are now perceived as fringe dwellers on the shores of nursing practice.

Street reminds us that this negative stereotyping is reflective of oppressed group behaviour and produces a fatalism which perpetuates accepted myths, rather than creating an environment whereby those involved can reflect on their reality and bring about change (Street 1988). 'The facts are seen and studied not as a reality which is becoming, but as something which is because it has to be' (Friere cited Street 1988).

The messages that are transmitted as a result of this are strong. Nurses are 'doers' not 'thinkers', they do not write or read, and they are a group who have separated out practice from theory and have undervalued their practitioners. Assuming that these are messages which the majority of nurses would not wish to transmit, I would argue that we need not only to uncover the myths but also to establish ways of ensuring that our story is told clearly and with care.

As more nurses take time to reflect on their daily activities and make them live through their rhetoric, the discipline we call nursing will develop out of practice. This move to praxis in itself insists on a dialectic relationship between the clinical practitioners and those who study and write about such things. Without this relationship, the findings of research will remain silenced rather than used to empower the performers and the viewers. In order to ensure clarity and congruence in our messages we must be careful that our rhetoric and research are true to those values and beliefs lived out in our praxis.

PRAXIS

What is it?

Praxis is dynamic in its evolution as well as its meaning. It has been written about and espoused by philosophers, educationalists and pragmatists throughout the centuries. For Aristotle, praxis was 'those sciences and activities concerned with knowing for its own sake' (Aristotle cited Pearson 1988); while Paulo Friere took this notion further by describing it as 'the action and reflection of people upon their world in order to transform it' (Friere 1972). Certainly Habermas saw it in a similar way as 'the centre of human activity' (Habermas 1965), and thus it has become an important component for those working within the Critical Theory paradigm. Empowerment of self and others by making values live through action is at the core of such an enterprise. In this way there is continual transformation occurring as our actions are altered by experience and reflection.

Prior to the Enlightenment, praxis was valued as an essential base in any community where the concept of knowledge emerging from and belonging to practice was seen as valid and important to everyday life. Socrates asserted that before understanding nature it was important to understand human nature. The philosophers of the day were also the scientists and Science was perceived as speculative, requiring long periods of reflection. Thus the relationship between scientific and humanistic understanding was symbiotic, which is in direct contrast to the present notion of such a relationship where the two are separated quite distinctly between disciplines, methods of study and professional status.

To understand the shift in thinking and relating, it is important to acknowledge the historical and social context in which it occurred. The Scientific Age or Enlightenment emerged from a need to reject metaphysics with its associated notions of the mystical and of sensory experiences. Comte wished to establish 'a science of stability and social reconstruction...whereby all the difficult and delicate questions which now keep up a perpetual irritation in the bosom of society...will be scientifically estimated to the great furtherance of social peace' (Comte cited Swingewood 1984). While an understandable hope in the era directly after the French Revolution, this is one which continues to be expressed by humankind in many ways as we attempt to understand our world and our purpose. Certainly Science has not solved all the problems of society, has not ensured peace, and indeed has created its own set of instabilities and irritations in the form of ethical, moral and social concerns.

The scientific movement which was spawned in some part by Comte was called Positivism and gave birth to the valuing of objectivity, causality and the reduction of the whole into parts. Knowledge from experience was no longer recognised as credible, thus devaluing praxis. Indeed knowledge gained from practice was seen as subjective and not real knowledge. This meant that those disciplines valuing such knowledge also lost credibility as agents of truth.

Praxis and Nursing

Although traditional healing and birthing were sometimes carried out by wise women prior to 'modern' medicine, nursing in most cultures was carried out by women who were not educated in any way but were perceived as the natural carers of the community. The thesis that women needed to care to achieve their femininity was very convenient, since it provided a pool of poorly paid labour to do those tasks least valued by the community in terms of status or remuneration. This expectation of women continues today where the majority of lay caring is done by women with limited financial remuneration. The effects of this on women and their families have been well documented (Spring Rice 1981). Chodorow asserts that while women are 'being', men are 'doing', since men gain their sense of identity by 'doing for and by themselves' (Chodorow cited Finch & Groves 1983). However studies by Margery Spring Rice (1981) have revealed that women care in order that children and husbands can survive. The role of women in caring within society has been revealed to be more an outcome of a society prescribed by males and capitalistic forces than women's inherent requirement for fulfilment (Grosz 1989). In more recent times males are slowly taking on some of these roles, although the continued use of gender characteristics as a measure of suitability for work has certainly been detrimental for women in terms of professional and political advantage.

This path of women in the workforce has some links with nursing which has historically been female dominated. Nurses have been thrice condemned, however, because of their roots in the church and army. Notions of selflessness and obedience have compounded the low self esteem felt by women in a society where value is placed on education, research and competition, all things which have been out of the reach or notion of nurses (say women) in the past.

Prior to passing on knowledge to others it is important that one perceives that what one believes in has external value in the world. For nurses who historically have learnt not to heed their own actions, not to interpret their actions as knowledge, and certainly not to feel empowered or empowering, the concept of praxis has not emerged as a possibility despite its inevitability.

The knowing that comes from nursing practice has been devalued in a health care environment where objective, scientific facts are identified as the only real knowledge and the purveyors of such precious commodities are those educated to understand the mysteries behind such truths. Indeed those who hold the keys to such truths have been granted the personae of tribal wise men. These are the scientists and doctors of Western society. Nurses have adopted the values of such an environment in an effort to gain credibility and status. The written language, behaviours and the research paradigms adopted by nurses reflect this transference. Such imitation of values has not only failed to achieve credibility and status, but has left nurses uncertain about the knowing that they develop as a result of their practice, and how to express this in ways that capture the richness of their experiences which then become the basis for their praxis. Denial of this knowing in turn stunts growth for the individuals involved in the group as well as growth of the group in terms of understanding and describing their practice.

Personal awareness is an essential component of praxis since it enables the identification of values, ethics and reasons behind an individual's or group's actions (Wheeler & Chinn 1989). Out of such awareness comes a knowledge of self and of the world in which one exists. The irony for nurses is that despite this lack of personal empowerment, nursing is about empowering others in their lives. The rhetoric of 'holistic' health care oozes such warm words. The jargon of primary health care incorporates autonomy, equity and empowerment. So if nurses are not personally empowered how do they manage this empowerment of others? And without personal awareness as a beginning step how does one move to the processes of reflection and critical enquiry in order to identify the practice, the conditions and the context, and to act upon them?

Knowledge from experience

More recently the knowledge that comes from experience is being identified as important and valuable even in scientific endeavours. Polanyi (1962) rejects the notion of impersonality as an essential of scientific knowledge by returning to the roots of scientific enquiry which are planted as the result of the wonder of our being in the world. After all, personal passion has always been an important element in intensive studies of any kind in order to sustain interest in the task at hand. There are many examples in science where the personal passion of the researcher was identified as madness by the community, but was the force which eventually led to a breakthrough. The discovery of an antivenene for the funnel web spider bite is one such example occurring in our own country where the scientist involved suffered personal hardship over years due to his passion for the search.

The move to value the knowledge gained from practice and experience emerged out of a general discontent with the scientific method of explaining knowledge and truth. In 1920, Max Scheler coined the phrase the 'Sociology of Knowledge' although it could be claimed that this had its roots in Marx's proposition that 'man's consciousness is determined by his social being' (cited Berger & Luckmann 1972). It was also influenced by other movements of the time including that of Historicism which emphasised the inevitable 'historicity of human thought' (cited Berger & Luckmann 1972). Scheler argued that society determined the presence (*Dasein*) but not the nature (*Sosein*) of ideas. Karl Mannheim (cited Berger & Luckman 1972), also a German, pursued this thinking further to assert that the social context of the time influences all human thinking. This view of the world made sense to those who perceived that everyday life informed their thinking and thus their construction of reality.

These notions were not new philosophically. Giambattista Vico in 1725 published the New Science in which he proposed a science of man. In this he argued that those notions identified as the myths of ancient cultures were in fact the perceptions of the people of the time, and were the ways in which they made some sense of their surroundings. It was their construction of reality. As man/woman constructs stories, institutions and societies, thus woman/man is in turn constructed. This move away from viewing the world as made up of separate entities acting independently from one another led naturally to an emphasis on the relationships of things. Indeed Structuralism led to Semiotics as the linguists began to move away from the notion of language as made up of individual words and examined more closely the relationship of language (*langue*) and speech (*parole*). Thus the emphasis moved to the linguistic sign as the structural relationship between the signified (i.e. the image or the concept) and the actual sound which represents that image (i.e. the signifier). The health care arena is a wonderful stage in which to test such concepts.

Language is a powerful tool in all this as it creates its own imagery and thus influences perceptions. The very dialectic nature of society means that each person participates not only in her/his own reality but also in the realities of others. Individuals involved in the close caring of other individuals must take this responsibility seriously. Nurses know all about misperceptions and the effect on individuals who have misread signs. They are also involved in the correction or interpretation of significations after the doctor has left the patient confused by the use of jargon and must in turn be aware of the danger of mimicing such jargon in an effort to be valued.

The concept of praxis while perhaps identified as jargonese by many nurses practising today is at the base of their being in the world of health care. If one were able to map the thinking of nurses as they make decisions with those for whom they care, then I believe that praxis would be the framework of their emerging and evolving practice. And if one follows those nurses into their recreational activities this praxis would emerge through language. Certainly Patricia Benner found that 'nursing theory has not been adequately shaped by the practice of nurses' (Benner & Wrubel 1989); and argued that nursing theorists have been constrained because of the positivistic 'received' view of the world and therefore have had difficulty in explaining the complex contextual issues which surround expert nursing care (Benner & Wrubel 1989).

Nursing literature still abounds with discussion on theory and practice...ways in which we must identify each...ways in which we must bridge the gap. It is time to stop using language which represents division. While we continue to write or discuss the issue in this way then that is exactly how it will be perceived both within and without nursing. If we value nursing for its practice centredness then knowledge comes from this arena and in turn informs the practice, thus ensuring an evolving dialectic occuring between those who care, those who are cared for and those who write and speak about such things. If praxis is 'values made visible through deliberate action' (Wheeler & Chinn, 1989) then we must begin to be aware of the way in which our actions in turn reflect our values through language and behaviours.

REFLECTION

What is it?

Thinking about the day that has just passed by is part of being human. Thinking of the day that is about to dawn is also part of our destiny. Many people also think about what they are doing while they are doing it. Others, particularly those involved in repetitive tasks, turn their thoughts to anything but what they are doing. So what part of all this is reflection? Reflection is an important part of praxis since it is only through this process that one is made aware of one's actions. It encourages a self consciousness which makes individuals aware of the way in which they make sense of the world in which they operate. This movement in focus from external forces creating one's world to the awareness of personal control is an important one for nurses. An obsession with the way in which things affect nurses and nursing is reflected in the literature on the occupation itself: the stressors, roles, attrition rates, staff selection as well as the education and management of nurses. Theories, conceptual frameworks, philosophies are written, debated and incorporated into every curriculum. Little has been done on the process of nursing itself. This move to self awareness and thus to a 'critical consciousness' offers great hope to a profession since it reflects a maturing and an openness to possibility. The ability to analyze critically the knowledge and the truth that surrounds an individual is a 'reflective awareness' (Thompson 1985), but it does require a commitment to reflection on practice.

Reflection on and in practice

It does seem that today one is asked to incorporate reflection into many spheres. Certainly this is so in the educational arena where there has been a strong move to encourage self appraisal in order to change practice where this is identified as appropriate and possible. Briefing and debriefing in the arena of clinical learning with students is now an acceptable form of encouraging reflection. This process explores the feelings of the students as a result of the experience, and incorporates questions such as what was worthwhile about the experience from the perspective of the individual, the patient and the group, what would one do differently and why. The purpose of this is to encourage the act of considering one's practice in order to make changes as appropriate and thus continue to grow as a practitioner. Valued at undergraduate level it is more likely to encourage continuing reflection in an individual's professional life.

Inherent in the act of reflection is the reflective nature of the process. Action informs reflection which in turn informs action. Schön describes the various types of reflection according to the time in which they occur. Reflection-in-action occurs during the performance, while reflection-on-action occurs at some stage after the event (Schön 1983). The length of time is also important since reflection-in-action may be more difficult for those involved in split second decision making.

The knowing that the public relies upon for expert advice is often that knowledge which has been developed 'in the field' not in the classroom. Recently a general practitioner talked to me of the hours spent in medical school learning about (or being spoken to about) systemic lupus erythematosis and other such severe immune disorders, and the fact that in his practice of over a decade he has yet to come across any of them. Instead he cares for many people who are severely immune depressed as a result of poor diet, hypersensitivities to chemicals (including food) and psychological stressors due to relationship breakdowns. He was not prepared adequately to treat people suffering from the stressors of life. Yet the majority of his time is spent with such people. He has learnt this 'on the job' through reflecting on the various techniques which he has adopted and identifying which ones seemed to be effective. As a result of his experience and his development of knowing-in-action—his 'intuition'—he has a variety of techniques which he uses according to the needs of his patients. These techniques vary from dietary regimes, homeopathy, hypnotherapy and psychotherapy. When asked how he chooses which to use, he talked of having a feel for the person at the time and what felt right after he had taken a good history.

Effective nurses do that all the time. The way in which they approach a relationship will be different according to the context, the person's cultural and social history, age, education and response to their illness. The techniques they use when attending dressings, bathing, positioning, giving medication will be adapted to take account of all these parameters. And how are these differences accounted for? How do practitioners learn these adaptations? Gilbert accounts for it by explaining that what distinguishes 'sensible operations from silly operations is not their parentage but their procedure' (Gilbert cited Schön 1983). It is the methodology not the method. The second can be learnt by rote, the first requires a knowing-in-action; a knowing which does not arise from an intellectual antecedent but is incorporated in the act so that the act becomes an intelligent one.

Nurses and their knowing

The concepts of praxis and reflection as active ingredients of intelligent and informed care are essential if nurses are to value their practice. As they make sense of what they do, nurses use a variety of ways of knowing. A study into the way in which nurses perceived holistic care, uncovered intuition as an important way of knowing (Agan 1987), while Carper described four ways of knowing in nursing, 'intuitive, aesthetic, personal and empirical' (Carper 1980). In describing intuition, a nurse in Agan's study described it in language that many nurses will immediately relate to:

> For me it's a physical sensation. I have two kinds of knowing. I have the knowing that comes out of my head that is subject to conscious awareness. And I have the knowing that, for me, comes out of my heart which is where I feel it—or maybe my solar plexus—that comes out of what I consider to be subconscious information, information that I'm taking in that I'm not aware that I'm even taking in and it comes out that way (Agan 1987).

Acknowledgement of a person's knowledge as valuable is the key to ensuring the continuation of the development of that knowledge through reflection. Intuition has been acknowledged as legitimate knowledge by others including Schön (1983) and Polanyi (1962) although they may use terms such as personal knowledge or 'tacit knowing'. It arises from an awareness of the situation over time and therefore is more likely to be interwoven through the practice of experts. As specialists in a field of nursing we identify with the notion of 'having a feel' for the way a patient is progressing without consideration of the physiological parameters. And we have all admired those people who are categorised as creative and are said to have a feel for words, colours or materials. Nurses on the other hand deny their art. This denial has been another reality forced upon nurses. They are the 'doers' and 'doers' do not have time for contemplative creation. In addition, the people taking up nursing have been classified into a certain personality type which does not incorporate an ability to be artistic.

Yet I see this art every time I walk into an environment where a nurse is busy 'creating' the day for another person. They are busy using light, space, sound, words, movement and touch to deliver the message of care. And like true artists they are willing, indeed they see it as essential, to share their performance with others. 'It is something to be able to paint a picture or to carve a statue and so to make a few objects beautiful. But it is far more glorious to carve and paint the atmosphere in which we work to effect the quality of the day...This is the highest of the arts' (Thoreau cited Donahue 1985).

Bendetti (1976) asserts that the art of acting is a 'rigorous discipline' requiring a knowledge of principles underlying the methodologies and skills involved, as well as an awareness of the job at hand. Isobel Stewart talks of 'the creative imagination and sensitive spirit' of nursing (Stewart cited Donahue 1985). Nursing is thus well described. Nurse's concerns about articulation of what it is they do should be tempered by the reassurance that in many judgements made by practitioners in a variety of disciplines 'we can recognise and describe deviations from a norm very much more clearly than we can describe the norm itself' (Vickers cited Schön 1983).

Since humans express their reality through the use of signs, mainly in the form of language, then language is the basis for our reflection. Through the use of self dialogue we begin to reason out our own actions and to place ourselves in society as individuals. Words influence thought and words in context, i.e. speech, can manipulate another's behaviour depending on the way in which they are received. Language is also the medium of our 'cultural tradition' (Mueller 1973) and this is recognisable in discourse involving nurses or nursing. But language in discourse also offers the possibilities of changing perceptions and social conditions for groups and individuals. It is one of the ways in which feminist writers have suggested changing the patriarchal views which permeate so much of our society (Jay, Lloyd, Iragaray cited Grosz 1989).

Reflection in or on action is more likely to be utilised if something occurs which is out of the ordinary. It forces one to consider the usual and to look at alternatives. In nursing where there is considerable change in any one day and where the environment is more likely to revolve around individual responses, the possibility of the unusual and/or the surprising is high. Listening to nurses talking about their daily activities at a handover is an experience filled with examples of reflection-in-action which produced alternative strategies. Assisting nurses to identify their reflective practice is more problematic because it is so much part of their 'being in the world', and because in their world of highly valued explicit knowledge and technical competence, reflection is regarded as non rigorous and subjective.

RHETORIC

What is it?

Listen to our rhetoric! It haunts our hospitals; it surrounds us in our social situations; it follows our families. It communicates our common cause of caring. And it is mainly a rhetoric of reluctance. The reluctance of a group who share opposing rhetorics. I will call these our rhetoric of reflection and our rhetoric of rationality. The reflective rhetoric is one which is confined to tearooms, to comrades, and occasionally to students. This is mainly oral. The rational rhetoric is that which is revealed to the public, to the journals and to the conference crowd. This is both oral and written.

Will the real nurse stand up? Or have we lost sight of the real nurse in our effort to be understood, to be valued, to gain entry to the world of real 'professionals'?

Rhetoric is described as 'the art of speaking or writing effectively' but it may also be defined as 'artificial or inflated language' (Australian Pocket Oxford Dictionary). Which definition do we follow or fall under when we address our role in terms developed by other disciplines and dance to the tune played by other professionals? More importantly how effective is our communication with colleagues and with the wider society? How well do we tell our story?

Beliefs, bodies and behaviours

The answers to the above questions can only be explored if we are clear about the message which we wish to transmit. Perhaps the confusion begins here and accounts for the confusion of our rhetoric. Perhaps nurses are divided about the way in which they view their role. Certainly different groups have different roles dependent on the client group and their particular needs. The other variable is the context in which the nursing takes place. The nurse who conducts a well baby clinic obviously requires a specialised knowledge base as well as different goals from those required of a nurse in a hospice for terminally ill people, or the nurse working with people with psychiatric disturbances. But it could also be argued that the philosophy behind all such actions and attitudes is similar; that all nurses require a knowledge base about people, their beliefs, their bodies and their behaviours. I have yet to meet a nurse who would deny the nature of nursing as emerging from a desire to care and assist people to meet their individual needs. So why does our public rhetoric and the discourse in which it occurs deny much of this?

While an easy explanation is the lack of political interest in 'caring' as a worthwhile or valid activity, this rhetorical dissonance is not new where women are concerned. Given that nursing tends to attract women to its ranks, analysing it from a feminist perspective explains some of our dissonance. The history of nursing is dominated by the church and army with the consequent essentials being altruism, selflessness and devotion, along with rigidity, cleanliness and order. Thus clothed in the asexual uniforms of conformity and obedience, nursing gave birth to large groups of suppressed women who in turn oppressed other groups of women. In all this the male dominated medical profession gained the upper hand through education, economy and empowerment via gender, social status and collaboration. And along with this domination came power through the rhetoric of science and male discourse. This discourse domination by the male is well documented (Marks & de Courtivron 1981). Discourse as the relation between language and the object to which it refers, structures the perceptions of society. Our values as a group in society are given meaning through the way we talk about our area of concern. Our discourse also prescribes what is permitted or prohibited to be talked about (Kress 1985). In the past the dominant discourse has been that of the male. Until recently women have rarely been published in popular or private text or exhibited in art galleries. Aristotle tells us that 'the female is a female by virtue of a certain lack of qualities; we should regard the female nature as afflicted with a natural defectiveness' (Aristotle cited Marks & de Courtivron 1981).

Discourse about nursing and nurses

Women's voices have been silenced and thus their influence on the common discourse. Those who wished to be heard in literature adopted masculine pseudonyms, e.g. George Sand and Daniel Stern. While they have certainly been portrayed in visual and written text, their portrayal has been through the eyes of the male. The binary opposites game, so well demonstrated in language, always defines the female in relation to the male; male/female, cure/care, he/she, rational/emotive, objective/subjective (Iragaray cited Grosz 1989). While the latter are open to interpretation, the majority of the population would equate objectivity and rationality with the male and subjectivity and emotion with the female. The first term dominates the second and defines it. However it was the male who developed these opposites. While feminine terms are invented to describe a woman involved in an activity, it is assumed that the norm is for males to be the sole proprietors, e.g. poet/poetess. 'In actuality the relation of the two sexes is not quite like that of two electric poles, for man represents both the positive and the neutral as is indicated by the common use of 'man' to designate human beings in general' (de Beauvoir cited Marks & de Courtivron 1981).

Women (say nurses) must claim the title of their energies. We see this now in medicine and law where the gender is not specified by title. In nursing the roots of our language hamper us if we wish to remove the gender bias. 'Nurse' comes from the Greek 'to nourish or to nurture' which was derived from breastfeeding and suckling the young. This is definitely a female activity and perhaps adds to the controversy surrounding males entering the profession, although this is mainly culture related and in Australia is diminishing to some extent. Indeed it may be the changing gender balance itself which has allowed the professionalisation of nursing to occur.

And so nurses wrote as they felt they should write. Having no language of their own, they imitated as they were used to doing. They had been taught well. Nursing literature emerged looking very much like that of the doctor and the scientist who were in turn already male influenced. Despite the difference in their roles and their approaches to their work, this did not live in their portrayal. In fact it reduced the nursing that occurred to a few basic concepts which could be written in text books. The richness of the practice was lost in the written word.

Simultaneously the public were bombarded with images of nurses as subservient angels of mercy, handmaidens to the doctor, dominating, rigid, asexual matrons, and senseless sex objects. While using the past tense here, these images are unfortunately not confined to the past but are presently available to viewers today. We must not be surprised that the public image of the nurse is that of a feminine, nurturant follower who is of average or less than average intelligence and requires only a moderate level of education (Lumby & Zetler 1990). All this in a time where the World Health Organization has acknowledged that the nurse plays a prominent part in positive health care outcomes, and where nurses are required to be the 24 hour companions of people undergoing life threatening procedures. This companionship requires the companion not only to be highly skilled in communication and counselling, but also learned in the latest technologies and their application in a complex context fraught with ethical and legal dilemmas.

The continuing battle about the Science or Art of nursing is one of many debates which one must question at this time in the development of nursing. After all does it really matter? Surely the important issue here is nursing knowledge. Yet nurses are locked into the game of matching and comparing with the traditional disciplines and the traditional ways of thinking. The outcomes of such exercises may of course have concerning consequences. Science faculties in universities may claim nursing as one of its derived disciplines as has already been done in some universities. And nursing care may become even more compartmentalised, may be submitted to rigorous experimental testing and the human component thus separated out. For some this would be welcome with open arms. I doubt however if those who have chosen nursing for the human element would change their caring. Of course this part of nursing could easily be taken over by others who do not need to undertake a university education but are 'caring individuals'!

The Art/Science debate takes on a particular significance at the level of discourse required for each to explain its unique knowledge and truth. It is at this point that confusion and misunderstanding usually occurs. If the world is seen from a purely biophysical perspective then the language and concepts used during discussion are quite different from those used if one views people from their experiences of life. This means that two levels of discourse are being used. While the two views of the world have some commonalities or at least links, the philosophical bases are quite different. And our reality is influenced by the values and beliefs underpinning our practice and reflected in our language.

Describing our practice

It is understandable that nurses are confused and disillusioned. Writers have identified this when they discuss the language of prescription and scientific method which nurses have used to describe their practice. Nursing care plans and nursing diagnosis have exemplified this. Nurses have felt limited in their language and power to express what they actually do. Walk into the tea room if you want to find this out. And if you do take this excursion, listen carefully. Nurses are incredibly articulate in such an environment. It is only when they are placed in an artificial milieu such as a lecture room, or with those who obviously do not appreciate what they do, that they become silent. After all how often does one read about the experience of illness in refereed journals? Yet pick up popular magazines and one will find many such articles. This is where the public wants to be heard. And who are we to decide that we are cut off from the real world? After all, aren't we in a position of accountability to the public? Placed in a privileged caring position we are also placed in an ethical position in relation to those for whom we care (Noddings 1984).

I have just completed a session with registered nurses enrolled in a graduate nursing programme. My involvement was in a unit called Advanced Nursing Care Management, a title which I remain confused about. It was my concern which prompted the teaching/learning approach which I ultimately adopted. This approach was to encourage the group to identify what advanced nursing care was; how it was different from other nursing care; whether we could observe the difference; whether the outcome was different; and whether it mattered. After initial silence one brave nurse offered the class a wonderful examplar. She did not name it as such. What she did say however was that the only way she could explain her patient care after 20 years in a variety of settings was to talk of experiences she had and how she handled them. Her story of a woman coming into Casualty with her baby who had just died, and the way that she had coped with the situation, was a special experience for us all but also one with which we identified. Once the ice was broken, the stories came with a rush. It was evident to all in the class that we understood advanced nursing practice compared to beginning practice. Would it have been evident to someone outside the nursing world? The stories were told in everyday language which was certainly understandable to all involved in everyday life. And it would be understandable particularly to those who had been through meaningful illness experiences. They talked of feelings; of observations which had meanings; of 'being' with the person; of touching; of using their experience in an intuitive way to make sense of what was happening.

The next week I asked the same group to take a prepared case study and in pairs to map the thinking that went on while working through the care required for the patient in the study. Feedback was fascinating. The language of presentation was quite different from that the week before, when the recall had been more reminiscent of story telling. Each couple talked of assessment, observations, planning and diagnosis. Even taking into account the simulated nature of the exercise, the way in which they described their practice was extremely structured in the language used and the way in which client and the context was discussed. The spontaneity had gone and despite my efforts to recapture it they felt comfortable in this rhetoric. If I had entered the tearoom during the break I would have heard it all expressed with spontaneity and 'everyday' language. The students, all experienced registered nurses, admitted that they had no other way of explaining their practice in a way which was 'advanced'. They also acknowledged the lack of structures to assist them to describe the dynamism and complexity of their practice. Yet this very thing is what has caused the silencing of our world of practice. As I considered the wealth of experience in the thirteen registered nurses in the room it became even more evident that it is imperative that we find ways of expressing what we do while still acknowledging the differences within the practice. While it is exciting and important to share with each other spontaneously, it is not enough for nurses or for explaining nursing practice.

The knowledge that expert nurses have about their practice has been handed down mainly by word of mouth. This has been condemned as inappropriate, and certainly it has meant that it has not been possible to collect knowledge in large texts and display it as a collection of the 'work' of nurses. Since Western society values such displays of knowledge and scholarship it has meant that nurses have not been regarded as true academics and ipsofacto their work not regarded as valuable. The knowledge that nurses have, however, has not been lost as claimed by many. Indeed quite the opposite. It has been passed down to the new practitioners by the elders. And despite the concern which nurse academics have expressed about reinforcing traditions and 'bad' behaviours, the art of passing down knowledge from elders by story telling and song is a much valued art in many societies. Oral transmission of knowledge is less able to be avoided than the printed word which offers a choice. Ignoring the knowledge offered by a colleague in daily interactions is almost impossible without direct confrontation. Reading a journal or listening to a lecture requires one to actively take steps and then to act upon the knowledge, which means that it must have some relationship to practice it if it is to have an impact. Working side by side with another nurse facilitates, indeed actively encourages learning if the activity is seen to be relevant and the outcome worthwhile. The discourse used in daily practice is heavily laden with knowledge about nursing's central focus—our relationship with people. Would it have made a difference if it had been written in texts over the centuries, given that this opportunity had been made possible through structures and access to the publishing arena?

Horton & Finnegan (1973) in their text emphasise the difficulty of avoiding contact with oral knowledge in a non-literature society. This in turn defines the nature of knowledge and truth in that society. In such a society nurses would be valued for their knowledge and their truth. In our society ,oral transmission of knowledge has been regarded as inconsistent, subjective and even mythical. Thus certain cultures, including the Australian Koori, have been disregarded as illiterate, relying on stories made up from the imagination. It is interesting to note, however, that this oral knowledge enabled life to be carried on from generation to generation in a way which ensured adequate nutrition and health practices, as well as appropriate social structures which accounted for issues of justice and morality.

Scientism ensured that only written knowledge was viewed as incorporating possibilities of truth and that the structure of the text was prescribed. This immediately isolated large groups of society even in the Western world, apart from all the societies with a tradition of other ways of determining knowledge and truth. Oral knowledge impregnated with ink somehow assumes a respectability not possible otherwise. Goody (1968) believed that writing should not be an alternative to oral transmission of knowledge but should be an addition. The problem in Western cultures is the relation between the written and the oral tradition.

Story tellers in non Western cultures have been held in high esteem and still are in cultures not transformed by Western ways of knowing. Micronesia is a society which Turnbull observed valuing oral knowledge as the elder men shared their navigational knowledge through talking and singing. In this way it was passed down to the younger men. 'The web of social, economic and political relations that provide for that valuation of navigational knowledge are quite powerful but not invincible' (Turnbull cited O'Brien 1990).

The handover is a tradition in nursing whereby knowledge is passed down orally and by short notes. This continues to be a ritual protected by nurses and one which has resisted change. During this time nurses engage in reflective practice by reviewing their care, passing on their experiences and strategies and making suggestions for change. This is Reflection-on-Action as described by Schön (1983), and may be initiated by a change in a person's health status, a change in a person's attitude, an expression of need or the presence of someone significant.

The passing down of therapeutic practices in nursing is often observable, and despite the move to throw out tradition there are many practices which remain effective and may be best passed down by oral transmission and role modelling. What is required is to separate these practices from those which have emerged for no better reason than expediency. Although formal evaluation of outcomes may not have been written down, nurses are usually able to know if their practice has been effective although the converse is more problematic. Nurses tend to talk about their work socially and in this way they review current practices. The contextual nature of the practice requires that individual cases need discussion. There is no way that all this could or should be written down but these conversations must be regarded as important rhetoric for the development of the discipline. Bart O'Brien (1990) discovered as he studied nurses in their transmission of knowledge that 'they would often find it necessary to tell their story even though they might have documented it explicitly'. He believes that this reinforces the need for the narrator to put her/his personality into the story thus making it uniquely his/her own creation (Horton & Finnegan cited O'Brien 1990).

Nurses' reluctance to transmit knowledge by written word may be due to lack of expertise or an inherent valuing of story telling. Is it that nurses fear the loss of important details if one is required to write things down? Often the need to be concise in a written report may not allow for the need to clarify certain points, particularly related to responses of individuals, to feelings or to intuition. Alison Kitson (1987) reinforces the importance of reflective practice in order to respond to and identify our gut reactions and hunches for effective practice. While set standards for quality nursing care are important as guidelines they should not replace 'stout hearts and gut reactions'. As nurses we all know we are not alone in the latter. Good medicine embodies such characteristics, but continues to be identified and valued for its scientific foundations and respectable research methods along the scientific inquiry mode. For doctors this is much more possible since in general they are not involved in responding to the individual encounter continuously over an eight to ten hour period or to physical needs of a very intimate nature.

Medicine has demanded that doctors in hospitals work more by remote control relying on written records and scientific data from investigation rather than 'hands on' clinical diagnosis. The latter encourages a more intimate relationship whereby the patient feels inclined to express needs and concerns. Specialisation has also compounded this distancing due to the dissection of the body into parts, thus further reinforcing a reductionist approach to people. Even the 'psyche' is removed and given to a specialist. The lack of satisfaction for both patient and doctor may be one of the motivating forces behind the move to alternative therapies and holistic healing centres.

Image as reality

The stereotyping which continues to date nursing is also a factor when considering the way in which nurses talk about their work. Despite tertiary preparation for practice and professional rates of pay, the image has not changed dramatically in the last decade. This of course has implications for entry to the profession given the opening of other careers to women, and the move to careers embodying the characteristics of competitiveness and high financial remuneration which reflect the values in our materialistic society. Imagery certainly plays an important part in influencing the way in which things or persons are perceived. Media bombardment both visually and by text ensures that information today is very much distributed by the use of imagery. This in turn involves assumptions about certain aspects of our society. And if these images are not challenged when they continue to invade the consciousness of society then the images become reality. Equally as important is the way in which those thus presented begin to accept the images rather than deny them. 'Man is a symbol forming organism. He has constant need of a meaningful inner forumulation of self and world in which his own actions and even his impulses have some kind of "fit" with the outside as he perceives it' (Lifton cited Markley & Harman 1988).

Nurses have been misrepresented for a long time particularly in the visual media with little challenge by the profession itself. Examples abound on the popular television channels with 'A Country Practice', 'G.P', and 'M.A.S.H.' as well as a recent addition to the screens of Australian viewers in 'Let The Blood Run Free'. The misrepresentations one views on these programmes must be challenged not only for the public's sake but also for nurses themselves if they are to develop Lifton's (cited Markley & Harmann 1988) 'meaningful inner formulation of self and the world in which they practice their art' and if they are to develop a rhetoric which reflects that world and that art.

RESEARCH

Our inheritance

While discourse signifies the values of a group to the public, the way in which a discipline communicates its values to other disciplines is mainly by the questions it asks, the methods it uses to explore such questions and the language it uses to explain the discipline which it espouses. Nurses in Australia have followed those philosophical underpinnings which have surrounded and controlled their practice. These have emerged from the empiricist philosophy which argues for the explication and classification of concepts in order to ensure clarification and prediction. Such fundamentals provided the foundations for future grounding of knowledge in the discipline. Nurses believed that this was the way to uncover nursing knowledge and truth since it appeared to uncover truths about medicine. And naively most nurses believed that this would be relatively simple given that it was merely a matter of writing down what it was that nurses did.

Such assumptions were built on practices based in the belief that the only truth is that which can be observed and measured. And this meant reducing the whole to measurable parts. For a practice involving a surgical technique or a drug regime this may be ideal. For a complex practice involving human relationships and human behaviours in health and illness this approach was neither appropriate nor possible. For a practice incorporating multiple therapies involving individuals with different values, histories and from a variety of socio-economic groups this approach was invalid. Yet validity was at the heart of much of nursing's explorations. We wished to be accepted and to be valued as a scholarly discipline. Indeed we hoped to 'come of age'. After all, it had been a long road with many obstacles in our path. We were mainly women not men; were 'trained' not educated; 'practised' rather than 'philosophised'; and did 'dirty work' (Lawler 1990). Our history haunted us and our devotion daunted us. We were the 'doers' not the 'thinkers' of the world.

The identification of nursing as a science, albeit 'applied', placed nurses further under the influence of scientists, their rhetoric and their research practices, while ensuring second class citizenship by the term 'applied' (say impure). As apparently emerging disciplinarians (despite our long history of practice) we followed rather than led. Was there ever a choice? Of course our behaviour was also related to our practice environment where decision making was not seen as part of our role despite the fact that it formed part of our existence.

Controlling nursing knowledge

The paradigms in which nursing research was situated up until the present day thus reflected these scientific influences. The rhetoric surrounding the theory explosion in nursing perpetuated the scientific approach to thinking about nursing, to educational practices and to the way in which nursing was studied. Nurses seized theories often developed by scholars removed from the practice arena. They manipulated conceptual frameworks in order to guide practice. Many such theories and concepts had not evolved from practice and many had not been refined to the stage of classification as a theory. Despite this, nursing pursued the hallmarks of scholarship in an effort to be validated. The controlling nature of this pursuit in itself can be concerning. Since conceptual frameworks represent a certain view of the world, then a model developed from such a framework continues to represent the social reality in the same way and so controls the outcome. The recent move to metatheories away from epistemology based on single theories may represent a new awareness of the need to test multiple models and to create possibilities, instead of narrowing our options and thinking.

Australian nurses are in their infancy in nursing research publications with only one journal in which to publish. However, already the research bias discovered in the United States is obvious here. This bias was disclosed when 23 journals were analysed for the methods used by nurses in their research. Between 1950 and 1982 nursing studies published were primarily based in the Positivistic paradigm (Reeder 1984). Since research funding tends to favour the experimental method in the academic and the political arena, and other methods are so costly in terms of human resources, this may be a strong influence. The lack of graduate studies in nursing in this country must have played a part in this trend since most nurses who moved into the academic circle and were doing research, were nourished in other disciplines, many of which used positivistic methods. It is no surprise that nurses were unaware that there were other methods and indeed thought that the experimental method was synonymous with the scientific method, which of course excludes any other method from being 'scientific'. Michael Foucalt, who believes that power is not held but is a 'strategic situation in a given society', would identify this as part of the power/knowledge hold which determines all that can and will be known (Foucalt 1976). Out of such supression comes change, however, due to the knowledge which results from discourse of the forbidden.

This discourse is one we are now seeing in nurses, in the way they describe their practice, and in the way they are turning to alternative paradigms which more accurately fit with the view of the world arising from their practice. It appears that nursing may be questioning its identify and its structuring. Acknowledgement of the need for nurses to pursue tertiary studies in their own discipline and to function in faculties of their own must encourage a self awareness not possible when nurses were still apprentices and the only health care group not 'educated'. An increase in the number of publications by women writers which acknowledge women's ways of understanding the world has also had an empowering effect (Belenky et al 1973, Cameron 1985, Gilligan 1982, Spender 1980).

These ways of understanding the world and the practice called nursing must be explored through appropriate ontological and methodological commitments. Only in this way will nurses change the way in which the discipline is understood and viewed. Research methods must be congruent with practices and with the questions that nurses need to ask and to explore. These questions involve values, preferred practices and beliefs.

The ontological debate in which nurses involve themselves on a daily basis both personally and vicariously, involves the question of what it is to be human. Daily they are dealing with people and responses of individuals to their state of health. Yet our funded and published research reflects a view of the world that appears to be separate from those for whom we care. It reflects a belief that experience, culture, history and language are unrelated to the person and their responses. While this may suit a group who wish to control and maintain the status quo or who wish research to be merely a technical activity, we claim that nursing is about assisting others to make choices about their health and the care they receive. Our research must be of a kind which explains, creates understanding and is shared. It must create the possibility for change.

A new look

The paradigms which offer such possibilities and which emphasise understanding rather than objective results include the interpretive, the critical theory and the feminist paradigms. Prior to moving into such paradigms and the resultant methods it is important to undergo considerable personal preparation if positivism has been the main framework used to study phenomena. There are many examples of research written in positivistic language but claiming to use a method in another paradigm. There is also widespread belief that if qualitative methods are used then the study does not have a positivistic stance. But quantitative and qualitative methods both fit happily in positivism. It is all in the way the researcher designs the study and the way the underlying philosophy is espoused both in overt and covert ways. While the qualitative method, influenced by German idealists in the 18th and 19th centuries, grew out of the belief that the world could be understood by other senses, the term is now used loosely to describe any method whereby other than statistical data is gathered.

The interpretive paradigm includes phenomenology which incorporates the 'being in the world' concept of Heidegger which negates the dualism of the positivists. Heidegger's freedom is about the self being in the world not isolated from it (Kaelin 1988). Nurses identify with this as they fight to assist people to choose alternatives or even to remove themselves to a context which provides greater possibilities. They see only too well how many people are a result of the world in which they exist socially, culturally, economically, and even genetically. This multidimensional view of people is also one that is found in nursing curricula throughout the country. Students of nursing are being encouraged to view people as individuals who respond to the world because of their history. Individuals are what they are because of the values and beliefs they hold and pursue. This *Dasein* (existence) as described by Heidegger must be studied in the situation in order to identify the significance for those involved in the experience.

If students are being encouraged to value the individual in this way and are then exposed to only the experimental method of research as is happening in some programmes, then nursing will continue to experience the confusion which has been felt by so many nurses in the past. Using methods which objectify components of the lived experience of a person will cause compartmentalisation and a loss of the whole. It will also create dissonance for the group and the public when our espoused values are not reflected in our studies.

The study of illness using a phenomenological method insists that the complete experience is part of the whole existence for that person, not just a snapshot in time. It involves the culture, the language and the context. It captures the complexity of humanity which nurses know and relate to daily. Those involved in such studies share in the 'validation' of the interpretation of the experience. This form of research is about studying 'with' a person or group not 'on' a person or group. Methods within the critical theory paradigm are those which incorporate notions of praxis and emancipation. Action research is one such method and is being explored by an increasing number of people studying phenomena related to health and illness. Essential to this form of study is the liberatory process which occurs for those involved. This arises from the practice orientation of the method. Thus it incorporates the praxis and empowerment spoken of by Habermas in his early writings (Habermas 1988).

The collaborative aspect of studies is given even more emphasis in methods which have a women-centred perspective (Reinharz cited Bowles & Klein 1989). The basis for using such methods in studying nursing and nurses is the assertion that research methods, and the language which has been developed to explain the outcomes, are male centred, which reinforces the objective (scientific), the domination by the researcher and the removal of context. Maria Mies argues for a 'view from below' to replace 'the view from above' (Mies cited Bowles & Klein 1989). She urges that we must use research to serve those that are exploited and dominated rather than 'as an instrument of dominance and legitimation of power elites' (Mies cited Bowles & Klein). Nurses are in a position to observe the power relationships played out through research in the name of health care and must be wary of playing similar games, particularly given the privileged position they hold in the relationship with those for whom they care.

Schön (1983) describes the dilemma we face by contrasting the high hard ground of manageable problems with the murky swamps of practice, where problems are more complex and less easily identified or explained. 'There are those who choose the swampy lowlands. They deliberately involve themselves in messy but crucially important problems and when asked to describe their methods of inquiry they speak of trial and error, intuition and muddling through. Those who stay on the high ground do so in order to remain protected from the unknown and to devote themselves to a narrow but safe world of 'technical rigor and solid professional competence' (Schön 1983).

OUR STORY

So do we need to tell our story in other ways than those already prescribed? And if we do, how are we to ensure that we do not perpetuate the 'fellowship of discourse' described by Michael Foucalt (Foucalt 1972). This fellowship perpetuates the use of symbols, circumstances and language in a closed community in a way that ensures exclusion of others by the determination of 'word choice, signification and impact' (Hays 1989). Hays believes that if we are able to 'achieve excellence in increasingly complex patient care, we can learn to describe it in words' (Hays 1989). She urges us to reject the notion that our only communication is a clinical record prescribed by others. We need to engage the patient as a full participant in the recording, acknowledging our ethical responsibility. While many nurses feel secure in their oral culture, it is important for us to realise the power of recorded language which enables reflection by and empowerment of a larger audience. 'The real power of Martin Luther King was not only that he had a dream but that he could describe it, that it became public and therefore accessible to millions of people' (Pondy cited Street 1988).

While alternative rhetorics can be a sign of healthy differences, we must ensure that our descriptions, our practice and our research present a united message: a message which fosters reflection and trust in our own valuing of the 'therapeutic use of self' (Peplau 1952). This is our only hope if we are to draw together the threads of our discipline: a discipline emerging out of practice and from which practice evolves.

REFERENCES

Agan R D 1987 Intuitive knowing as a dimension of nursing. Advances in Nursing Science 67 (October): 63-70

Belenky M F, Clinchy B M, Goldberger N R, Tarule J M 1973 Women's ways of knowing: the development of self, voice and mind. Basic Books, New York

Bendetti R L 1976 The actor at work. Prentice Hall, New Jersey

Benner P, Wrubel J 1989 The primacy of caring. Addison-Wesley, Menlo Park, p 5

Berger P, Luckmann T 1972 The social construction of reality. Penguin , Harmondsworth, p 17,18,21

Bowles G, Klein R D 1989 Theories of women's studies. Routledge and Kegan Paul, London, p 123,162

Cameron D 1985 Feminism and linguistic theory. MacMillan Press, Hong Kong

Carper B 1980 Fundamentals of knowing in nursing. Advances in Nursing Science (1):13-23

Donahue M P 1985 The finest art. C.V. Mosby Co, St Louis, p ix, 467

Finch J, Groves D (eds) 1983 A labour of love: women, work and caring. Routledge and Kegan Paul, London

Foucalt M 1976 The will to know. Paris Gallimard, p 21

Foucalt M 1972 The discourse on language. In: Sheridan Smith A M The archeology of knowledge. Harper & Row, New York, p 215-237

Friere P 1972 Cultural action for freedom. Penguin, Harmondsworth

Gilligan C 1982 In a different voice. Harvard University Press, Cambridge

Goody J (ed) 1968 Literacy in traditional societies. Cambridge University Press, London

Grosz E 1989 Sexual subversions. Allen & Unwin, Sydney

Habermas J 1965 Knowledge and human interests (Translated 1986 Jeremy Shapiro). Polity Press, Cambridge

Habermas J 1988 On the logic of the social sciences (Translated Nicholen S W & Start J A). Polity Press, Cambridge, in association with Basil Blackwell, Oxford

Hays J C 1989 Voices in the record. Image. Journal of Nursing Scholarship 21(4) (Winter):200-203

Horton R, Finnegan R (eds) 1973 Modes of thought: essays on thinking in western–non-western societies. Faber & Faber, London

Kaelin D F 1988 Heidegger's being and time. University Presses of Florida, Florida

Kitson A 1987 Raising standards of practice—the fundamental issue of effective nursing practice. Journal of Advanced Nursing 12:321-329

Kress G 1985 Linguistic processes in sociocultural practice. Deakin University, Geelong

Lawler J 1990 The body, dirty work and nursing: towards understanding the invisibility of nursing care. Presented at 'Nursing in the Nineties'—12th National Conference, Royal College of Nursing, Australia, Sydney, 24,25 May

Lumby J, Zetler J 1990 The image of the nurse—1890's or 1990's? Royal College of Nursing, Australia, 12th National Conference, Sydney

Markley O W, Harman W W 1988 Changing images of man. Permagon Press, Oxford, p1

Marks E, de Courtivron I 1981 New French feminisms. Harvester Press Ltd, Sussex, p 43,177

Mueller C 1973 The politics of communication. Oxford University Press, New York, p 15

Noddings N 1984 Caring: a feminine approach to ethics and moral education. University of California Press, Los Angeles

O'Brien B 1990 Unpublished paper, doctoral student, School of Nursing, Deakin University, Geelong, p 13

Pearson A 1988 Theorising nursing: the need for multiple horizons. In: Expanding Horizons in Nursing Education. Proceedings of the National Nursing Educational Conference Perth, Western Australia, December, p 210

Peplau H 1952 Interpersonal relations in nursing: a conceptual frame of reference for psychodynamic nursing. Putnam, New York

Polanyi M 1962 Personal knowledge. Routledge and Kegan Paul, London

Reeder R 1984 Nursing research: holism and philosophies of science. Points of congruence between E Husserl and M E Rogers, dissertation. New York University, University Microfilms No. 84-21 466

Schön D 1983 The reflective practitioner. Basic Books New York, p 43, 51, 53

Spender D 1980 Man made language. Routledge and Kegan Paul, London

Spring Rice M 1981 Working class wives. Virago, London

Street A 1988 Nursing practice: high, hard ground, messy swamps and the pathways in between. Reflective Processes in Nursing Course Guide. Deakin University, Geelong, p 23-38, 223

Swingewood A 1984 A short history of sociological thought. MacMillan Education, London, p 42

Thompson 1985 Practical discourse in nursing: going beyond empiricism and historicism. Advances in Nursing Science 7 (4):59-71

Wheeler C E, Chinn P L 1989 Peace and power: a handbook of feminist process, 2nd ed. National League for Nursing, USA, p 2

Epilogue

Genevieve Gray   Rosalie Pratt

Before you close this volume, please join us in reflecting on the stage we have reached on this journey-within-a-journey towards a discipline of nursing, and on the way in which the pattern of the tapestry is evolving.

Given that the crucial element of the discipline is its body of knowledge and ideas viewed from the unique perspective of the profession to which the discipline applies—in our case nursing—what have the authors in the book suggested in this regard? They have indeed taken us down many highways and byways, and as predicted we have reached a rise which is enabling us to command a 360 degree view of the Australian nursing landscape at this time. And the landscape before us is already richly patterned.

As we contemplate this view-in-the-round, we see that it is comprised of a foreground, a middle distance, and further horizons. A consideration of these three aspects of the landscape around us enables us to summarize the journey so far and what is perceived to lie beyond. The foreground is clearly discernible. Despite the diversity of their perspectives, our authors display considerable agreement in relation to caring as the essence of nursing; the necessity for grounding our theory in practice; and the accompanying shift in ways of knowing, from positivist through to interpretive and critical theory, and beyond. The colours are vivid in the pattern of the tapestry here, with contributions woven from the varying threads of clinicians, scholars, researchers, and educators. As we ponder the foreground it is important to bear in mind, with Parker, the 'post modernist understanding that there is no objective reliable universal foundation for knowledge...theory development is seen to be possible for nursing to the extent that it is constituted through practice and claims to be no more than a set of viewpoints at a particular time, justifiable only within its own time'.

In the middle distance the focus shifts, and one is able to perceive the greater utilization of the interpretive, the critical, and the feminist paradigms in the generation of nursing knowledge. It appears that these ways of knowing will be complemented by new concepts such as Lawler's somology and by the reinvigoration of the concepts of caring and healing. As Lawler describes it, somology 'allows an integration of the physical with the socio-cultural and personal aspects of being but it is only possible if the nurse is concerned for the experience of "the other"—a situation which is typically called caring and which is universal and fundamental in nursing'. There in the middle distance too, but less focused, is the sense that nurses are prepared to recognize and acknowledge that there is no one right viewpoint.

There is a stirring of excitement as we shift our gaze towards the horizons and realize the vista of possible worlds that promise adventure in awaiting our discovery. We share with Parker 'a sense of mystery, awe and wonder' which she perceives, together with a 'moral stance moved by passions and purposes', as contributing to 'the achievement of health and wholeness and the resacralizing of being and nature...[which is] the goal of discipline development and practice in nursing'. And there is a gathering sense in the authors' work of nursing as moral art and aesthetic activity. At the same time, there is an anticipation that complementing nursing as an aesthetic activity will have to be an actively grounded pursuit of political and social relevance.

The opening up of our possible worlds is dependent upon our willingness to not only deconstruct and understand, but also to reconstruct and transform, our lived-world. Crucial to this transformation will be a milieu which is characterized by a 'connected' profession where uncertainty, tentative thought, and conflict will be expected, ambiguity tolerated and a diversity of viewpoints accepted as a part of the pattern of progress and as a basis for growth.

It is a measure of the distance we have travelled between the pages of this book that we will never again be compelled, as we were in the Prologue, to draw upon largely imported ideas (however pertinent). It is clear that unique ideas and thus a unique discipline 'emerging out of practice and from which practice evolves'—are blossoming in the Australian context. Those of us who have always believed that Australian nursing has much to offer the world and its peoples can feel vindicated by the outpourings of mind and spirit evident in the writings of this book.

As together we continue on this journey towards a discipline of nursing may the richness of the tapestry increase and the vision of our possible worlds be realized.

Index

Index by Juliet Richters